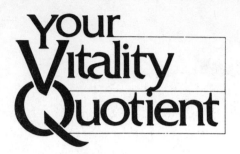

Your Vitality Quotient

THE CLINICALLY PROVEN PROGRAM THAT CAN REDUCE YOUR BODY AGE – AND INCREASE YOUR ZEST FOR LIFE

Richard Earle, Ph.D., David Imrie, M.D.,
with Rick Archbold

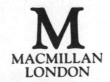

MACMILLAN
LONDON

This book is *not* intended as a substitute for the medical advice of physicians. The reader should regularly consult a physician in matters relating to his or her health and particularly in respect to any symptoms that may require diagnosis or medical treatment.

The authors gratefully acknowledge the following:

The "Body Age Test" in Chapter 3 is based on the work of Dr. Robert Morgan and is used by permission.

The questionnaire "Are You Ready for Exercise?" in Chapter 11 is used by permission of the Province of British Columbia Ministry of Health.

The grading table for the "Arm and Shoulder Strength Test" and the charts "Calculate Your Target Heart Rate for the Training Effect" and "A Picture of a Complete Aerobic Workout" in Chapter 11 are from *The Canadian Standardized Test of Fitness* developed by Fitness Canada, Government of Canada, and are reproduced with the permission of Fitness Canada.

The "Frame Size Measurement Chart" and the "Metropolitan Height and Weight Tables," which appear in the Chapter 12 section "Your Ideal Body Weight," are reprinted by permission of Metropolitan Life Insurance Company.

The table of positive and negative beliefs under the section "My Roadblocks" in Chapter 12 is adapted from J. W. Farquhar, *The American Way of Life Need Not Be Hazardous to Your Health*, © 1987 by Stanford Alumni Association. Reprinted with permission of Addison-Wesley Publishing Co., Inc., Reading, Massachusetts.

First published in the USA 1989 by Warner Books.

Published in the UK 1989 by
Macmillan London Limited
a division of Macmillan Publishers Limited
4 Little Essex Street London WC2R 3LF
and Basingstoke

Associated companies in Auckland, Delhi, Dublin, Gaborone, Hamburg, Harare, Hong Kong, Johannesburg, Kuala Lumpur, Lagos, Manzini, Melbourne, Mexico City, Nairobi, New York, Singapore and Tokyo.

ISBN 0-333-49930-1

A CIP catalogue record for this book is available from the British Library

Printed by Billings of Worcester

Designed by Giorgetta Bell McRee

To the memory of Hans Hugo Selye,
medical pioneer and founder of the Canadian Institute of Stress

CONTENTS

INTRODUCTION

Aging is a fact of life. But the aging process isn't something that just happens to you; it's something over which you can exert considerable control. Both the way you age and how rapidly you age are determined to a surprising degree by your behavior and attitudes, especially as these affect the way you deal with stress. Premature aging is preventable, and to a significant degree, its signs and effects are reversible.

This book is based on the results of a ground-breaking study of the relationship between aging and stress, the first large-scale, long-term clinical study of aging in humans. The Body Age Study was conducted between 1981 and 1984 under the auspices of the Canadian Institute of Stress, founded by stress-research pioneer Dr. Hans Selye. It involved 623 subjects, 336 men and 287 women. Of these, 602 completed the full eight-month program—an unusually low rate of attrition for a voluntary study group of this size. This is the first time the study's results have been published in any form.

Here are some of its striking findings:

Many people are "older than their years." We chose 623 study subjects from a group of 1,868 applicants. Those who entered the program all tested biologically older than their chronological or calendar age— many by 10 years or more. To measure their biological age as opposed to their chronological age, we gave our subjects the Body Age Test, a form of which you'll take in chapter 3.

You can reduce your biological age, or body age, in as little as four months. The study participants were able to reduce their body ages by an average of 8.2 years—and in many cases by much more. The single greatest body age reversal was experienced by a woman architect who entered the program at age 35, but with a body age of 62. At her eight-month checkup, she'd gained 25.5 years of biological age—her new body age was 36. The majority ended up "younger than their years," testing at body ages younger than their chronological ages.

You can look younger. Our Body Age Study subjects showed dramatic improvements in their physical appearance, as assessed by a carefully trained panel of judges. A high percentage who were overweight reached the ideal weight range in eight months. Skin tone, the number and depth of facial wrinkles, and posture were markedly more youthful at the end of the study period.

You can feel better. A great number of our study subjects entered the program complaining of fatigue, low energy, insomnia, minor aches and pains, and frequent short-term illnesses. Almost without exception, these symptoms had largely disappeared at the end of the study: Our subjects invariably reported more energy and enthusiasm for life. A clear indicator of this, apart from the testimony of the subjects themselves, was the sharp reduction in the number of visits to the doctor, which dropped by 53 percent, and in days absent from work, which dropped by 58 percent.

Although premature or accelerated aging can take place at any stage of life, it is most prevalent among people in their prime. Both men and women tend to experience more rapidly accelerated aging between the ages of 40 and 50. According to our research, during this "decade of vulnerability" the average North American male ages 15.2 years and the average female 18.6 years. However, premature aging can strike at any time, and its behavioral seeds are sown in your twenties or thirties, or even earlier.

People in their fifties and sixties are as able to lower their body ages as people in their thirties or forties.

The results of the Body Age Study have made it possible for us to provide the first customized prescriptions for combating stress and aging. These prescriptions are geared to your particular behavioral type, or stressotype. The study identified six basic stressotypes: Speed Freak, Basket Case, Cliff Walker, Drifter, Worry Wart, and Loner. At the same time, we identified five effective anti-aging interventions, or Vital Life

Skills: Values/Goals Clarification, Effective Relaxation, High-Performance Nutrition, Self-Affirming Communication, and Essential Exercise.

All five interventions turned out to be more successful when used in combination with a mind technique called autogenic training, which involves a simple form of self-hypnosis (done with the aid of a relaxation tape) along with the use of verbal affirmations and mental images, or visualizations. You will learn this technique at the beginning of Part Two.

Your Vitality Quotient allows you to benefit from what the Body Age Study revealed about stress and aging, as well as from the individual experiences of the 623 people who entered the program. In particular, you will learn about the following:

- Your body age versus your chronological age: Are you younger or older than your years?
- Your Vitality Quotient (V.Q.), a measure of your current level of vitality and your current rate of aging.
- Your stressotype profile: How much of each behavioral/lifestyle type (stressotype) is part of your individual makeup?
- Your personal vitality prescription: the specific Body Age Program that is right for you—a mix of the three Vital Life Skills that will work together most powerfully to lower your body age.

The book is divided into two parts. In Part One, "Your Vitality Prescription," you'll learn about aging and stress and the key role that stress plays in the aging process. We'll explain the six stressotypes and how each one is susceptible in different ways to premature aging. You will also take the Body Age Test and the Vitality Quotient Test. Finally, you'll write your personal prescription for change.

In Part Two, "The Body Age Program," we will describe in detail each of the five proven anti-aging interventions, or Vital Life Skills. In each intervention chapter, you will start by rating your existing strengths and weaknesses in a particular area. Then we'll teach you the key techniques for putting the intervention into practice. Finally, we'll provide you with a structured four-week start-up program to make it as easy as possible for you to phase the intervention into your ongoing lifestyle.

We believe that *Your Vitality Quotient* presents something new in the fields of stress and aging. Many books have dealt with stress and stress management. An increasing number have talked about how to minimize the cosmetic effects of aging, wrinkled skin, hair loss, and loss of muscle mass. This is the first approach to explore the link between the way you handle stress and how rapidly your whole body ages, including the many body systems and functions most of us take for granted.

The Body Age Program is based on our success in reducing the biological ages of more than 96 percent of those who participated in the

Body Age Study. It is simple and straightforward, consisting of small, concrete behavioral changes that anyone can make. It is customized to meet your individual needs, and it works.

If you follow the logical steps outlined in this book, you will be able to slow down your rate of aging and increase your energy and zest for life.

Richard Earle, Ph.D.
David Imrie, M.D.
September 1988

AN INVITATION TO OUR READERS

This is your invitation to become part of an ongoing Body Age Study. Once you've written your personal prescription for change, we'd like to know about your progress so that we can continue our research. We learned a great deal from our 623 original study subjects, but we want to learn more. Your insights and questions will help us refine our program.

In Appendix D, "How to Join Body Age II," you'll find the details of how you can become a participant in Body Age II: An International Study of Body Age Reversal, our ongoing investigation of the most powerful techniques for lowering your biological age. With your help, perhaps we can discover even more powerful strategies for coping with stress and aging.

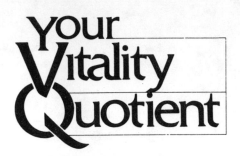

Part I

Your Vitality Prescription

CHAPTER 1

Premature Aging
(The Vitality Drain)

Our research at the Canadian Institute of Stress indicates that premature or accelerated aging is the number one degenerative condition in North America, possibly affecting as much as one-quarter of the adult population. If you've got it, it saps your vitality and weakens your immune system—making you more susceptible to illnesses and diminishing your quality of life. If you're in a demanding job, premature aging decreases your ability to achieve at top levels. If you lead an active life, it reduces your level of performance in every area from sex to softball. Nevertheless, if you have a case of premature or accelerated aging, you probably don't know it. In all likelihood, you dismiss its symptoms as merely the inevitable side effects of growing older. They aren't.

The symptoms are part of many people's lives. Here are some of them: frequent fatigue, dragging yourself through the day and then collapsing when you get home from work; feeling old; aching joints; stiffness; loss of body flexibility; frequently feeling "tense." Perhaps the single most prevalent symptom is a generalized feeling that your reserves of energy just aren't what they used to be—a sense of lost capacity.

Almost everyone who entered the Body Age Program was experiencing some of these symptoms.

Larry, age 38, was a national organizer for a large labor union. For some time, he'd been suffering from constant fatigue and daily headaches; he was taking roughly 200 Tylenol a month. "Some days I feel like my body has formed a union and all the parts are on a slowdown," he told us. "And by evening I feel like every one of them is out on strike."

3

Referring to his chronic headaches, he added, "And the grievances are piling up."

Joyce, a 35-year-old legal secretary, was acutely aware of the difference a few years can make. "Five years ago, it took me ten minutes to 'get beautiful' in the morning," she told us, in describing her daily application of makeup. "Now it takes an hour . . . which means less time for my 'beauty sleep.' There must be a better way."

George, age 46, had been a small-town minister for nineteen years. When he came to us, he was fifty pounds overweight and suffering from ulcers, and five or six times a year he was immobilized by lower-back pain. He felt pulled apart by the demands of home and congregation, and realized he had to learn to budget his time better. "When all I could think about was making it to the end of the week, I realized I was shortchanging not only my congregation, but my family—and myself," he said.

We don't all feel as old as Larry, Joyce, and George, but most of us "feel old" some of the time, even if we don't think of ourselves as aging unduly fast. We may play a hard game of tennis and discover we are stiff for days. Or go out with friends, have a few too many drinks, and wake up the next morning with a hangover that seems out of all proportion to our indiscretion. These and a hundred other commonplace irritants are messages from our bodies that we are growing older.

Accelerated aging affects the quality of your life. And it affects you most when you are in your prime—at peak performance levels in your professional and personal lives, when you should be enjoying those lives to the fullest. Jonathan, a lawyer age 39, commented as he entered the program, "I used to worry about getting turned down by a good-looking woman. Now I worry she'll say yes."

Some people who entered the program were practically paralyzed by the effects of premature aging. One of these was Susan, age 38, a mother of two who in her mid-thirties had returned to the work force as a radio producer. When we met her, she said she "felt like a woman whose future was all behind her." No wonder. Susan suffered from almost crippling arthritis; some days it was a heroic struggle for her to walk three blocks or to use a keyboard or pen for more than five minutes. During other weeks, she could function almost normally. But her symptoms always intensified in step with her stress level.

Crippling arthritis (by the end of the program, Susan's had subsided to occasional mild twinges) is an extreme manifestation of premature aging. More often, people who suffer from this debilitating condition are frequently tired or tense and lack motivation. Many are prone to minor chronic injuries or illnesses, and complain of insomnia or recurring headaches. Almost all say that they don't have as much energy as they used to. In fact, fatigue is one of the most common complaints heard in doctors' offices, yet it defeats most medical investigations and treatments.

No age group is immune to premature aging—even children and teens can show its signs. Whether or not you are in your forties, the decade of vulnerability, you may be a sufferer. Premature aging can strike whether you're in your twenties, your thirties, or your sixties (many people experience accelerated aging when they reach retirement age). As it takes its toll, you may experience more and more difficulty in dealing with the ordinary demands of daily life. And the decade-of-vulnerability aging rates we quoted in the introduction—15.2 years for men and 18.6 years for women—are the averages based on our research. Other studies suggest that the average rate may be even higher.

On the other hand, we all know people who seem younger than their years, who have boundless energy and who use it efficiently, with lots of time and oomph left over for leisure pursuits. George Burns is almost as legendary for his youthful vigor as for his skills as a comedian. Now in his nineties, Burns makes many 60-year-olds seem over the hill. Former Canadian Prime Minister Pierre Trudeau is another striking example. In 1971, when he married the young Margaret Sinclair, few would have guessed his age—52. Margaret was reputed to have said that her husband, "has the body of a 27-year-old." And a 70-year-old woman we know organized a grocery delivery business; because many of her friends "just couldn't make the grade anymore," she started a company to do their shopping for them. Such people are proof that individuals age at widely differing rates and that you can live a fast-track, highly demanding life without being hobbled by fatigue and other premature aging symptoms. Unfortunately, such slow agers are rare. Fortunately, you could be one of them.

WHAT IS AGING?

Scientists are only beginning to understand the physiological process that is aging, but many believe that aging is not biologically inevitable. For instance, Nobel Prize-winning biochemist Linus Pauling has said, "Death is unnatural. . . . Theoretically man is quite immortal. His body tissues replace themselves. He is a self-repairing machine." Even those scientists who believe we are programmed to age admit that there is no inevitable biological reason for us to age as quickly as most of us do. Our research supports the view that there is no internal biological clock ticking away at one predetermined rate, telling your eyesight when to dim and your blood pressure when to rise. Your body ages because certain of its systems begin to lose efficiency over time in response to external factors, such as disease, injury, lack of exercise, or poor diet. All these factors are what Hans Selye, the father of modern stress research, called stressors; they all cause a stress reaction in your body.

Aging is simply the progressive loss of efficiency in all bodily systems. That means, for example, that your heart doesn't pump as efficiently, your bones and joints aren't as resilient, your muscles aren't as strong, and damage to your tissues is not repaired completely. Some aspects of this degenerative process are more apparent than others. For instance, older people often begin to suffer hearing loss and diminished eyesight. As many people age, their sense of smell and taste narrows and fades. Above all, those who are older—as well as younger people who experience accelerated aging—are more susceptible to degenerative diseases, whether colds, viruses, cancer, or heart failure. If the aging process can be slowed, then the "diseases of old age" simply don't have to happen. As a physician who entered the Body Age Program put it, "You can die young at an old age, rather than old at a young age." Or, as so many people do today thanks to the life-extending "miracles" of medical technology, instead of very old at an old age.

If genuine aging is a gradual loss of the body's efficiency, then good health is the opposite—a high level of bodily efficiency. So the more slowly you are aging, the healthier you are and the healthier you feel. Vital health means you feel great, have lots of energy, and are ready to take on the world. If you think of health and aging in these terms, then a disease or illness can be thought of as a usually transitory but significant drop in your body's overall efficiency. In most cases, almost all of the lost efficiency is recoverable; you get well, although there is a net loss each time you suffer a serious sickness. For instance, a liver that has had hepatitis rarely functions as efficiently again; after a heart attack, the heart muscle will never again be as strong. This doesn't mean that if you've had a serious illness the Body Age Program won't work for you. Just the opposite is true. After you've been sick, you can use the program to get your body back to optimum operating efficiency—in many cases to a much more youthful state than before you became ill.

Your rate of aging is the result of many factors, some of them beyond your control. Genetic predisposition, for example, is a significant factor in degenerative ailments. There are more pollutants in city air than in country air, so city folks likely have to fight off more toxins than do their country cousins. If you are too poor to afford good nutrition or if you make poor nutritional choices, you will probably die younger. And people who live in the Third World generally have shorter lives than North Americans. But many of the factors that affect aging are at least partly within your control.

If you escape fatal injuries or terminal infections, you will eventually die from the progressive accumulation of small biochemical imbalances in the body. These imbalances result from poor nutrition, accidents, illnesses, and toxic substances that enter your system. The degree of danger from each of these factors is influenced by how you deal with the countless stressors in your daily life. Eventually, this gradual accumulation of biological damage weakens your body to the point that one or another degenerative disease will surface. The result is either a quick death—for example, a heart attack—or an illness that lingers until one or more essential organ systems fail.

But premature aging is present long before the acute symptoms of a disease occur. Long before "horizontal illness" strikes, many people are "vertically ill"; they are walking around upright, but they are not well and often don't feel up to par. A heart attack doesn't come from nowhere. It is the sudden, sometimes fatal, evidence of a degenerative process that has been going on for years. These vertically ill people are the "revolving door" patients who crowd the average doctor's office with undiagnosable complaints and account for 28 to 35 percent of all visits to physicians. According to the American Academy of Family Physicians, two-thirds of all visits to general practitioners are stress-related.

The key to premature aging is the human mind. We all know that people react differently to similar events. Some people seem able to mourn the death of a beloved parent or child and then get on with their lives. Others are immobilized by grief for months or years, or even die within hours or days of the loss of the loved one. Some people thrive on challenge and excitement. Others have nervous breakdowns when faced with too-rapid change. To these commonsense examples can now be added mounting scientific evidence that how you deal with what Selye called "the stress of life" has a great deal to do with how quickly you age.

BODY AND MIND

Until recently, modern Western medical science treated the body and the mind as two separate and independent entities; it looked on physical health as unrelated to psychological well-being. But recent medical research increasingly shows that "psychological factors can cause disease in themselves and significantly influence disease caused by other factors." Today, more and more doctors are treating the whole person, not just his or her medical symptoms.

Boston researchers Joan and Myrin Borysenko, who wrote the words quoted above, are at the forefront of a growing field known as psycho-neuroimmunology, the investigation of how the body's immune system is affected by psychology. They and many other researchers are convinced that a person's health is closely tied to things like positive or negative attitude to recovery from an illness, or a person's ability to cope with stress.

There is increasing laboratory evidence to back them up. Research in this area is being conducted in many medical faculties in Canada and the United States, among them the Harvard Medical School, the Tufts University School of Medicine, the Salk Institute, the Linus Pauling Institute, the Washington University School of Medicine, the University of Rochester School of Medicine, St. Luke's Medical Center (in Chicago), the University of Southern California, Carleton University (in Ottawa, Canada), and the University of Toronto. All this scientific evidence confirms what your mother probably told you years ago: You're unlikely to get sick unless you're "run down." In the simplest terms, high stress levels cause your immune system to become less effective.

When the immune system is working properly, it protects the body in two basic ways. One is the production of B cells, which form antibodies when they meet a virus or bacterium. These antibodies are cells custom-designed to neutralize or destroy specific enemy invaders. (Vaccines stimulate antibody production by the injection of a small amount of the weakened disease agent.) The other basic defense reaction involves what are known as killer T cells, the white blood cells that are a primary defense against infection. These multiply in number and attack all poisonous or foreign material, including cancer cells.

Similarly, there are basically two ways in which the immune system can malfunction. In the first, the body is not under attack, but for some reason the B cells start to produce antibodies that are directed against your own body; they actually begin to attack healthy cells as if they were enemy invaders (this is the part of the immune system that rejects a transplanted organ). In a sense, the body is attacking itself, giving rise to the auto-immune diseases, which are believed to include multiple sclerosis, systemic lupus, Sjogren's syndrome, and rheumatoid arthritis.

In the second type of immune malfunction, the body's T cell defense forces are suppressed and fail to effectively fight off diseases or toxins that enter the body or that are already present. They also fail to play their central role in regulating your total immune response. Your immune system is weakened, and you become more susceptible to disease. This explains why one person in a family can get a cold or the flu while the others don't, and why one person can become very ill or die of an illness that another person can recover from quickly.

Researchers in the field of psychoneuroimmunology have documented many impressive examples of negative psychological factors causing suppression or malfunction of the immune system. For instance, it is well known that people with a genetic predisposition to the auto-immune disease rheumatoid arthritis tend to develop the disease when certain psychological factors (the distress of bereavement or depression) are present. These psychological factors also indicate that the symptoms will be more severe and will occur more often.

The incidence of lung cancer is also closely related to emotional factors. It's generally accepted that cigarette smoking is a direct cause of this disease, but if that's true, why do only some smokers get sick? Studies suggest that your likelihood of getting lung cancer is sharply increased if you are emotionally repressed (that is, if you have difficulty expressing your emotions) or if you have suffered a traumatic bereavement, such as the loss of a loved one, in the five years previous to the diagnosis of the cancer. One study conducted by Margaret Linn at the Veterans Administration in Miami, Florida, found that the heavy smokers who developed lung cancer usually perceived such life events as marriage, divorce, and family illness as stressful. The smokers who showed no symptoms generally had less difficulty with such events.

Other kinds of cancer also seem to be triggered by your emotions. In a 1981 study of more than one hundred cancer patients and their families, family therapist Michael Kerr found that "in the majority of instances a period of increased, intense, and sustained anxiety lasting from several months to a year or more preceded the cancer diagnosis." He concluded that people are most at risk when these high stress levels occur in the absence of a solid support system of interpersonal relationships.

In a large number of studies, emotional factors have been strongly linked to how fast cancer spreads. And there are some remarkable examples of complete cancer remission that resulted from an apparently purely psychological approach. Perhaps the most famous of these was recounted by Norman Cousins in his bestseller *Anatomy of an Illness*, in which he describes how he cured himself of terminal cancer by reading every funny and upbeat book he could find.

Dr. Selye provides another example. At age 65, he was diagnosed as having reticulum cell sarcoma, a type of cancer from which recovery is rare. He was given six to nine months to live. Here is how he described his response: "I was sure I was going to die, so I said to myself, 'All right now, this is about the very worst thing that could happen to you, but there are two ways you can handle this; either you can go around feeling like a miserable candidate on death row and whimper away a year, or else you can try to squeeze as much from life now as you can.' I chose the latter because I'm a fighter, and cancer provided me with the biggest fight of my life. . . . A year went by, then two, then three, and look what happened. It turned out that I was the fortunate exception." His cancer went into remission and did not recur. Selye continued to live a very active and productive life until his death ten years later at age 75.

Dr. Bernie Siegel, author of *Love, Medicine & Miracles*, uses Selye as an example of what he calls an "exceptional patient." In his words,

"Exceptional patients refuse to be victims. They educate themselves and become specialists in their own care. They question the doctor because they want to understand their treatment and participate in it. They demand dignity, personhood, and control, no matter what the course of the disease." In his experience, it is these "fighters" who are the ones who experience "spontaneous remission" of "terminal" cancer. Siegel is convinced that it is a patient's conscious and unconscious attitudes to his disease that largely determine the success of the treatment.

One of the best-known investigations of the relationship between distress and susceptibility to disease was the research that identified the Type A personality, a character type that emerged in the 1950s in the course of a study by Meyer Friedman and Ray Rosenman. When they investigated what behavioral profiles were most likely to lead to heart disease, they found that certain individuals otherwise at low risk (for example, those with no family history of heart disease and in generally good physical health) were very prone to coronary problems. These were aggressive, fiercely competitive people who never stopped their relentless race for success and status. Subsequent researchers have found that similar behavioral patterns lead to immunity suppression. And it has become clear that prolonged periods of high stress weaken the immune system. It's as though the body, in its attempt to muster maximum resources to meet one kind of demand (a stressor), withdraws support from another area (the immune system), temporarily reducing its ability to deal with a very different demand.

The symptoms of chronic fatigue syndrome, or yuppie flu, are usually those of a flulike illness and, beyond unrelenting fatigue, can include frequent headaches, muscular pain and weakness, the inability to concentrate, and acute distress in family and work life. Many people suffering from this extreme form of chronic fatigue become incapacitated. Others are absent from work frequently and, when on the job, perform at 50 percent of their normal productivity levels. The symptoms may disappear for as many as several years, but seem almost inevitably to recur.

The deciding factor in chronic fatigue syndrome seems to be stress. Women in high-stress jobs are especially vulnerable; two to three times as many women as men fall prey to the disease, which is thought to be caused by the same bug that causes mononucleosis: Epstein Barr virus (EBV). The syndrome appears after periods of intense, chronic stress, and it recurs after another high-stress period or highly stressful event. It often follows a death in the family, a job loss, relocation or promotion, a financial setback, or even a marriage or the birth of a child. The severity of the symptoms seems to fluctuate along with stress levels. Ongoing research at the Canadian Institute of Stress is beginning to show that the symptoms disappear as the immune system is strengthened by the Body Age Program.

Chronic fatigue syndrome appears to be at an epidemic level in North America. According to one impressive study conducted at a large general practice in Boston, 21 percent of 500 patients experienced a debilitating form of chronic fatigue that could be explained by no other known disease factors. While no definite link to EBV has yet been established by this or other studies, a higher than normal level of EBV antibodies has been found in a significant proportion of patients exhibiting the symptoms of yuppie flu. While 90 percent of the adult population carries this virus, a much smaller percentage actually develops chronic fatigue syndrome. Like many "germs" that float around in our bodies, EBV is normally kept in check by a healthy immune system.

There's no doubt that stress can be bad for your health. The other side of the stress-immunity coin is that positive psychological experiences can actually strengthen your immune system. This helps explain why exceptional patients such as Cousins and Selye get well. One recent study by David McClelland at Harvard Medical School involved a number of college students who were asked to watch a videotape of Mother Teresa, the revered Catholic nun who ministers to the poor of Calcutta and who has been a spiritual inspiration to millions. The scientists measured the students' level of immunoglobulin A before and after this experience. Found in saliva, immunoglobulin A is a protein that plays an important role in the mouth's immune system. After viewing the tape, this group of students showed a marked increase in the levels of this protein in their saliva. Their immune responses had become stronger.

In 1983, at Toronto's Wellesley Hospital, over the course of a four-week relaxation-training program, researchers measured the level of killer T cells in their study subjects. Between the beginning and the end of the experimental period, the subjects' average level of these cells increased 30 percent.

The power of the mind to help in the healing process is being explored successfully by a number of pioneering medical practitioners. Dr. Carl Simonton, Dr. Bernie Siegel, and others have had remarkable success in using positive mental imagery with cancer patients. Dr. Nicholas Hall of George Washington Medical Center, in Washington, D.C., discovered an increase in levels of killer T Cells in cancer patients who used similar imaging techniques. He also noted an increase in a hormone secreted by the thymus gland, an organ that plays a key role in the immune system.

We've described only the tip of an iceberg of evidence that suggests a direct link between excessive stress, immune suppression, and the onset of disease—and of the opposite, the power of positive feelings, thoughts, and images that enhance your immune response. As the evidence continues to mount, the field of psychoneuroimmunology is bound to grow in importance.

But what does all this have to do with aging? In essence, the immune system is the body's first line of defense against aging, the progressive loss of efficiency in the body's various systems. High stress levels weaken the immune system, making disease or dysfunction more likely. And without a strong, healthy immune system, aging is bound to be accelerated.

When the average person reaches the age of 70, he has lost 60 to 70 percent of his ability to ward off disease. Yet there are 80-year-olds with 80 percent (or more) of their immune system in full fighting trim. These octogenarians are better able to fight off sickness than many a young child. With almost the immune capacity they had in their twenties, they probably feel better than many 50-year-olds. One of the main differences is how they have dealt with stress over the course of their lives. Dr. Siegel puts it this way: "In particular, the onset and course of disease are strongly linked to a person's ability and willingness to cope with stress. Stresses that we *choose* evoke a response totally different from those we'd like to avoid but cannot."

Dr. Selye's favorite commonsense definition of stress was "that which accelerates the rate of aging through the wear and tear of daily living." He believed that your stress level and the way you handle stress determine how and how quickly you age. When he wrote those words, the field of psychoneuroimmunology hadn't been invented. But he would not have been surprised at its discoveries. His pioneering research had already revealed how the way your body performs under stress is closely tied to your overall bodily efficiency, including the effectiveness of your immune system.

Selye understood that the physiological process he called the stress reaction releases enormous energy; in effect, stress can be thought of as a source of energy. How well—how efficiently—you use this energy determines not only how good you feel hour to hour and day by day; it also directly influences your rate of aging.

The theme of this book can be encapsulated as follows: How efficiently you use your "stress energy" determines your vitality and your rate of aging. The more efficiently you use this energy, the greater your vitality and the slower your rate of aging—and the better you will feel.

CHAPTER 2
Stress Is Energy

Your body's energy comes from the food you eat. But the way you experience this energy—for instance how available it is when you need it—is primarily due to a bodily process called the stress reaction. The stress reaction mobilizes and channels your available energy to meet any challenge you face. And it is this high-performance form of energy that we call stress energy.

The biochemical reaction that causes this energy release is a normal and necessary physiological process your body goes through over and over again each day as you deal with the fluctuating demands and challenges of your life. In simplest terms, stress is a heightened state of bodily functioning triggered by the release of certain hormones, especially adrenalin and noradrenalin. It allows you to cope with or adapt to changing circumstances, which is why Hans Selye referred to stress as adaptation energy. You experience stress whether you are the president of General Motors or the resident of a senior citizens home.

Human stress is neither good nor bad in and of itself. The bodily process is the same whether it leaves you feeling great or lousy. What then is the difference between good and bad stress experiences (sometimes referred to misleadingly as "good" stress and "bad" stress)? Although scientists may eventually discover some minute biochemical distinctions between the two, there is only one apparent difference: Stress you experience as positive is accompanied by a low level of perceived uncertainty. Simply put, you experience stress as positive when it is stress that you want—for example, a sky dive, good sex, an exciting play-off game. As Selye and many researchers since have noted, positive stress experiences tend to take place when you have some sense of control over your environment. This is possible even under very adverse circumstances. For example, one of the American hostages in Iran hoarded bits of food from each meal and then offered these scraps to his rare visitors, including his captors. He thus managed to turn his cell into his home and himself into the host, rather than a helpless prisoner.

By contrast, stress you experience as negative or unpleasant is stress in the face of which you feel ambivalent or uncertain or powerless. Such stress always brings with it additional or secondary stress that compounds and prolongs the stress reaction. For example, if you find your job stressful and unpleasant, even a small added irritant—perhaps a sick subordinate —may cause your stress level to jump sharply. Negative stress is stress that you don't want, or are uncertain how to handle, or feel unable to control: getting fired, getting stuck in a traffic jam, spraining your ankle.

Given this basic distinction, the same external event can result in either a positive or a negative experience, depending on how you take it—not everyone enjoys sky diving!

Selye liked to recount a story that nicely illustrates this fact. As a young medical student at the University of Prague in 1926, he was, in his own words, "a man in a hurry." Even during vacations, he would rise at 5 or 6 A.M. to study all day in the garden. His mother warned him that if he kept it up he would soon break down in nervous collapse or exhaustion. Fifty years later, despite his brush with "terminal" cancer, Selye was still keeping much the same schedule (usually working even on weekends and holidays) with little sign of diminished energy.

Some of the best things in life are extremely "stressful," that is, they produce a lot of stress energy—joy, love, sex, excitement, inspiration, and creation, to name a few. They are accompanied by exactly the same internal bodily process as some of the worst things in life—physical threat, psychological trauma, real sickness. Selye used the word *distress* to describe the feeling of unpleasantness or unwellness that is the negative result of stress. He called the positive state *eustress*. Eustress is very close to what we call *vitality*, namely, maximum stress-energy efficiency that produces a minimum rate of aging.

STRESS-ENERGY EFFICIENCY AND
RETURN ON INVESTMENT

The key to the difference between people who mostly experience stress as something good, and people who mostly experience it as something bad, is the idea of stress-energy efficiency. Because this is not the way most people talk about stress, this concept requires some explanation.

One day in 1982, Dr. Earle was trying to describe the concept of stress efficiency to a group about to begin the Body Age Program. Tom, a professional actor, put up his hand and said, "Doc, we actors experience what you are talking about every time we give a good perfor nance. And we have a saying that puts it well: 'If you don't have butternies in your stomach, you'll give a rotten performance. But the secret is to get the butterflies flying in formation.' " Tom had hit on a perfect image for optimal stress efficiency. When the butterflies are flying in formation, you are experiencing stress at its best, stress that makes for peak vitality.

When we talked to our 623 Body Age subjects about stress efficiency, we often spoke of a person's stress-energy investment. How much stress capital (precious energy) are you spending to get the benefits you desire? Are you spending much more than you need to at the moment? Is the stress energy you are spending appropriate to the challenge or demand you face? You may experience this energy surplus as "nervous" energy, muscular tension, an inability to concentrate, or anxiety: all examples of a poor return on your stress investment.

A high rate of return means that you get the results you want from the stress energy *you choose* to spend—and you feel good. A low rate of return means you've wasted stress energy; you feel bad and over time pay a bodily price. David, a 41-year-old stockbroker (initial body age 48) who successfully completed the Body Age Program, put it this way: "There's really no such thing as 'bad stress,' only investments of stress that yield a very poor return. And as with your financial portfolio, the aim is to get as much back from the stress you spend as you possibly can." David learned this lesson well. At his eight-month checkup, he tested 11 years younger—a body age of 37.

George, age 46, is a graduate of the Body Age Program who provides a perfect example of a good return on a stress-energy investment. Recently he wrote to us to say he was resigning his cushy government job to work with a group of missionaries helping to feed starving children in Africa. In his letter, he said that the transition was bound to be very stressful, but that short of a heart attack or serious illness, it would be "stress well spent." Six months later, when he was back in North America for a visit, he requested a new assessment of his body age. He felt great but wanted to find out if our instruments agreed. In spite of his stressful career change, George tested a full 14 years younger than his chronological age—and 5 years below his score when he'd graduated from the program. He had spent his stress very well indeed.

DISTRESS

When most of us use the word *stress*, we are talking about the negative effects of stress poorly invested and inefficiently spent—what Selye called *distress*. All those who entered the Body Age Program were suffering to some degree from chronic distress. The following examples provide a taste of their experience of this widespread modern condition.

Michel, age 47, body age 55, was the admired coach of an NHL hockey team when his physician referred him to the Body Age Program. Distress warning signals had begun to interfere with his job. That April, when his team had made the Stanley Cup finals, he began to have recurring migraine headaches and frequent diarrhea. His condition got so bad that he could barely manage to stand behind the bench for the length of a twenty-minute period without literally seeing double. As it turned out, the play-offs (which his team failed to win) were only the final chapter in a saga of stress inefficiency that each year began in mid-summer when he started to "gear up" for the season. From August until the following May, Michel operated, in his words, "at fever pitch," reaching a stress boiling point during games. By the end of his third week in the Body Age Program, the headaches and diarrhea had disappeared. After eight months, his body age was down to 44.

Linda, age 34, body age 38, a marketing executive for a large food-processing firm, was able to use the energy of stress to get terrific results whenever she made a sales presentation to a client. But by the end of most days, she had little or no energy left to do the necessary follow-up that would turn a first sale into a repeat client. When she entered the Body Age Program, she told us that this energy shortfall was beginning to reduce the intensity she could bring to her sales pitches. And her failure to follow through was affecting her sales performance: After becoming one of the company's top guns, her yearly sales total was slipping. Four months after entering the program, she reported that she had more energy; as a result, she was spending more time on follow-up. By her eight-month graduation, her body age was down to 30. The next year, she won her company's client service award and had a higher sales total than ever before.

You'd probably feel somewhat silly if, after a rough day at the office, you heard yourself say, "Boy, I'm really aging fast today!" Yet you and almost everyone else you know talks about distress—of "feeling stressed," of "stressful situations," of "stress overload," of "high-stress jobs," of "being under a lot of stress," of feeling "stressed out." And sooner or later most people feel the effects of inefficient stress expenditure in terms of lower performance and the other symptoms of premature aging. A 1986 Louis Harris Poll conducted for *Prevention* magazine found that 89 percent of adult Americans say they periodically experience negative stress symptoms and that 59 percent admit they experience unpleasant stress at least once a week.

These figures, while high, seem very conservative to us. Consider these 1979 statistics from the U.S. Surgeon General. Americans consume nearly 1.5 million tons of aspirin a year, well over ten *pounds* for every man, woman and child! One out of every six Americans takes some form of tranquilizer at least three times per week; the most-prescribed drug in the United States is Valium, the second, Librium. A conservative estimate is that 10 percent of the work force can be labeled as either alcoholics or problem drinkers. All these figures indicate higher than healthy stress levels in the general population. And it's safe to say that they haven't improved during the past decade. In a 1983 cover story on stress, *Time* magazine reported that, along with Valium, the two best-selling drugs in North America were Tagamet, an ulcer medication, and Inderal, a medication for hypertension (high blood pressure). The same article estimated that one in five *Fortune* 500 companies had some sort of stress-management program. That number is growing.

YOUR BODY'S STRESS REACTION

In essence, stress is a very primitive bodily reaction that provides you with the energy to either fight or flee. You can also think of it as the body's built-in mechanism for adapting to unexpected changes in the world around you.

Dr. Selye identified three basic stages the body goes through each time it experiences a stress reaction. He named this three-stage model the General Adaptation Syndrome (GAS), and it remains the basis of all modern discussions of biological stress. The three stages are: the alarm reaction; the stage of resistance (or adaptation); and the stage of exhaustion (in biochemical terms, an enforced recovery through a depression of resistance). The GAS is a very primitive response mechanism, the body's attempt to deal with a threat and then get back as quickly as possible to normal operational equilibrium, or homeostasis, what Selye characterized as the normal or healthy level of resistance. During the resistance phase, it's as if your body temporarily turns up its stress thermostat. As soon as possible, it turns it back down to normal.

As the two diagrams on the next page show, the GAS has two distinct patterns. The first diagram shows an acute, or short-term, stress reaction, with a short resistance phase, that quickly returns the body to normal. A good example of this is when you run to catch the bus: You see it's about to pull away; you put on a burst of speed and just make it; then you find a seat and relax. Your resistance phase—the actual dash for the bus—lasted a short time and came to a clearly defined end.

The second diagram depicts a prolonged stress reaction. Here the stage of heightened resistance is stretched out over a period of minutes, hours, days, or weeks—or it may even be the way you live your entire life. This second diagram is a picture of many of us over the course of a normal working day. Dr. Selye was fond of saying that the major cause of distress in modern man was frustration, the cumulative effect of the many difficulties and annoyances of daily life. Because of them, most of us spend most of our time in a prolonged resistance stage, on top of

HANS SELYE'S GENERAL ADAPTATION SYNDROME

An Acute, or Short-Term Stress Reaction

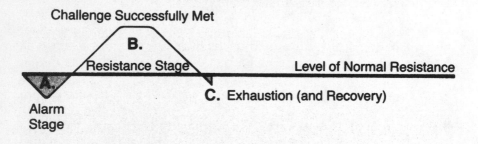

A Prolonged Stress Reaction

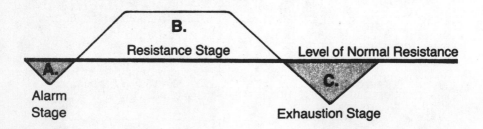

which we experience intense stress reactions of shorter duration, such as running for the bus or getting into an argument with the boss.

Stage 1: The Alarm Reaction. In this intial response stage, the body calls on all its resources to be available for immediate action, mainly by releasing hormones that trigger specific changes in the body. It is during this stage that you feel that surge of adrenalin and your heart begins to pound.

Stage 2: Resistance (or Adaptation). This stage occurs as long as heightened readiness or actual action seems necessary. (This perception has a lot to do with psychological factors.) During this stage, you are adapting, successfully or not, to changed circumstances. Unfortunately, many people stay in this high-stress resistance stage long after a particular challenge has passed. Their hearts keep pumping overtime, their muscles remain tense. These people, sometimes referred to as "hyper," often complain they have trouble relaxing after a tough day or a big meeting.

When Jim, age 38 going on 50, entered the Body Age Program, he was a self-confessed stress junkie, a vice cop who loved his job and hated vacations. His fellow cops, however, didn't seem to understand the importance of "being ready for anything—at all times," as Jim put it. They accused him of creating emergencies for the sheer excitement they provided. Jim had become increasingly aware that he was revved up and ready for action whether he wanted to be or not. Eventually he decided he wanted to "kick the stress habit," and the police psychologist referred him to our program.

People like Jim are actually addicted to the natural drug the body produces during the resistance phase of the stress reaction. The beta endorphins, designed by nature to dull your sense of the pain of battle, produce a natural high (sometimes called the runner's high). Jim not only needed to kick his stress habit, he also needed to get off the uppers and downers he'd been using more and more frequently. When he graduated from the program eight months later, Jim reported that he had been promoted to the rank of lieutenant, a position for which he'd been passed over several times because his superiors felt he was too prone to "knee-jerk responses under pressure." And his body age was down 10 years, from 50 to 40.

Stage 3: Exhaustion. This stage happens once you perceive the threat to have passed or when you run out of available stress energy. It provides a necessary period of recuperation for the body.

Spending too long with your stress thermostat turned up leads to periods of paralytic exhaustion as your body requires more and more time in stage 3. Betty, age 38, a supervisor of airline flight attendants for a major international airline, complained of frequent bouts of fatigue and depression after working a series of fourteen-hour shifts. Although during these shifts she often had a number of hours of "down time just sitting in the stew lounge" between flights, she couldn't relax. She was still "on the job." But once she recognized that she had a choice about how long she stayed in the resistance stage—that she could learn to relax during her breaks instead of "stewing in the stew lounge"—she suffered less and less from the crippling exhaustion that had been eating up her leisure life. By the end of the program, Betty's body age was down from 43 to 34.

Unless you have stayed in the resistance stage until all your stress-energy resources have run out, you won't experience the exhaustion stage as complete physical depletion. But after any intensely stressful experience—a demanding meeting, a fight with your spouse, watching the seventh game of the World Series, or making love—you will at some point be aware of a letdown, often characterized by a feeling of deep relief or pleasant lethargy. Your body is seizing this much-needed opportunity to rest and recuperate. People who spend a lot of time in the resistance phase often resort to drugs such as alcohol to get them out of stage 2 into stage 3; these are the people, for example, who fall asleep at parties. They are also likely to use caffeine or other stimulants to prolong the resistance phase long after their body says "enough," just in order to get through the day. This was why Jim, the vice cop, was becoming dependent on uppers and downers.

Every stress reaction, at whatever level of intensity and whatever its duration, goes through all three phases. But one of the key things we'll teach you in Part Two is how to short-circuit the resistance phase by recognizing and regulating your stress reactions. This means giving you a choice of how you "spend" your stress energy, including whether or not to spend it in ways that may be positive or negative.

In the modern world, we are not usually faced with such a simple choice as fight or flight. Our lives are filled with a thousand frustrations and uncertainties, small and large. If your boss criticizes your work, you don't either punch him in the mouth or run out of his office. If your spouse seems to have lost interest in sex, if one of your kids is in trouble at school, or if your best friend is inexplicably giving you the cold shoulder, a simple solution is not always obvious or even possible. As a result, your body is often unnecessarily in a state of red alert, pumping adrenalin and producing unnecessary stress energy for unnecessarily extended periods.

Psychologists have studied the effect of this state of red alert, or "chronic vigilance," in people ranging from jet fighter pilots to staff members of hospital emergency rooms. One of the most famous of these was the study of the incidence of "blitz ulcers" among residents of London,

England, during World War II. (Peptic ulcers are a direct result of the shutting down of the digestive system during the stress reaction.) Six months after the German blitz ended, the incidence of peptic ulcers in the Greater London population increased by approximately 300 percent. But those who lived in the London city core, where they knew bombs would drop every night, showed only about a 50 percent increase in ulcers, while those on the outskirts, where bombing was unpredictable, got 500 percent more ulcers than normal. It seems that the less sure a person was about the likelihood of being bombed, the higher the level of chronic vigilance, and this extra uncertainty caused a higher stress level.

THE PHYSIOLOGY OF THE STRESS REACTION

Through the work of Selye and others, the physiology of the stress reaction is now well understood. The following capsule summary describes the sequence of chemical and physical events your body goes through during the three stages of the GAS. This sequence makes even clearer the pivotal role stress plays as a link between mind and body.

The Alarm Stage

1. Your body perceives a stressor—something new or unusual that seems to represent a challenge or a threat. A stressor may be psychological (that person looks angry; this meeting is really important and I've got to perform at my best), physical (a heat wave or very cold winter day; stubbing your toe or falling hard on the pavement; a hard hit in a football game), or biological (a disease or virus; poor nutrition; the ingestion of a toxin). Regardless of the kind of stressor, your stress reaction is essentially the same.

2. Your hypothalamus triggers a series of chemical and electrical changes in your body. The hypothalamus is the primitive base of the brain, a tiny area that regulates the majority of the body's unconscious processes, including temperature, heart rate, water balance, breathing, and blood pressure. Its job is to maintain homeostasis, or functional balance, so that, for instance, you sweat when it is hot and shiver when it is cold. The response of the hypothalamus to a stressor is to attempt to return your body to this normal, balanced state. One of the ways it does this is through the autonomic (automatic) nervous system, which has two branches: the sympathetic nervous system and the parasympathetic. Another of the ways is through the endocrine system, comprised

STRESS AND YOUR IMMUNE SYSTEM

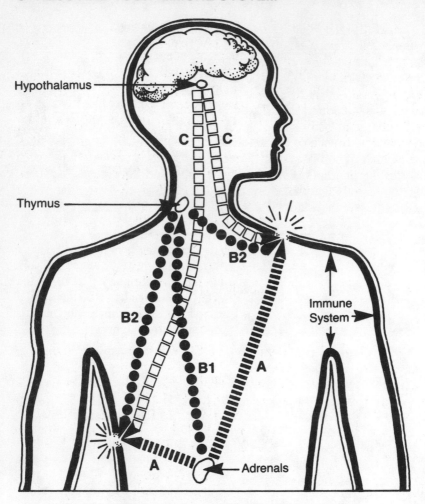

Hypothalamus

Thymus

C C

B2

B2

Immune
System

B1 A

A — Adrenals

As your stress level rises, your immune system becomes less effective.
The diagram shows the three basic immuno-suppressing pathways:

A. Direct suppression of immune cell activity by stress hormones
released from your adrenals.

B1, B2. Stress hormones cause your thymus to shrink, killing immune
cells or leading to their release at a premature (weaker) stage
of development.

C. Beta endorphins activated by your hypothalamus suppress immune
cell activity as well as acting as your body's natural painkillers.

The thick line that follows the outline of the body represents your immune
system. In the diagram, we have shown the immune system being weakened in
two specific spots by the combined effect of these three pathways. In reality, your
whole immune system becomes less effective as a result of these three types of
immuno-suppression.

of the various organs that secrete hormones, ranging from adrenalin to testosterone, into your bloodstream. The hypothalamus is also closely linked to the functioning of the immune system.

As soon as a stressor is perceived, the hypothalamus causes three things to happen. First, stress hormones are released into the body (especially adrenalin and noradrenalin). These temporarily suppress your level of killer T cells, your body's first line of defense against infection. Second, the sympathetic branch of the autonomic nervous system begins to stimulate a number of bodily systems, including the blood vessels, the smooth muscles of the internal organs, various glands, and the digestive system. When your pupils automatically adjust to changes in light, that is the autonomic nervous system at work. Finally, the hypothalamus triggers the release of the beta endorphins, the body's own painkillers that are opiates identical to morphine. The beta endorphins raise your pain threshold, allowing you to withstand a prolonged physical attack and to tolerate higher levels of emotional tension and physical discomfort (for example, muscle tension). This is why you don't feel a cut or bruise incurred during intense physical exertion until much later. As a by-product of the release of these natural painkillers, your immune cells become less effective.

3. *The package of stress hormones combined with the stimulation of the sympathetic nervous system triggers a multitude of other bodily reactions.* Taken together, these reactions are similar to a military general marshaling his troops for an expected attack. He concentrates his forces and puts them on high alert. Your body's metabolism—the rate at which you burn fuel—speeds up. Your heart beats faster, your blood pressure rises, you begin to perspire, your lungs take in more air, your eyes dilate, your mouth goes dry, the hairs on your skin stand on end. All of these symptoms, including the "butterflies" in your stomach, are familiar to the athlete, the actor, and the speechmaker just prior to a performance. To some degree, you experience them every time you feel "stressed."

4. *Blood begins to flow away from peripheral areas and nonessential organs in order to maximize the effectiveness of your more essential organs, such as the heart and lungs.* As a result, your skin begins to pale, and your digestive system starts to shut down. That's why your stomach often becomes queasy and you may get a stomachache if you try to eat when under stress. Your voluntary, or skeletal, muscles become tense, ready to fight off an attacker. Finally, the stress hormones affect glandular activities; you sweat more, for example. In combination with decreased blood supply, this causes your skin to become cold and clammy.

Blood also flows away from areas of your brain responsible for problem solving and information processing, impairing these faculties. And because of the increased adrenalin flow, you will start to have trouble concentrating and difficulty staying still.

The Resistance Stage

5. The stress reaction continues as long as you stay in the resistance phase—that is, as long as you perceive a threat and your body is able to maintain itself in this heightened state. But you may not be aware you are in a stage of heightened resistance. It can become a familiar, rather featureless, plateau.

This never-ending "readiness for the worst" is a rapidly growing phenomenon in the North American corporate landscape. Following the recession of the early 1980s came much company downsizing and many an organizational "rationalization." Often these actions were taken in ways that left employees feeling betrayed and unable to predict when or why the next reorganization or mass firing would happen. In human terms, this meant that a formerly secure environment became extremely insecure, and stress levels rose. As a result, millions of workers ranging from tenured professors and civil servants to production-line veterans now live in a constant resistance phase, waiting for the other shoe to drop.

If the resistance phase is prolonged, a key part of your immune system is affected. Within forty-eight hours of the onset of an acute stressor such as disease, injury, or psychological shock, the thymus shrinks to half its normal size, effectively neutralizing millions of B cells and T cells.

The Exhaustion Stage

6. The exhaustion phase is triggered by a rapid increase in the release of cortisol, a steroid hormone produced by the adrenal gland. This action has a damping-down effect, reversing the stress reaction and returning the body to normal. The stimulating effect of the sympathetic nervous system is now supplanted by the calming effect of the parasympathetic branch of the autonomic nervous system. Among other things, it causes the blood to flow back to the skin surfaces, the digestive tract, and the brain.

As a side effect of the release of cortisol, the immune system is again suppressed. Also known as hydrocortisone, cortisol is often used as an anti-inflammatory drug for the treatment of auto-immune diseases such as skin rashes and rheumatoid arthritis.

7. Ideally, after the exhaustion phase, your body returns to a healthy level of resistance. However, it may damp down only to a lower set point—a lower but less than ideal setting of the stress thermostat. This means that you remain at a higher degree of alertness than is necessary or efficient, given the situation. People who have trouble relaxing, or "coming down," after a high-stress experience are having trouble turning down the stress thermostat. They end up expending a lot of unnecessary stress energy and have less available when a real challenge comes along.

Normal body mechanisms that restore balance following a short-term challenge become a problem when prolonged at elevated levels. The longer or more intense a stress reaction is, the more wear and tear it will inflict on your body. Chronic (long-term) stress in effect turns the body against itself.

More important in terms of the aging process is the way stress affects the immune system. The short-term suppression, or loss of efficiency, of your immune functioning is not a problem. The problem, if you are continually in a state of heightened stress, is the long-term reduction of your ability to fight off disease. And it is immune system malfunction that makes you more susceptible to infections ranging from the common cold to Epstein-Barr virus and more vulnerable to auto-immune diseases such as rheumatoid arthritis and multiple sclerosis.

REGULATING YOUR STRESS FOR MAXIMUM PERFORMANCE AND MINIMUM AGING

The key to mastering stress is learning to budget your stress energy for maximum return—for vitality, not distress. The potential of this energy is evident from all the amazing feats accomplished by mere mortals in extraordinary circumstances, from taking on and beating the schoolyard bully, to performing some astonishing act of strength or courage on the battlefield, to breaking the world record in the 100-yard dash. But not every challenge, or stressor, requires the same degree or duration of response.

The person who masters stress is like the driver of a finely tuned car with a full tank of high-octane fuel. He has his foot on the gas pedal, his hands are firmly on the steering wheel, and he knows when to shift gears or go into highly efficient overdrive. Some people are born with bigger gas tanks than others, tanks that can hold bigger supplies of immediately available stress energy. But assuming that you have a healthy diet and are physically fit, the key to having stress energy available whenever you need it is to not use it when you don't. In other words, you don't rev the engine when your car is in neutral, but you put your foot to the floor when there's a long steep climb ahead. Just as important, you know how to ease up on the gas when the road is straight and level.

Like every car, every person has an optimum operating level. An engine gets its best gas mileage at certain speeds, and your body functions the same way when it comes to stress. Every body is unique. Its optimum stress-energy efficiency is a function of body age and other factors, such as genetics, nutrition, and physical fitness. The basic return you get on your stress-energy investment can be shown graphically by means of the stress-performance curve.

As every athlete knows who has gotten psyched up for a big game, your level of performance rises as you increase your expenditure of stress energy—up to the point of maximum efficiency. After this point, you get a diminishing return on your stress-energy investment; you suffer from a gradual loss of efficiency. As with athletes who have overtrained, at a certain point on the graph your energy efficiency plummets, along with your ability to perform. At this point, you enter the zone of overstress, expending great amounts of energy for very little return and feeling worse and worse as you do. You find that you are unable to concentrate, have a very short fuse, and are accident prone. What puts you over the edge may be a crisis—a fight with your spouse, an emergency at the office, a traffic jam—or it may just be that one additional small stressor that tips the balance. Whatever the trigger, it's at this point that you are likely to crack up your car or sprain your ankle just walking down the stairs. As insurance actuaries know, in the six months following a marriage breakup, the risk of automobile accident doubles.

Before you can learn to stay out of the danger zone of overstress, you need to learn to monitor your position on your personal stress-performance curve: to recognize your stress level and the return you are getting for the energy you are investing. Is your stress level interfering with your ability to function well at an important meeting, or to respond sympathetically to your kids, or to discuss an issue with your spouse? Or is it giving you the edge you need to function at the peak of your form in a demanding situation? As you gain skill at monitoring your personal stress-performance curve, you'll know when you need to slow down (or get a good night's sleep) rather than speed up (or go for a two-mile run).

One of the participants in the Body Age Program was Sharon, age 34, body age 38, a high-flying executive who believed firmly in the power of positive thinking. But when she arrived at the Institute, she reported she had just had her first "less than excellent" performance appraisal in her twelve-year business career. It turned out that she'd been operating at close to her optimum stress-performance level at work when her marriage began to run off the rails. Then she added the stress of a night-school course (at least it got her out of the house). Without really understanding why, she'd gone into chronic overstress. At the time she entered the program, almost all of her stress energy was spent in fending off "any more disasters" (real or imagined) at home or at work. Her ability to run meetings, formerly a strong point, suffered—especially

THE STRESS-PERFORMANCE CURVE

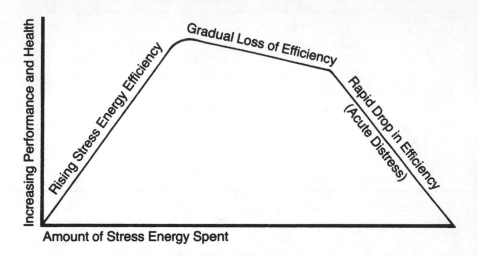

when senior management was present. She found herself "constantly in arguments" with her co-workers. In short, she had her foot to the floor all the time and was no longer steering the car.

During the Body Age Program, Sharon decided to stage a "strategic retreat" at work. This meant "not trying so hard," being satisfied with "adequate" job performance for several months, and renegotiating her targets and time frame accordingly. Almost immediately, she was back in the efficient part of the curve and enjoying her work once more. And after eight months, her body age had been lowered to 28.

THE FIVE PHASES OF DISTRESS

We all experience distress from time to time. However, many of us have gotten so used to some of its symptoms that we've simply accepted them as part of a demanding job or getting older or raising children or battling rush-hour traffic. The following checklist is by no means a complete accounting, but it includes most of the common signs of chronic distress.

Your Personal Distress Checklist

Check each item that is frequently true for you, particularly during a working day or in a demanding or difficult situation.

Physical Signs

_____Your heart pounds or skips a beat for no apparent reason.

_____Your throat and mouth are dry.

_____You find yourself clearing your throat.

_____Your muscles are tight, especially in the neck and shoulders and in the lower back. You may complain of chronic neck and back problems and suffer from sore, tight muscle knots.

_____You get headaches, especially when you are letting down after a tense or stressful period or gearing up for one.

_____You have indigestion or queasiness in your stomach.

_____Your hands tremble.

_____You have muscular tics with no obvious cause.

_____Many of your illnesses turn out to be difficult to diagnose. You're told you "just have to live with it."

_____Insomnia is an increasing problem. The quality and quantity of your sleep go down.

_____You are tired, even if you sleep through the night, and you have less and less energy to get through the day.

_____Your blood pressure is higher than it should be.

_____You develop some of the following problems: allergies, skin rashes, asthma, colitis, ulcers, frequent colds, and flus.

Mental/Emotional Signs

_____You have trouble concentrating, particularly when you most need to.

_____You are emotionally tense, all keyed up.

_____You are easily startled.

_____You find yourself daydreaming.

_____You are prone to excessive worrying and negative thinking.

_____You find yourself brooding, and you may even go into an emotional depression.

_____You experience anxiety (knots in the stomach, tight chest muscles, pounding heart, shallow breathing), with no specific cause.

_____You are subject to feelings of worthlessness; you lack self-esteem.
_____You are forgetful.

Behavioral/Lifestyle Signs

_____You become irritable, easily annoyed.
_____You feel restless. This may be expressed by pacing about or drumming your fingers or feet.
_____You become more impulsive.
_____Your judgment is poor and you make mistakes.
_____You experience difficulty making decisions.
_____You smoke, or drink, or use other drugs—to calm yourself down or keep yourself "up."
_____You mistrust others.
_____You have difficulty getting along with people.

If you checked ten or more of the above twenty-eight items, you are probably going through one of the five phases of chronic distress. These are distinguishable stages as your distress escalates from a minor but annoying fact of life into a major emotional or physical crisis.

At the Canadian Institute of Stress, we have evaluated thousands of individuals who complained of distress symptoms. The five phases emerged from a careful statistical analysis of their responses to our Stress Inventory System questionnaire (a version of the Vitality Quotient Test you'll take in chapter 5). Practically everyone passes through these phases as he or she becomes less and less able to cope with the stressors of life. People continue to experience the symptoms of the earlier phases once they've passed into the later ones, and quite often they cycle through the five phases over and over again. However, different types of people tend to get stuck at different spots in the continuum.

Phase 1: Chronic Mental or Physical Fatigue

At age 42, Bill was an executive on the fast track. Admired for his physical and mental energy, he was always brimming with ideas and the ability to see them through. For as long as anyone could remember, he'd been the life of the party and a fierce competitor in sports. But unknown to most of his friends, Bill had regular spells of exhaustion, of extreme and crippling fatigue. During these periods, he had to sleep longer and didn't have the energy for his usual round of work and socializing. When he finally went to see his doctor, exhaustion was starting to take over his life. He was tired all the time and couldn't get through the day without at least ten cups of coffee. His two packs of cigarettes "helped" him calm down. He couldn't get a good night's sleep. Not even regular exercise worked anymore.

His physician followed standard medical practice and took a comprehensive medical history, conducted a thorough physical exam, and ran an extensive and expensive series of tests. But he could find no evidence of organic disease. Because stress was clearly the underlying problem, he suggested some lifestyle improvements, including a lower intake of coffee, tobacco, and liquor. He also advised Bill to watch his diet and to take some vitamins.

Bill knew he "should" try to change his bad habits. But since there was nothing really wrong with him, he couldn't bring himself to give up his drugs or to eat more sensibly. He didn't want to change, so he rationalized that his problems were just part of growing older.

Early in phase 1, you need a coffee or a strong cup of tea to get started in the morning. You may get through the day okay—probably with the help of several hits of caffeine—but even so you probably suffer an energy low in the middle to late afternoon. When you get home from work, all you want to do is collapse; the hormone cortisol kicks in and you enter an extended exhaustion phase. At night, you tend to sleep poorly and wake up tense, or you sleep soundly but don't wake up refreshed. In the evening, you may feel the need of a drink to unwind, but find that it knocks you flat. Over time, the onset of your daily collapse seems to come earlier and earlier, until one morning you wake up and can barely drag yourself out of bed.

Phase 2: Interpersonal Problems/Withdrawal from Others

When Susan went to see her family physician, it quickly became clear that the problem wasn't her, it was her husband. At age 30, Brian was losing his grip. What's worse, he wouldn't admit there was anything wrong, refused to take any steps to change, and wouldn't consult a doctor. He couldn't see it, but he was about to lose his wife, his two kids, and a six-year-old marriage that had started out solid and loving.

Brian was a handsome, physically powerful man, with a good job as a construction foreman. On the surface, there was no reason for the most important relationship in his life to be going sour. But he had always had a short fuse, and now the fuse was getting shorter and shorter. The whole world had become his enemy—the driver who cut him off on the freeway, the waitress who was slow adding up the bill, the co-worker who looked at him the wrong way. He walked around like a clenched fist aching to land a punch. He'd even gotten into a shoving match with his boss.

When he arrived home at the end of each day, Brian was ready to explode. On a few occasions, he actually blew, physically assaulting his wife. He didn't mean to hit her, he just lost control. As a result, Susan had learned to keep the kids away from him and to keep her troubles to herself. He was okay as long as dinner was on time, the kids were quiet, and everyone left him alone in his favorite chair with a beer and the sports section or his favorite television program. Susan was becoming terrified of him. She was afraid to leave but afraid to stay.

In the second phase of distress, you begin to have problems relating to other people—your co-workers, family, friends, even strangers. Increasingly you withdraw from stabilizing and rewarding contacts with others, even the social anchors of friendship and family. You become suspicious of the people around you or feel hostile toward them. You walk around with a chip on your shoulder, and your boiling point gets lower and lower. You get angry or upset for little or no reason. You spend less time on relationships, put less energy into them, and get less out of them. As a result, the quality of your interactions with people and your sense of satisfaction and support go down. You may, for example, seem to be spending the same amount of time with your spouse, but increasingly you are two separate people who happen to inhabit the same space. More and more, you withdraw into yourself, hoarding your remaining energy for essentials, like just getting through the day at work. Small problems become insurmountable.

Phase 3: Emotional Turbulence

At 29, Marlene's emotional life was on a roller coaster, with wild swings up and down. She enjoyed her job as an executive secretary, but whether at home or at work she was hyper one minute, depressed the next. Lately the swings had become more extreme; she felt as though she had completely lost control of herself and her life. She was buffeted by every little gust of circumstance: the weather, the traffic, her kids' report card, her husband's moods, her boss's demeanor. She loved the highs—all that energy—but the price was becoming too high: The lows were becoming deeper and more debilitating, simply too much to bear. It never occurred to her that there was something in between. If she had once experienced it, she had forgotten the feeling.

In phase 3, the low boiling point of phase 2 has become an almost constant boil, and the churning cauldron of emotions inside you is no longer mainly directed outward but is pandemic: You are filled with self-doubt, unable to focus, arrange priorities, or make decisions. Your interpersonal problems become even more pronounced. Your emotional anchors, your relationships, become more and more tenuous. Now you find that your ability to maintain emotional balance is diminishing. That feeling of stability, of emotional equilibrium, becomes more and more precious as it becomes less and less frequent. You may become easily depressed or find yourself blowing up with no warning. Your reaction to something someone says or does or even how a person looks at you is often out of all proportion to the event that caused it. You are increasingly either hyper or depressed or swinging wildly between these extremes. Your performance at work suffers noticeably. You may have crying fits or fly into rages. You become psychologically worn out. You have totally lost control of your life: It seems directionless, without purpose. Your life is controlling you. Your important relationships—those that remain —become rigid and unsatisfying.

Phase 4: Chronic Physical Discomfort

Marie was 28 years old and had been married for six years. Everything had been fine until her pregnancy four years before, during which she'd developed lower-back problems. After the baby was delivered, the problem remained, gradually becoming worse. She was coping with a newborn and trying to hang on to her part-time job, but she was spending more and more time flat on her back. She quit work. Her friends began to shun her, bored with the main subject of her conversation: how lousy she was feeling. Not surprisingly, she'd become more and more depressed.

When the doctor examined her, he found no serious structural problem. Her back muscles were very weak and imbalanced, and she had numerous muscle knots in her shoulders, down her back and in her buttocks, a condition known as fibrositis. These problems can be treated with acupuncture and massage, and the back muscles can be stretched, balanced, and strengthened through a proper exercise program. But with Marie none of these things would have worked until she could first learn to relax.

In phase 4, your body starts to inform you loudly that you are spending far too much of your time in the second stage of the GAS, the stage of resistance—a state of chronic vigilance. The most obvious symptom is chronic muscle tension, notably in the neck and shoulder area, the lower back, and across the forehead. You may find that you clench your jaw a lot, and you may grind your teeth at night. You may even develop an unpleasant dental condition called bruxism or problems with your jaw joint, a condition called temporal mandibular joint syndrome. You may be subject to chronic headaches, and migraine headaches may occur whenever you do a bit of letting down, for instance on Friday evening or Saturday morning after a long week. In fact, migraines really are "relief headaches." The pain is caused by the rapid relaxation of the constricted blood vessels in your forehead as you let go of stress-induced tension.

Phase 5: Stress-related Illness

When Michael graduated from law school, he'd expected to be able immediately to set up a lucrative practice. He craved material wealth and wanted to be seen as successful by his wife and peers. Instead, he found it wasn't easy for a young lawyer to set up practice in a large metropolitan area and just rake in the dough. Many of his classmates who'd moved to smaller urban centers or specialized in other legal areas seemed to achieve success much more quickly than he. He took a job teaching night classes at the university; it didn't pay much, but he thought it looked good. He worked harder and harder, and went ever more deeply into debt in order to create the appearance of the success that he so desired: the house in the country, the fancy car, the expensive suits, the exotic vacations. He seemed to have everything, and he liked to show it off; he always seemed to be bragging about his latest expensive toy.

But underneath the almost aggressively arrogant manner was a profoundly unhappy man, a person out of tune with himself. The gap between the genuine success he craved and the facade of success he'd created was taking its inexorable toll. In his early thirties, he began having an affair with one of his night-school law students. He thought he loved her, but he was simultaneously wracked with guilt (his wife had quit school and gone to work to put him through law school). His new girlfriend wanted him to move in with her. It was at this point that he was diagnosed with ulcerative colitis.

A serious operation was decided upon, to remove the affected portion of the bowel, but it was only a partial success. The ulcerated bowel was cut out, but the healthy section could not be reattached to the rectum, and Michael ended up with a colostomy. For the rest of his life, his bowel would empty by way of a tube through his skin into a bag attached to his waist. And his sex life would be severely curtailed, since the operation had severed a nerve in the pelvic area.

How did Michael get this way? It wasn't some inherited intestinal defect. There were no discernible organic explanations. A look at the last few years of his life supplied the only possible answer: distress caused by chronic foot-to-the-floor stress-energy expenditure. Perhaps if he had learned to recognize the early warning signs of chronic stress and set more realistic goals for himself, he would not have reached the stage he did. But by the time Michael was ready to do something for himself, permanent damage had been done.

Phase 5 is when you have left the stage of chronic resistance and have entered a chronic version of the exhaustion stage (often referred to as burnout). The accumulated invisible damage to your body manifests itself in specific illnesses, many of them the result of the long-term suppression of your immune system: colds, flus, ulcers, colitis, asthma, high blood pressure, and some cardiovascular disorders. And when you do relax, as on a vacation, your body goes through rapid hormonal changes that can trigger an event as catastrophic as a heart attack. Doctors have traditionally tried to deal with people in this phase by treating only the specific disease. But we are now realizing that without recognition of the underlying cause—stress—and real changes in behavior to combat it, the specific complaint, or another stress-related illness, will soon recur.

As the stress reaction subsides and exhaustion sets in, accumulated physical damage begins to show up. Selye compared this exhaustion phase to the human phase of senile old age. Indeed, as our Body Age research showed, the fifth stage of distress is synonymous with rapidly accelerated aging.

Some interesting research has recently been conducted on the relationship between a chronic phase 5 illness, the common cold, and chronic distress. Studies at several centers, including the Cold Research Center in Bristol, England, have investigated the factors that make people vulnerable to one of the more than one hundred viruses that can cause the common cold. In a study of married couples one partner was deliberately infected with a cold virus while the other was not. In only some cases did the noninfected partner catch the cold. When the results were analyzed, it became clear that the single most important factor in accounting for the difference was the person's distress level.

Doctors now pay much greater attention than they used to to lifestyle as a contributor to disease, and many recognize stress as an underlying cause of many of the complaints people bring into their offices. But doctors lack a framework for helping a patient deal with his particular stress. They can give good general advice, for example, telling a patient to cut down on coffee or cigarettes, or to eat better and take some vitamins, and in general to "take better care" of themselves. How many of you have been advised by your doctor, "You've got to learn to relax more" or "You need a vacation"? This may be good advice, but it usually isn't enough to overcome deeply ingrained habits and behaviors.

Particularly difficult for doctors to deal with are patients with the symptoms of the first three phases of distress, patients with a "vertical illness"—the ones who are walking around with no specific organic disease that can be "cured." Their aches and pains are real, but they have nothing really wrong with them. Even a person who has reached phase 4 is basically "healthy," in the sense that he or she shows no organic pathology. Fatigue, low energy, and insomnia aren't considered treatable conditions unless they are the result of an organic disease. Interpersonal difficulties are often dismissed as character defects in the patient that can be helped only by counseling or psychotherapy. Emotional turbulence might be damped down with tranquilizers or referred to a psychiatrist or psychotherapist.

All five phases of distress are indicators of accelerated aging. But, as the Body Age Study showed, the combination of specific lifestyle changes that's right for you will "cure" your distress and bring down your body age.

THE STRESS MASTER

People who cycle through the five phases of distress are playing a dangerous game that might be called the poker game of stress: They are gambling with their well-being. The poker game takes many forms, but it is always costly and sometimes fatal. Yet as the stakes go higher, it becomes more and more difficult for the player to leave the table.

The workaholic is an example of a chronic stress gambler. But as with Jim, the ever-ready cop who entered the Body Age Program wanting to "kick his stress habit," it's not really work he's addicted to, it's the beta endorphins, the high produced every time he has a stress reaction. The workaholic keeps needing more of these self-produced opiates just to maintain his high, to dampen his withdrawl symptoms when demands decrease, and to relieve or mask his physical discomfort. Every time he gets close to the exhaustion stage of Selye's General Adaptation Syndrome, he raises the adrenalin stakes to keep the stress reaction going and to get more of this drug for his system.

The result of the poker game of stress is that the body "forgets" what it is like to operate at normal, healthy stress levels. Accustomed to this higher stress set point, it forgets how to turn down the thermostat. It wastes enormous amounts of energy trying to maintain internal balance while in a hyped-up condition. It spends little or no time in a truly restful and restorative state. It has become recalibrated to ever-higher levels of stress.

Not surprisingly, this style soon becomes counterproductive. The workaholic spends more and more time getting the same quantity of work done. Meanwhile, his overall quality of life diminishes as he withdraws from other pursuits. Sooner or later, he will pay the price of accelerated aging. By contrast, many people who are really successful are not workaholics but *stress masters*. They may work long hours and use a lot of stress energy, but they are focused and efficient. Their return on their stress-energy investment is high. They also know how to relax—even in the midst of a "stressful" day—and how to choose and vary their stressors, mixing work and play.

Dealing yourself out of the poker game of stress may be your first step toward becoming a stress master, toward using stress energy to achieve optimum vitality instead of letting it use you up. Alternatively, you may be suffering from too little stress (are you sure you're still breathing?) and need to add some well-chosen stressors to your existence, such as regular physical exercise, a more stimulating job, a challenging hobby. The stress master isn't afraid of stress; he welcomes it because he knows, in Selye's words, that "stress is the spice of life."

But the stress master realizes when he (and his body) have had enough. As a result, he seldom goes over the top of the stress-performance curve; before he's even close, he takes remedial action. He achieves not only stress-energy efficiency, but a total efficiency of his physical and emotional systems in harmony with the challenges and opportunities of life.

Much international research, notably that of Sweden's Karolinska Institute, highlights the fact that the average worker spends as much as two and a half times the amount of stress energy he needs to reach the level and quality of output he is currently achieving. In truth, most of us are highly stress inefficient. We never seem to have the time or enough energy for everything we want to do.

In some ways, the stress master resembles a household cat. Sitting below a window ledge, it is perfectly at ease, at rest. Next it eyes the window and seemingly the thought gradually forms that it would like to be up there. Then, in one swift and elegant motion, it jumps, landing perfectly on the ledge. Immediately it relaxes, so completely that the recent expenditure of energy seems a distant event. Like the cat, the stress master fits his energy expenditure to the task; he doesn't waste energy when it's not needed. He knows what his goals are, and he achieves them.

Mastering stress allows you to exert conscious control over invisible and primarily reflexive bodily functioning. It allows you to make stress work for you, to experience stress as something positive, to increase your overall sense of well-being.

Your body constantly seeks to return to a steady, healthy state. It is a naturally health-seeking mechanism always striving for maximum efficiency—as long as you don't undermine it. What we traditionally have called disease or sickness is really a temporary loss of operating efficiency while the body attempts to return to a state of balanced functioning. What we have traditionally called aging is the progressive loss of efficiency over time in many bodily systems. Stress mastery, which makes for the efficient use of your body's resources, slows the aging process and promotes vital good health. We like to think of this as living in harmony with the laws of nature.

CHAPTER 3
Test Your Body Age (The Body Age Study)

Your chronological age, or calendar age, tells you how many years you have lived on this earth. Your body age tells you your biological age—how old your body really is. Body age is the key to a clinical measurement of aging. In other words, your chronological age may be 40, but your body age, as measured by certain key body functions, may be 60 or it may be 23. That is, at age 40, you may have the bodily efficiency of a 23-year-old, that of a 60-year-old, or any age in between.

In the 1950s and early 1960s, researchers in the field of aging found that more than forty measurable physical characteristics changed progressively and reliably with adult aging. These characteristics included blood pressure, body flexibility, finger-tapping dexterity, glucose tolerance, and cholesterol level. However, measuring all forty was a cumbersome and time-consuming process. In the late 1960s, a Canadian researcher, Dr. Robert Morgan, came up with a standardized test for body age, using only three physiological characterstics: blood pressure; high-frequency hearing, and near-vision blurring. He picked three variables for which the level of efficiency was relatively easy to measure and which closely correlated to the loss of overall bodily efficiency, or aging. Morgan called his test the Adult Growth Examination (A.G.E.). It was one of the earliest satisfactory tests for individual body age and is today the most widely used of the twenty most common aging tests. In fact, everyone who participated in the Body Age Study we conducted at the Canadian Institute of Stress took Morgan's A.G.E. test—at the beginning of the program, halfway through, and at the end.

We've modified and slightly expanded the test for our readers, adding several items not used by Morgan that we've discovered are excellent indicators of body age. For instance, we've eliminated the test for high-frequency hearing, which can be conducted only with expensive laboratory equipment.

With the possible exception of the measure of blood pressure, you can do the whole test at home with the help of a friend. Here is the equipment you'll need to take the Body Age Test:

a blood pressure monitor (optional)
a watch with a second hand
a yardstick or meterstick
a vision card (see test #5 for details)
a metal tape measure (the kind that scrolls in and out).

If you have a portable electronic blood pressure monitor (available commercially), you can accurately measure your blood pressure yourself. If you don't have one of these or don't have a recent blood pressure reading from your doctor, make it part of your next checkup. Although a blood pressure reading is helpful, you can take the test without it.

Take the test when you are well rested and aren't on medication of any kind. Make sure the room you are in is at a comfortable temperature and that your last meal was at least an hour earlier. Don't smoke or take caffeine, alcohol, or other stimulants for at least fifteen minutes before you take the test. Before you begin, spend a few minutes resting comfortably in a chair. Stay seated throughout the test, unless instructed otherwise.

A separate Body Age Score Sheet is provided for each subtest. As soon as you have a score, you can look it up on the sheet and find your Body Age Score for that particular test. For the most accurate results, do the whole Body Age Test more than once during the space of several days. Then take the average of your scores.

If you get a reading that seems way out of line, check the calculations again. This home version of the the Body Age Test is accurate 19 times out of 20 within a range of plus or minus 3 years. In other words, if you test within 3 years of your calendar age, there is probably no significant difference between your chronological age and your body age. The Body Age Test is most likely to give a good measure of body age for people between the chronological ages of 30 and 60.

Don't worry if you are unable to perform every subtest. Because each is in itself a valid measure of body age, as long as you do several, including the test for near-vision blurring, your body age score will be accurate. However, the more subtests you do, the more valid your score will be.

THE BODY AGE TEST

Blood Pressure

Make sure you are seated in a comfortable chair and are relaxed. You will be measuring your systolic blood pressure, the maximum pressure in the arteries when your heart is contracting to pump blood.

Place the blood pressure monitor cuff over the bulge in your upper left arm (the bicep). Plug the cuff into the instrument case, switch the machine on, and close the air valve by rotating the cap clockwise with thumb and forefinger. Pump the hand bulb to inflate the cuff to a pressure point that equals the normal systolic blood pressure for someone of your sex but 20 calendar years older (but no higher than 160 mm/hg). You'll find these figures on Body Age Score Sheet #1: Systolic Blood Pressure.

Slowly deflate the cuff by gradually opening the air valve (turn it counterclockwise). Your partner can help you to read the pressure the moment a flash occurs on the control dial: That's your systolic blood pressure reading. Once you've finished deflating the cuff, record your number in the space provided below.

To ensure accuracy, we recommend that you measure your blood pressure two more times during the Body Age Test, once in the middle of the test sequence and once more at the end. Then take the average of the three readings.

If you have recently had a physical examination, a phone call to the doctor's office should get you the information you need. Your blood pressure will read in the form that follows: 102 over 74, or 102/74. The first number is the only one you need to remember. Once you find it on Body Age Score Sheet #1, you have your first body age measure.

FIRST BLOOD PRESSURE READING _____
SECOND BLOOD PRESSURE READING _____
THIRD BLOOD PRESSURE READING _____

AVERAGE BLOOD PRESSURE READING _____
BODY AGE IN YEARS _____

Resting Heart Rate

Place a watch with a second hand in front of you where you can read it easily. Breathe normally. Place your middle finger on the big artery in the side of your throat so that you can feel the pulse. Another good spot is the wrist, but any place you can feel a strong pulse will do. Count the

BODY AGE SCORE SHEET #1:
SYSTOLIC BLOOD PRESSURE

Systolic Blood Pressure SBP mm. Hg.	Men: Body age in years	Women: Body age in years
0–110	19 or less	19 or less
111	19 or less	20
112	19 or less	21
113	19 or less	23
114	19 or less	25
115	19 or less	28
116	19 or less	30
117	19 or less	32
118	19 or less	33
119	19 or less	35
120	19 or less	36
121	20	37
122	21	39
123	24	40
124	27	41
125	30	42
126	32	43
127	35	44
128	38	45
129	40	46
130	42	46
131	44	47
132	46	48
133	48	49
134	50	50
135	51	52
136	52	53
137	53	55
138	54	56
139	55	58
140	56	59
141	57	59
142	58	61
143	59	61
144	60	62
145	63	62
146	65	63
147	67	63
148	69	64
149	71	64
150	72	65
151	73	65
152	74	66
153	76	66
154	77	67
155	78 or more	67
156–157	78 or more	68
158–159	78 or more	69
160	78 or more	70
161 or more	78 or more	71 or more

number of pulses over a twenty-second period. Repeat several times to ensure accuracy. Multiply the average number by three, and enter the resulting number in the space below. Then consult Body Age Score Sheet #2 for your score.

RESTING HEART RATE: BEATS PER MINUTE
(Pulses counted × 3) _____
    BODY AGE IN YEARS _____

Reaction Time

Stand up. Have your partner suspend the yardstick vertically in front of you. Hold your thumb and forefinger on either side of the ruler so that they are lined up at the 12-inch mark, and be ready to grasp the ruler as soon as your partner lets go. Keep your thumb and forefinger at least 1 inch apart, but not much more.

Your partner's job is to release the ruler unexpectedly. When he does so, grab it between your two fingers as quickly as you can. Measure the number of inches the ruler falls with as much precision as possible. Do the test three times with each hand, then take the average. Enter this below, then look at Body Age Score Sheet #3 for your body age equivalent.

    AVERAGE REACTION TIME _____
    BODY AGE IN YEARS _____

Skin Elasticity

Place one hand, palm down, on a flat surface. Be sure the hand is relaxed. With the thumb and forefinger of the other hand, take a large pinch of skin in the *middle* of the back of the hand. Hold the pinch firmly for five seconds. When you release it, count the number of seconds your skin takes to resume its normal shape. Either hand will do. Do this two or three times, then enter the average below. Your body age score is on Body Age Score Sheet #4.

    SKIN ELASTICITY READING (RECOVERY TIME) _____
    BODY AGE IN YEARS _____

BODY AGE SCORE SHEET #2:
RESTING HEART RATE

Heart rate: Beats per minute	Men: Body age in years	Women: Body age in years
50 or less	19	19
51	19	19
52	19	19
53	19	19
54	19	19
55	19	19
56	19	19
57	19	19
58	19	19
59	19	19
60	19	19
61	20	19
62	21	19
63	24	20
64	27	22
65	30	25
66	32	27
67	35	30
68	38	33
69	40	35
70	42	37
71	44	39
72	46	41
73	48	43
74	50	45
75	51	46
76	52	47
77	53	48
78	54	49
79	55	50
80	56	51
81	57	52
82	58	53
83	59	54
84	60	55
85	63	58
86	65	60
87	67	63
88	69	63
89	71	64
90	72	64
91	73	65
92	74	65
93	76	66
94	77	66
95	78 or more	66
96	78 or more	67
97	78 or more	67
98	78 or more	68
99	78 or more	69
100	78 or more	71 or more

BODY AGE SCORE SHEET #3:
REACTION TIME

Reaction time in inches	Men: Body age in years	Women: Body age in years
1.0–1.25	19	19
1.26–1.50	19	19
1.51–1.75	19	19
1.76–2.00	20	19
2.01–2.25	21	19
2.26–2.50	22	19
2.51–2.75	22	20
2.76–3.00	23	21
3.01–3.25	25	23
3.26–3.50	26	24
3.51–3.75	28	25
3.76–4.00	29	26
4.01–4.25	30	27
4.26–4.50	31	27
4.51–4.75	33	29
4.76–5.00	34	30
5.01–5.25	35	31
5.26–5.50	36	32
5.51–5.75	36	32
5.76–6.00	38	32
6.01–6.25	39	33
6.26–6.50	39	33
6.51–6.75	40	33
6.76–7.00	42	34
7.01–7.25	44	36
7.26–7.50	45	37
7.51–7.75	46	38
7.76–8.00	46	38
8.01–8.25	47	39
8.26–8.50	49	40
8.51–8.75	50	41
8.76–9.00	50	41
9.01–9.25	51	42
9.26–9.50	53	43
9.51–9.75	54	44
9.76–10.00	54	45
10.01–10.25	55	46
10.26–10.50	56	46
10.51–10.75	57	47
10.76–11.00	59	48
11.01–11.25	60	49
11.26–11.50	61	50
11.51–11.75	62	52
11.76–12.00	63	53
12.01–12.25	64	54
12.26–12.50	65	55
12.51–12.75	65	56
12.76–13.00	66	58
13.01–13.25	68	60
13.26–13.50	70	61
13.51–13.75	71 or more	63
13.76–14.00		66
14.01–14.25		68
14.26–14.50		71 or more

BODY AGE SCORE SHEET #4:
SKIN ELASTICITY

Skin elasticity in seconds	Men: Body age in years	Women: Body age in years
2–	19	19
2–4	30	30
4–6	40	40
6–8	45	45
8–10	50	50
10–12	60	60
12–14	70 or more	70 or more

Near-Vision Blurring

This is a test of how closely you can see printed material without blurring. If you wear corrective lenses of any kind, remove them before taking the test. Whether you are nearsighted or farsighted, this test is equally accurate. For this test, you'll need to make a vision card that exactly matches the illustration below. The accuracy of the test depends on type size; most normal 10-pitch (pica) typewriter type will do. The simplest method is to type the phrase ''Vitality Is Efficiency'' onto a blank index card. Use upper- and lower-case letters rather than all capitals.

To prepare to do this test, tape the card to the end of a metal tape measure (the kind that scrolls and unscrolls) so that it stands vertically. Make sure the lighting in the room is excellent, with no glare.

```
                Vitality Is Efficiency
```

BODY AGE SCORE SHEET #5:
NEAR-VISION BLURRING

Near vision in inches	Men and women: Body age in years
0.0–3.9	19 or less
4.0–4.1	20
4.2	21
4.3	22
4.4–4.5	23
4.6–4.7	24
4.8	25
4.9–5.0	26
5.1	27
5.2–5.3	28
5.4	29
5.5–5.7	30
5.8–6.1	31
6.2–6.5	32
6.6–6.8	33
6.9–7.1	34
7.2–7.5	35
7.6–7.9	36
8.0–8.2	37
8.3–8.5	38
8.6–8.9	39
9.0–9.5	40
9.6–10.1	41
10.2–10.7	42
10.8–11.3	43
11.4–11.9	44
12.0–12.5	45
12.6–13.1	46
13.2–13.7	47
13.8–14.3	48
14.4–14.9	49
15.0–17.3	50
17.4–19.7	51
19.8–22.1	52
22.2–24.5	53
24.6–26.9	54
27.0–29.3	55
29.4–31.7	56
31.8–34.1	57
34.2–36.5	58
36.6–38.9	59
39.0–41.3	60
41.4–43.7	61
43.8–46.1	62
46.2–48.5	63
48.6–50.9	64
51.0–53.3	65
53.4–55.7	66
55.8–58.1	67
58.2–60.5	68
60.6–62.9	69
63.0–65.3	70
65.3 or more	71 or more

Ask your partner to begin with the card 6 feet from your face and gradually scroll it toward you. Hold the tape casing firmly in place, touching the cheekbone below your right eye, and cover your left eye. Your partner should keep the tape measure as level as possible as he slowly moves it closer. Stop your partner as soon as the letters begin to blur. If you're not sure, ask him to move it back and forth slightly until you have a precise fix on your near-vision blur point—the point when the letters are not sharply defined at the edges. Now test your left eye while covering your right eye. Average these two measures. Record this measurement to the nearest tenth of an inch. Then look at Body Age Score Sheet #5 for your score.

NEAR VISION BLURS AT _____
BODY AGE IN YEARS _____

Take the average of your body age scores. If there is a range of more than fifteen years in your results, eliminate the lowest and highest score. But don't eliminate your near-vision score. Then take the average of the scores you are counting. This will give you the most accurate at-home measure of your body age.

AVERAGE OF BODY AGE SCORES _____

Even if you've been unable to do all five tests, your result is still valid. In fact, the most sensitive of all is near-vision blurring, and this score alone is a good measure of your body age. Near-vision is a very demanding body age measure. As we age, we lose flexibility and elasticity throughout our bodies as a result of disuse and ongoing molecular changes. Since you are using your eyes all the time, lost elasticity in the lens of the eye, which is measured by near-vision blurring, is a very precise indicator of body age.

You now know whether you are biologically older or younger than your years. The difference between your calendar age and your body age is called the body age gap. We'll talk about this in some detail at the end of chapter 5, after you've taken the Vitality Quotient Test. But in general, the wider the gap, the more likely it is that you are aging either faster or more slowly than the average person.

If you scored more than three years above or below your chronological age, then your body is significantly older or younger than the norm for your age. If you scored significantly older, then you likely have been aging at an accelerated rate, and remedial action is called for. Pay particular attention to those subtest scores that are ten or more years older than the norm, especially the score for blood pressure. If your blood pressure score is ten years or more above your chronological age, it's probably time you had a medical checkup.

If you scored more than three years younger than your calendar age, congratulations! You should feel good about yourself. But your body age at the moment is only part of the aging story.

The Body Age Test is only a snapshot. It doesn't tell you how fast you're aging, only what your physical age is right now. The *rate* at which you are currently aging is much more important than this snapshot, useful as it is. It is quite possible, for example, to score a low body age but in fact to be aging rapidly, which means that your favorable body age gap is closing fast. If you've suddenly taken on a high-stress job or are going through a prolonged distressful period, you are probably aging at an accelerated rate. You may still be benefiting from body age years in the bank, but you are now spending them recklessly. And no matter how young you tested, you can feel younger still. Your vitality challenge is to see how low you can go.

Testing much older than your age is no cause for despair. Our study showed that people who are older than their age can make dramatic improvements in as little as a few months.

THE BODY AGE STUDY

In the late 1970s, Dr. Selye and Dr. Earle, the director of the Canadian Institute of Stress, noted that there was a major gap in the existing research on the relationship between stress and aging. There was ample evidence that heightened stress levels cause more rapid aging in animals. And there was growing scientific research suggesting that the same thing was true of human beings. But very little was known about which specific remedies for premature aging were effective for which sorts of people.

The Basic Study

Dr. Earle designed a research program to investigate the relationships between stress and aging by testing various existing stress-management techniques for their effectiveness in lowering body age. During the study, we referred to these techniques as anti-aging interventions. Each subject who entered the Body Age Program signed on for a period of eight months, so that his or her progress could be charted over an extended period of time, although four months is long enough for significant body age reduction to show up.

The program had three basic elements: assessment, training, and remedial action. Each participant agreed to return to the Institute for reassessment after four months and after the full eight months. Of the 1,868 who applied, we chose 623 who tested at body ages significantly higher than their calendar ages. They complained of the whole range of symptoms characterizing the five phases of distress. Because they were suffering from a self-reinforcing chain of negative biochemical events that is difficult to reverse, positive results would be difficult for them to attain but would be dramatic if they occurred. We excluded anyone from the test group who was currently in medical treatment for any chronic physical disorder, as well as anyone in psychotherapy or on continuing medication.

Upon entering the program, each subject underwent a comprehensive physical and behavioral assessment that went beyond the usual preventive medical examination, which is mainly concerned with detecting diseases already present before their more serious symptoms appear. In addition to body age, this assessment was designed to reveal the subject's cardiovascular capacity, stress-control and recovery capacity, physical conditioning, nutritional efficiency, and general psychological hardiness.

During assessment, each subject underwent physical and psychological tests, including Morgan's A.G.E. test to yield a measure of body age; a comprehensive medical examination by a physician; a detailed life-events questionnaire measuring behaviors, attitudes, and quality of life (the basis of the Vitality Quotient Test you'll take in chapter 5); a physical fitness assessment (including a cardiorespiratory test, a measure of body fat as a percentage of total weight, and a measure of body flexibility); and a stress-reactivity profile (measuring baseline stress levels, reactivity to stressors, stress-reaction patterns, and stress recovery time). After the various tests, each participant had a private interview with a staff member at the Canadian Institute of Stress. This was a chance to go over the results, congratulate the subject on areas of strength, flag areas requiring priority action (for example, high blood pressure or high cholesterol levels), and encourage full participation in the program.

After the assessment, the participants were trained in ten stress-management anti-aging interventions:

Self-hypnosis and anti-aging imagery
Nutrition
Values/goals clarification (career and leisure)
Relaxation
Physical conditioning (exercise)
Cognitive reappraisal
(a technique for rethinking high-stress situations)
Personal goal setting and motivation
Communication and conflict resolution
Managing decisions, priorities, and time
Budgeting stress energy

After the skill-training sessions, each participant began a personal eight-month program. The requirements were simple and straightforward. Each person undertook to use certain of the skills learned in the training sessions to make concrete changes in his or her lifestyle. We encouraged everyone to work with a partner, preferably someone in the program, who could provide informed support and act as a sounding board. Progress was to be recorded daily in a written diary that would allow the staff to monitor how closely each anti-aging intervention was followed. The diary was also a useful tool in keeping the participants committed to the program, providing them with a concrete sense of progress that reinforced their behavior changes.

Four months later, each subject returned to the Institute for a checkup, including a new test of body age and a progress interview keyed to the diary record. At the second interview, changes and ways of overcoming problems in an individual's program were discussed. Almost all of our study subjects (602 out of 623) continued on for the second four months, a low rate of attrition for a voluntary study group of this size. At the eight-month final checkup, all 602 remaining subjects were again tested for body age and overall progress.

As the study progressed, it quickly became apparent that our subjects were making remarkable progress. The average of the subjects' chronological age upon entering the program was 36.4 years; their average body age—according to Morgan's A.G.E. methodology—was 42.1. They ranged from a calendar age of 28 to a calendar age of 52, but their body ages ranged from 30 to 68. Many showed an alarmingly wide gap between chronological age and body age. The widest gap was a 35-year-old woman who tested at a body age of 62, a full 27 years older than her calendar age. A number of complaints and conditions were widespread, including borderline high blood pressure, serious overweight, chronic fatigue, and frequent energy deficits. Some people reported periodic bouts of depression.

When the 623 subjects were reassessed at four months, they showed an average 2.4-year reduction in body age. At eight months, the 602 subjects who completed the program had lowered their average body age by 8.2 years: The average body age had gone down from 42.1 to 33.9. Women, with an average improvement of 8.7 years, did slightly better than men, who averaged a 7.8-year reduction in body age. In other words, more than 80 percent of our subjects, all of whom had entered the program "older than their years," were able in eight months to lower their body ages to points below their calendar ages, and more than 96 percent of those who completed the full eight months were able to lower body age significantly. More than half showed a body age reduction of 9 years or more, and 208 of the 602 lost 10 or more years of body age.

Although first impressions are often misleading, in the case of Marion, the study participant with the widest body age gap, they were quite accurate. When she walked into Dr. Earle's office for the entry interview, he thought this bleary-eyed woman must be looking for the Sleep Disorder Clinic on the next floor. She had large, dark circles under her eyes and appeared to find it difficult to keep them even partially open. Her face was deeply lined, her knuckles were swollen in a way typical of longtime arthritis, and she was markedly underweight (100 lbs. on her frame of 5' 5"). Although she spoke deliberately and quickly, her voice sounded as though it belonged to either a chain smoker or someone who'd been up all night. Dr. Earle would have guessed her age at somewhere in her early to middle fifties, rather than her calendar age of 35. Testing revealed her body age as 62.

By training, Marion was an architect. Married at 21 to a rising member of the diplomatic corps, she had put her career and ambitions on the back burner while she followed her husband from one foreign posting to another. When the couple eventually returned to Canada, she was in her middle thirties, had practiced her profession for no more than a few months, and was possessed of a deepening sense of personal failure that further fueled her desire to succeed as an architect. She and her husband had put off having children until they were "more settled."

Marion borrowed $35,000 to start her own architectural consulting business for interior designers, but the business had quickly failed, mainly because she "hadn't paid enough attention to details." The business failure had only increased her sense of being hopelessly out of control of her life. A prime example of this was that she now accepted as normal the fact that she woke up every morning at 4 A.M. and couldn't get back to sleep, a syndrome that had been going on for three years. Dr. Earle remembers thinking to himself during the interview that although Marion's career had yet to start, her body was reaching retirement age.

At her eight-month checkup, Marion's body age improvement was nothing short of astonishing. She tested at a body age of 36.5 years—a 25.5-year improvement and almost down to her calendar age. She now slept regularly and deeply, her appetite had improved, and her weight was up from 100 pounds to 120. And she looked as young as her new body age: The dark eye circles were gone, her skin tone had improved markedly, and her posture was confident and communicated energy.

In accomplishing this turnaround, one area Marion focused on was exercise: first some walking, then hiking with her husband, and finally, near the end of the eight-month period, aerobics classes. She also went through the unsettling process of looking at her values and goals, in her career and family life. This led her to stop putting off starting a family (her husband agreed to refuse further foreign postings) and to make a more realistic entry into the work force (she got a part-time teaching position at a community college). The job gave her a great deal of satisfaction, and, although she failed to get pregnant, she recognized that in a sense she now had a baby: "After a dozen years of pregnancy, I finally gave birth to a career—one I wanted and had the energy to manage."

We witnessed many other examples of dramatic improvement in body age. Study participants invariably reported that they could feel the difference: They were less on edge, more in control, had more energy, were sleeping better, and felt better about themselves. They looked better and were much closer to their ideal weight. In short, everyone who completed the program showed a dramatic gain in their physical and psychological capacities. They had all increased their "positive health"—their vitality.

The following chart shows the main clinical results of the program, broken down by key health variables. All the figures are averages. The asterisked items show the average improvement of the study group, expressed as percentage changes from average baseline scores. In other words, if a participant tested a stress recovery time of 3 minutes at initial assessment and a recovery time of 2 minutes at final assessment, this is expressed as a 33 percent improvement.

Some of the items in the table of results require explanation.

Triglycerides are the form in which fat is stored in the body, so they constitute a measure of the body's fat content: The lower your triglyceride count, the better. They are released into the bloodstream as a negative side effect of medium- or long-term stress. At initial assessment, we assigned each subject a target triglyceride count, based on age and ideal

PROGRAM RESULTS AT FOUR AND EIGHT MONTHS

	At 4 months	At 8 months
Body Age Decrease	2.4 yrs	8.2 yrs
Doctor's office visits decrease*	22%	53%
Days absent from work decrease*	42%	58%
Below target blood pressure	49%	91%
Weight within 10% of norm	67%	86%
Cholesterol within target range	50%	74%
Immunoglobulin A increase*	24%	31%
T cells increase*	16%	28%
Triglycerides within target range	43%	61%
Stress hyper-reactivity down*	41%	46%
Stress recovery time down*	28%	36%
Ability to relax at will increase*	17%	31%
Physical strength increase*	26%	39%
Body flexibility increase*	18%	32%
Percent body fat decrease*	22%	36%
Oxygen uptake increase*	32%	47%
Forced expiratory volume increase*	16%	27%

body weight. Then we compared this target with the subject's actual triglyceride level.

Immunoglobulin A (found in saliva) and *T cells* are both standard measures of the effectiveness of the body's immune system. The fact that both increased by roughly 30 percent over eight months is striking evidence of the Body Age Program's effectiveness in strengthening the body's immune response.

Stress hyper-reactivity and *stress recovery time* are measures of a person's stress response: how fast he or she heads for the danger zone of overstress, and how quickly he or she can recover from a high-stress reaction. These measures were made by comparing a subject's baseline levels for EMG (muscle tension measured by electromyography) and heart rate with levels during and immediately after various stress-stimulating exercises.

Oxygen uptake is a measure of how efficiently the lungs oxygenate the blood. It can be estimated accurately by monitoring changes in heart rate.

Forced expiratory volume is tested by having a subject breathe out as much as he can into an inflatable sac. The bigger the volume he can inflate, the greater lung force he has.

Noticeable improvement was registered in every area and quite remarkable gains were made in several. For example, by the end of the eight-month study period, 91 percent of the subjects had reached or were below their target blood pressure. This surprised many of them, who believed that they were stuck with elevated blood pressure for the rest of their lives.

Another striking result is the program's success at reducing (or increasing) body weight to near ideal. It supports the growing belief among health professionals that the best way for people to lose weight is to think of themselves in a more positive light—a clear side effect of following the program. "Thinking lean" is increasingly accepted as a vital ingredient in sensible, permanent weight loss. This result is just one example of the effectiveness of self-hypnosis, combined with positive affirmations and visual-imaging techniques, in helping our study subjects achieve their goals.

Physical Appearance Change

In addition to our scientific measures of body age and the other physiological tests we did, we conducted a carefully controlled study of the change in physical appearance of our subjects over the eight months of the program. While a person's inner well-being is more important than his or her outer appearance, looks are still extremely important to most of us. Not surprisingly, one of the most common themes expressed by those entering the program was a desire to look better as well as feel better. While many of the cosmetic aspects of aging, such as balding and skin wrinkling, are only partially or peripherally related to the underlying loss of bodily efficiency, we were nonetheless interested to discover how much these inner changes would be mirrored by changes in physical appearance.

We needed to come up with a set of physical characteristics that could be assessed accurately and objectively by a group of trained apperance judges. So we asked three physicians (two men and one woman) and three physiotherapists (one man and two women) to make independent evaluations of the apparent age of a test group of fifteen men and fifteen women corresponding in age and general health to our study participants. These experts developed a set of twelve reliable age "appearance criteria": skin tone; number of facial wrinkles (within a preselected 4-inch square); depth of facial wrinkles; appropriate eye movement (while tracking changes in the position of the interviewer); degree eyes were fully open; energy level (appraised on the basis of speed and smoothness of movement); dark shadows under eyes; uprightness of sitting posture; length of facial wrinkles; graying hair (men only); balding hair (men only); eye-hand coordination (when picking up a pen and clipboard).

We used these twelve indicators to train our panel of age-appearance judges, four nurses (two men and two women) who would be with us for the duration of the program. The judges used a 0-to-10 rating scale, in which 10 equaled the most extreme manifestation of the criterion (for example, very deep facial wrinkles) and 0 equaled no evidence of the criterion (for example, no visible facial wrinkles).

When each subject entered the Body Age Program, his or her physical appearance was appraised by two of the four age judges. At the end of the eight-month study period, the other two judges conducted a second appearance appraisal.

The table below summarizes what our judges saw.

PHYSICAL APPEARANCE AGE APPRAISAL RESULTS

(0 = youngest appearance; 10 = oldest appearance)

Criterion	Average score at entry	Average score at 8 months
Skin tone	7.1	4.2
Number of facial wrinkles	6.4	5.1
Depth of facial wrinkles	5.9	3.7
Inappropriate eye movement	7.4	3.2
Degree eyes not fully open	7.6	3.1

	Average score at entry	Average score at 8 months
Fatigue level	6.8	3.4
Dark shadows under eyes	5.1	1.9
Slouched sitting posture	4.4	3.7
Length of facial wrinkles	6.1	5.7
Graying hair	5.6	5.5
Balding hair	5.5	5.7
Eye-hand coordination	5.3	3.6
Appraised Age-Appearance (in years)	46.2	33.4

NOTE: The final item is a summary of the twelve appearance criteria that gives extra weight to the more important items.

The results confirm what our sophisticated instruments so carefully measured in terms of body age. On average, the appearance age of our subjects went down 13 years in eight months. Even facial wrinkling was less apparent after eight months in the program. And for many criteria, the improvement was quite dramatic. For instance, skin tone was markedly more youthful, and our subjects looked more awake (eyes more open, dark shadows mostly gone), acted more energetically, and had better coordination. Significantly, the only two criteria that showed no improvement—hair balding and hair graying—are the only two almost entirely genetically programmed, so we didn't expect the Body Age Program to have much impact on these.

The Vitamin-Mineral Supplement: A Double-Blind Test

An important and fascinating subproject in our Body Age Study was the testing of a vitamin-mineral supplement. We had no conclusive evidence that supplementing your diet with vitamins and minerals has any short-term effect on your ability to cope with periods of acute stress, but there was some evidence that chronic high stress levels could significantly lower the levels of certain nutrients. And there was considerable laboratory evidence that, over a period of three or more months, nutritional supplementation can improve functioning at the cellular level, notably in oxygenation and energy production. But, because of the difficulty in getting large groups of healthy people to take part in a long-term nutrient study, there was virtually no research documenting vitamin deficiencies in people showing signs of lifestyle-induced stress. The research that has been done mostly deals with people who are sick, for example, vitamin C deficiencies in people who have just had major surgery. Since regulation of energy efficiency was at the heart of the Body Age Study, we decided to simultaneously conduct what turned out to be ground-breaking vitamin-mineral research.

In 1979, about fifteen months before the main Body Age Study was to get under way, we tested a separate group of 227 adults for vitamin deficiencies, using repeated blood tests. All those chosen for the study group exhibited chronically elevated stress levels and had body ages 8 or more years above their chronological ages. Overall, ten vitamins were found to be consistently below normal levels: A, B_1, B_2, B_3, B_6, B_{12}, C, E, folic acid, and biotin. We did not test for mineral deficiencies because of the questionable reliability of the testing methods that existed in 1979.

Of even greater interest than the deficiencies was the fact that the ratios among these ten deficient vitamins were highly consistent. In other words, whether a subject's overall level of deficiency was moderate or high, the ratios between these depressed nutrients were remarkably similar. These "deficiency ratios" pointed us toward the "supplementation ratios" promising the greatest benefits.

We were now ready to test a vitamin supplement on our original study group. Because we did not then find a commercially available product that met our precise specifications, we developed our own formula.

This second part of the vitamin study lasted eight months. Each of our 227 subjects took tablets containing our formula of vitamins and minerals. This supplement was the only anti-aging treatment received by the group. After eight months, 93 percent of our subjects showed normal levels of the previously deficient vitamins, and their average body age reversal was 3.19 years. As far as we know, this is one of the only longitudinal studies to track the results of vitamin-mineral supplementation in a large group of subjects.

Apparently, the right vitamins alone could lower body age. We were now ready to conduct an even more rigorous clinical test, this time on those participating in the main Body Age Study. First we refined our formula based on what we'd learned from the original study about minimum dosage levels. Then we did a double-blind test of this revised formula on our 623 Body Age Study participants. Double-blind means that half of the study group received a placebo and the other half the actual supplement. In addition, the person dispensing the formula was unaware whether he was dispensing the placebo or the real thing. Such a double-blind format is generally accepted as a prerequisite for scientific accuracy.

And at the end of eight months, the participants receiving the vitamin-mineral supplement showed an additional body age reduction averaging 2.62 years.

VITAMIN-MINERAL SUPPLEMENT BODY AGE RESULTS

Body age reversal achieved	Number of subjects using placebo (Total 297)	Number of subjects using active formula (Total 305)
10 or more years	40 (13%)	168 (55%)
7 to 9 years	153 (52%)	134 (44%)
6 years or less	104 (35%)	3 (1%)

We were particularly struck by the fact that the supplement made little difference in the area of disease prevention, as indicated by the frequency of visits to the doctor. Where it proved its mettle was in the health-enhancement categories: stress hyper-reactivity and the two immune function measures (immunoglobulin A and T cells)—most important for indicating body age, which measures physiological efficiency, that is, health.

No one who took the supplement experienced a body age reduction of less than 6 years. And more than half (55%) of the 305 who used the supplement showed a reduction of 10 years or more. By contrast, of the 297 who used the placebo, only 13 percent were able to reduce their body ages by an equal amount. In short, the supplement had considerable positive impact on the body age reduction of all those who used it, regardless of the anti-aging interventions they were working on.

What all this told us is that good eating habits alone aren't enough to guarantee high performance. The use of a vitamin-mineral supplement is one of our recommendations in chapter 12, "High-Performance Nutrition."

Summing Up the Study Results

Looking at the results of the Body Age Study as a whole, it's clear that the participants became remarkably healthier in an eight-month period. Not surprisingly, they reported how much better they felt. A company president from Montreal, who entered the program along with three of his top executives, commented, "A number of our key people were simply 'older than their years.' And their performance and satisfaction with the company were suffering. But each one of us wrote it off as part of the cost of doing business. We figured the fatigue and the blood pressure pills went with the territory. At least that's what we assumed until we felt the increased energy and balance that accompanied the decrease in our group's body age.''

A corporate executive from New Jersey echoed these comments in even stronger words: ''After our apparently healthy comptroller died suddenly of a heart attack two years ago, I wondered, 'Do the members of our executive team have what it takes to keep making the grade in a business world that sure isn't getting any easier?' Going through the Body Age assessment was a rude awakening for some of us, even though we knew the Institute's program could help our team regain the competitive edge, that ability to bounce back, that some of us had lost.''

Here is Dr. Earle's more detailed assessment, drawing on his opening and closing interviews with one person who entered the the Body Age Study. His name and various other details have been altered to protect confidentiality.

''When I met Peter at the clinic for pretesting, I formed an immediate first impression of his age. I remember thinking, 'For a man close to sixty, he's in pretty good shape: flat stomach, good posture, expressive face, neatly cropped white hair, well groomed and well dressed.' In sum, Peter was the picture of the successful older executive five or six years away from retirement.

''Then he spoke. His voice was a clipped staccato with little modulation; it was emotionless. As he talked, his pupils remained constantly dilated: They seemed to have a preset focus only somewhat related to our conversation. It seemed highly possible that he was on drugs. (He wasn't.) Then I asked him his age. He was 42.

''During our initial interview, Peter gave me an earful. Sleep was a major problem—always fitful, never long enough. His sex life was a long-standing trouble spot because of his inability to maintain an erection. He had an ulcer that prevented him from really enjoying food. This was ironic, since he was something of a gourmet, having joined a wine club and taken cooking courses. His blood pressure was up to a level that indicated borderline hypertension. His business consumed his life. 'My wife says that if I let myself,' he told me, 'I'd be at work all the time.' During a typical weekend at their country property, he was frequently on the phone to his partner and would often cut his holiday short to return to the city to work on Sunday. Not surprisingly, at the end of such a weekend he felt as if he'd 'had no time out.'

''Eight months later, Peter was a different man. It was almost as though a third dimension had been added to him. His skin tone (elasticity) was improved. His speech was easier, and he sat in the chair in a much more relaxed way. Somehow I could just tell that he had more energy, yet felt less need to be in constant motion. His blood pressure was down, and his body age score was about twelve years below his original test. 'I have the energy I had back in my twenties,' he told me. He reported progress in every aspect of his life."

Here are Peter's own comments.

On work: "For the first time, I'm making real choices about what's important to me, on my terms. I'm making my energy count for me. Although I still put in at least fifty hours a week, I'm getting twice as much back as I used to. Now I go into meetings not at my old minimum speed of 60 m.p.h., but more at about 20 m.p.h., just keeping the engine turning over smoothly. But I know I've got my foot on the accelerator. When I need to, I can put my foot to the floor, do what I need to do, and then use the Sigh of Relief technique to get unwound. At the end of the day, I don't just crawl into my car exhausted. Sure I still sometimes come home drained, but ten minutes with the relaxation tape and I usually get my second wind."

On his leisure time: "I have to confess that I was initially frightened when you told me that I could take charge. I realized that I'd been kidding myself: I pretended I was running things, but really I felt I was just swimming as hard as I could to keep up. So I tried not taking my briefcase home one weekend—and I began to feel a little freer . . . after I got over my panic."

On his sex life: "Our relationship in bed has gotten a lot better. I find my mind doesn't wander like it used to when we were making love. I guess I never realized that you have to really want it, that you have to put your whole self into it, if you're going to really enjoy sex."

On the stress-management anti-aging interventions: "One of the best things about this program is that the techniques I've learned make sense to me. I know they work. And I know how they work. So I use them."

Comments like these reinforce what the Body Age Study results suggest—that there is a close link between the aging process and vitality, both physical and mental. You and the people around you want to perform at your best all the time. That's when you enjoy your work and your play. That's when you feel good. That's when the years seem to "just drop away." As the study showed, it's within your power to increase your vitality, your zest for life, "to be old enough to know what you want . . . and young enough to enjoy it."

CHAPTER 4

The Six Stressotypes, or Six Scenarios of Accelerated Aging

One of the main reasons we conducted the Body Age Study was to find out which stress-regulation, anti-aging techniques worked best for which types of people. In order to do this, we needed to divide our study subjects into meaningful subgroups, identified by behavioral and lifestyle characteristics. This meant analyzing the results of the Stress Inventory Questionnaires filled out by each participant. This questionnaire forms the basis of the Vitality Quotient Test you'll take in the next chapter.

We identified groups of questions that received high scores on a single questionnaire. If a person scored high on a particular question, he or she usually scored high on certain other questions. For example, people who said they believe that worry is the price of success also believed, paradoxically, that worry was a major barrier to accomplishment. These same people also usually reported that they had trouble turning off their thoughts, and that they found it hard to take their own advice. When these and other strongly correlated responses were clustered together, a lifestyle or behavioral profile emerged—in this case, the chronic worrier, or Worry Wart.

Our analysis of the questionnaire answers led us to identify six distinct types, which we dubbed stressotypes: lifestyle profiles that are particularly prone to distress and accelerated aging. Each stressotype is stress-energy inefficient in different ways. In our training sessions for the program participants, we talked about the ways a person can "leak" stress energy. This can also be thought of as a "vitality drain" or a "stress-energy drain." Identifying your particular stressotype profile allows you to zero in on the particular ways in which you are inefficient at using stress.

Of course, no one person perfectly fits any of these six stressotypes, although some people, particularly if they have reached an advanced phase of chronic distress, may have gotten pretty close. The stressotypes are extremes, but anyone who has experienced distress at some time or other—that is, almost everybody—will recognize his or her distressed self in one or several of the types described. Even if you never get close to one of these extremes, your stressotype subscores on the Vitality Quotient Test in the next chapter will help you focus on the precise areas of your life that will most benefit from change.

This chapter is divided into two parts. The first consists of thumbnail descriptions of the salient symptoms and typical behaviors of each stressotype. The second part consists of six case histories of individuals who entered the Body Age Program. Each of the six is a good example of a person with a very dominant stressotype.

The people described in our stressotype case histories are real people in distress. We've chosen them to demonstrate vividly what can happen if you let stress inefficiency get the upper hand. These are actual people who entered the Body Age Program. Every one of them chose to change—and did change.

MEET THE STRESSOTYPES

Some stressotypes are more common than others. We present them here in the order of the frequency of their occurrence in our study group: Speed Freak, Basket Case, Cliff Walker, Drifter, Worry Wart, and Loner. The people who entered the Body Age Program may not be a perfectly representative sample of the general population; nonetheless, the order in which their stressotypes ranked in the study group is suggestive of the ranking of the categories among people in distress.

The Speed Freak (or Stress Hyper-Responder)

Mental/Emotional Characteristics: Impatient, easily irritated; represses feelings; general state of emotional turbulence (gets stuck in distress phase 3; see chapter 2).
Physical Symptoms: Sweats easily; has disturbed or shortened sleep (wakes early); may experience chronic physical discomfort (phase 4).
Behavior Symptoms: Interrupts; critical; frequently gets into arguments; tries to do two or three things at once.
Typical Examples: The workaholic; the superwoman.

Early Warning Signs: Diminished stamina; occasional bouts of debilitating fatigue.
Long-term Consequences: Total exhaustion; ulcers, heart attack, colitis.
Commonsense Solution: Learn and practice relaxation techniques.

───────────────────────────

Speed Freak behavior was the most common cause of accelerated aging in our study group. It was the dominant stressotype for 22.3 percent of those who entered the Body Age Program and the second most important vitality drain for another 11.1 percent. Speed Freaks usually also scored strongly in the Basket Case or Drifter categories. A full 32 percent had Basket Case as their second most dominant stressotype, and 24 percent were secondary Drifters.

We all know Speed Freaks—whether they are constant speeders or people who go through speedy or manic periods. They seem unable to slow down and are always two steps ahead, even of themselves. Often they are outwardly successful people who seem to be on the top of their particular world. But although Speed Freaks are people on the move, they often don't have a clear idea where they're going or why they're heading there so fast. They are often workaholics, but whether working or playing, they do it with intensity, seemingly unable to distinguish between what is important and what isn't. They are often physically fidgety, unable to sit still. Many have the habit of anticipating others in conversation and finishing their sentences for them; they interrupt often and frequently change the subject. They are annoyed or irritated easily, are often critical of others (though usually keeping their true feelings to themselves), and tend to get into arguments. They are extremely impatient when waiting—in line, in traffic, for a friend who's late. At work, at home, at play, they tend to try to do two or three things at once.

Speed Freaks are usually restless sleepers, waking once or twice during the night or rising early with an immediate charge of adrenalin before they've had a good night's sleep. They may be subject to periods of total collapse, but tend to hide these from even their most intimate circle. Apart from these occasional letdowns, they don't seem to know how to relax. Their idea of recreation is strenuous physical activity or perhaps a vacation itinerary as tightly scheduled as a typical business day. They must have projects to fill their leisure time.

Since the Speed Freak is such a common creature, a number of scientific studies have been done of this personality type. People with a high susceptibility to heart attacks or other cardiovascular problems—what has been called the Type A personality—are invariably Speed Freaks.

More than any other stressotype, the Speed Freak wastes his stress energy needlessly by keeping his body in a heightened state of red alert. A graph of his daily stress-energy expenditure would show an elevated baseline and frequent spikes up into the danger zone of overstress. Relaxation techniques would be effective in helping Speed Freaks lower their body age.

The Basket Case (Chronic Energy Impairment and Minor Illnesses)

Mental/Emotional Characteristics: Depression; lack of drive or staying-power.
Physical Symptoms: Chronic fatigue; lower-back pain, poor circulation, tension and migraine headaches; chronic muscle stiffness; highly susceptible to low-grade infections, including flus and colds; frequently suffers from allergies; gets stuck at two of the five phases of distress, either phase 1 (chronic fatigue) or phase 5 (chronic illness).
Behavioral Symptoms: Chronic complainer ("my back is killing me"); increasing use of stimulants to get through the day.
Typical Examples: The absentee employee (too many sick days and low on-the-job productivity); the doctor shopper.
Early Warning Signs: Increasing fatigue or lack of energy.
Long-term Consequences: Poor performance in all areas.
Commonsense Solution: Better diet; more exercise.

Basket Case behavior was the dominant factor in the accelerated aging of 19.6 percent of our study subjects. It was the second most important vitality drain for another 22.8 percent. A high percentage of Basket Cases (38 percent) show the Loner as their second most dominant stressotype. The other important secondary types are Drifter (20 percent) and Worry Wart (22 percent).

The Basket Case is a person who always feels drained at the end of the day and is often tired before the day begins. At work, he is constantly fighting low energy and tires easily; he is someone for whom it takes a mighty act of will to function in the workaday world. He is often a drain on co-workers or friends. He frequently complains of tension and migraine headaches, pain in the lower back, cold hands or feet, and tight aching muscles—all arising from no specific medical cause. If a doctor suggests more exercise, he will beg off, saying he's too tired for additional physical exertion. He seems especially prone to low-grade infections, colds, flus, and allergies. With friends, he often talks about how tired or lousy he feels. He can easily go into a vicious downward spiral leading to the loss of his job, the breakup of his relationship, or both.

The Basket Case leaks stress energy by being physically unfit. His body isn't capable of spending much stress without either going over the top of the stress-performance curve or exhausting itself. Common sense suggests that this type needs to get better prepared physically for his life, which means introducing some exercise and improving the diet.

The Cliff Walker (High Physical Vulnerability and Aging Risks)

Mental/Emotional Characteristics: Is either cavalier about all kinds of risks—from health to money to driving his car ("If I'm going to die or get sick, I'm going to enjoy getting there")—or knows he's "living on borrowed time" but at the same time feels invulnerable or immortal.
Physical Symptoms: High blood pressure; heart disease; gout; diabetes; arthritis; migraines; back problems.
Behavioral Symptoms: Diet probably high in caffeine, fat, salt, sugar, and refined food; likely a smoker and alcohol abuser; possibly a high aspirin intake; gets little or no exercise; may try fad diets but doesn't stick to them.
Typical Examples: Someone who is obese and may have sloppy dressing and grooming habits; the couch potato.
Early Warning Signs: Blood pressure rising above safe levels; visibly older than his calendar age; poor skin tone; slouched posture; dark circles under the eyes.
Long-term Consequences: Stroke, heart attack, premature death.
Commonsense Solution: Improving diet and exercise.

Among those who entered the Body Age Study, Cliff Walker behavior was the main contributor to accelerated aging for 17.2 percent. It was the second most important stress-energy drain for another 13.6 percent. Not surprisingly, given their close relationship, 40 percent of Cliff Walkers showed Basket Case symptoms as the second most important factor. Another 20 percent were secondary Drifters and 20 percent were secondary Speed Freaks.

As the name implies, the Cliff Walker is a marginal person, someone who lives on the edge; his lifestyle is one of chronic self-abuse and self-indulgence. Along with the Speed Freak, he is the most likely candidate for a fatal heart attack in his thirties or forties. He is susceptible to a host of other illnesses and complaints: migraine headaches, hypertension, ulcers, smoker's bronchitis, gout, diabetes, arthritis, and serious back problems. His health and eating habits are a mess: He probably smokes and drinks too much, is overweight (or on a fad diet), uses tranquilizers and antacids frequently, exercises never or erratically, and has little recreational or family life. His diet is most likely a disaster—high in fats, refined foods, and refined sugar. Because he simply doesn't take care of himself, it's impossible to know where, when, or how the Cliff Walker will fall off the cliff.

Superficially, the Cliff Walker and the Basket Case seem similar; in fact, they are quite distinct. The Basket Case is characterized by a progressive erosion of efficiency: He is a car gradually running down. By contrast, the Cliff Walker has already broken down, or is about to. If the Basket Case is physically unfit, the Cliff Walker is a physical wreck, leaking stress energy like a sieve. His stress-energy reserves are adequate until he springs a major leak, for example, a heart attack. He is an accident waiting to happen—his body keeps functioning, but it is only a matter of time before his weakest body system fails. The simplest challenge of daily living may be the straw that breaks the camel's back. Common sense suggests that improved nutrition and exercise are the keys to reversing the vitality drain of the Cliff Walker.

The Drifter (No Satisfying Life Purpose or Direction)

Mental/Emotional Characteristics: Unhappy, depressed, hopeless; lacks drive and feels a strong sense of falling short, of underachievement; doubts existing goals and is keenly aware of a gap between his current life and the way he'd like to be.

Physical Symptoms: Low energy; insomnia; frequent colds and minor illnesses.

Behavioral Symptoms: Puts most of his diminishing energy into nonwork areas; seeks short-term gratification (food, entertainment); relationships often become unstable, wavering between one extreme and another; may suddenly make a major change in direction, such as a big career or life change (ending a marriage, dropping out to find himself) in a vain attempt to "start fresh."

Typical Examples: A teenager or young adult who can't decide on education or career (for example, the "professional student" who is still in school at age 30); the 30- or 40-year-old in mid-life crisis; the recent retiree at loose ends, suddenly with no purpose; the homemaker suffering from the "empty nest" syndrome.

Early Warning Signs: Increasing alienation or dissatisfaction at work (even as outward success escalates); less and less energy for friends and family.

Long-term Consequences: Emotional disorders or eccentricities; higher risk of suicide or accidents.

Commonsense Solution: Get in touch with underlying values ("just what do I really want?") and start finding ways to live life more in tune with these.

For 15.4 percent of our study subjects, the loss or blurring of a clear, deeply motivating life purpose was the primary source of premature aging. For an additional 21 percent, it was the second most important stress-energy drain. Drifters tend to score highly in one of three other categories: Speed Freak (28 percent), Worry Wart (24 percent), and Loner (22 percent).

There are two main types of Drifters. The more obvious one is the person who never really seemed to find a goal or direction. He may have made it through college but subsequently drifted from one job to another, never finding his feet. Equally common, however, is the person prone to the classic mid-life crisis. These are frequently very successful people who reach a stage at which they begin to question their goals and the sacrifices they've made to achieve them. There are two other critical ages when Drifter behavior is likely to take over: The first is the late teens or early twenties, the age when people are first starting out on a career path; the second is upon retirement, when many people literally feel as though they've been cut adrift.

Most people, perhaps especially those who have achieved career success, at some point hit a stage of profound doubt and questioning of the personal value of what they have accomplished. (The career referred to here could be that of a housewife whose children have left the nest or a corporate executive whose "success" no longer satisfies.) These life crises can go on for months or years, and are marked by poor or uneven productivity and creativity, volatile interpersonal relationships, and lack of commitment to co-workers and to the job itself. As the gap between "career success" and "personal success" becomes more pronounced and more acutely felt, it can lead to deep depression, personal paralysis, and sometimes an impulsive life change that can have disastrous consequences.

Whether the crisis comes in mid-life or at some other time, the typical Drifter feels blocked from becoming the ideal person he dreams he can be. He believes that his creative self is being stifled and that he is making little of his talents or using his talents in inappropriate ways. He doubts the goals, especially the career goals, he has chosen, and feels that the way he is using his time doesn't reflect himself or his true interests. He feels that other people see him as being more successful than he really is. He isn't clear about what he wants; he's only sure that he doesn't want what he's got: His values and his actions are out of phase, and this is his major vitality drain.

The Drifter's existence resembles the plight of the mythical Sisyphus, who was condemned forever to roll a rock to the top of a hill, only to have it roll back down again. Since he expects nothing to satisfy him, he never stays with any course long enough for it to pay off. Yet he has invested so much energy in his life that he believes there must be something worthwhile out there. Otherwise why would he have tried so hard for so long?

The Drifter wastes stress energy through psychological uncertainty. He never applies himself wholeheartedly to any one job or life project; instead he rather haphazardly and halfheartedly approaches many different challenges, undermining himself through self-doubt. Common sense suggests that the Drifter's key to reducing body age is for him to get in touch with his underlying goals and values, and then to behave in ways that express those values in his daily life.

The Worry Wart (Chronic Worrier)

Mental/Emotional Characteristics: Has trouble "turning off" his thoughts; pessimistic attitude (expects the worst); lots of self-blame stemming from low self-esteem; frequent anxiety; believes that, if he just thinks (that is, worries) enough about things, somehow a solution will appear.

Physical Symptoms: Slowness in recovering from high-stress events; tension headaches, lower-back pain, difficulty getting to sleep; rapid weight loss or gain.

Behavioral Symptoms: Has a reputation as a worrier; fails to follow through on career and relationship opportunities.

Typical Examples: The boring friend who talks only about his problems; the chronic job switcher (career stops and starts); the person who is immobilized by fear of making the "wrong" decision.

Early Warning Signs: Becomes very agitated if there is not enough "time to worry"; often feels others are cold and heartless because they are not worrying about him.

Long-term Consequences: Never gets anywhere in his career; may have serious psychological problems, such as clinical depression and periods of "manic denial," in which various self-destructive enthusiasms (especially regarding changes in job or relationship) are vain attempts to lift depression.

Commonsense Solution: Learn to value himself more; learn to quiet the mind (mind-focusing relaxation techniques).

Chronic worry was the primary factor contributing to accelerated aging for 13.5 percent of those who entered the Body Age Program. This figure is quite close to the findings of Dr. Thomas Borkovec, a psychology professor at Pennsylvania State University. According to Borkovec's research, roughly 15 percent of adult North Americans are chronic worriers. Among our study subjects, Worry Wart behavior was the second most important vitality drain in another 13 percent. Worry Warts also score strongly as Basket Cases (28 percent), Drifters (22 percent), and Loners (22 percent).

A certain amount of worrying serves a useful function: It helps us anticipate and prepare for problems that lie ahead, in the sense of "putting your worry to work," as opposed to just plain wheel-spinning worry. But the act of thinking anxiously about the future or anguishing over the past has virtually taken over the Worry Wart's internal mental processes. He worries into existence problems that aren't there and makes small concerns into life-and-death issues. He expends so much energy in worrying about himself, his health, his relationships, and his job that he has little vigor left for living and working. He is in the driver's seat of his car, constantly revving the engine but rarely putting it into gear. He uses lots of energy going nowhere.

The Worry Wart either feels that worry is the price of success or that worry is a barrier to accomplishing more. He can't turn his thoughts off, and the same worries keep coming back. He is an obsessive or circular thinker who tends to blame himself for his problems but can't take his own advice about how to change. He is often of a pessimistic disposition and recovers very slowly from a stressful experience.

The Worry Wart is the sort of person about whom friends say, "If he weren't worrying, I'd be worried." He's likely become very absorbed in his health. Perhaps he devours self-help books (but doesn't act on their advice for long or worries about whether or not to try it), takes self-improvement courses, or is in and out of psychotherapy but never stays with a therapist long enough to make any real changes. His relationships suffer; for one thing, he starts worrying they'll end before they've begun. His career is likely to be characterized by many promising starts that soon fizzle out, by much potential that is always unfulfilled. For him, worrying has become a way of life.

The Worry Wart leaks stress through worrying, that is, by expending unnecessary energy on an internal debate, or "self-talk," that gets him nowhere. Common sense suggests that one of the keys to reducing body age for this type is to quiet the inner chatter by means of mind-focusing relaxation techniques. Another is to learn to value himself more—blaming himself less for his failures and finding more opportunities to experience himself as a successful person.

The Loner (Relationship Malnutrition)

Mental/Emotional Characteristics: Lonely and often depressed (although this feeling is often well masked by a smile, a brisk gait, and a superficially cheery hello for everyone); feels uncomfortable with others; has difficulty giving or receiving intimacy; has interpersonal problems (distress phase 2).
Physical Symptoms: Few distinct or overt physical symptoms, but a tendency to have a very erect posture and a stolid, serious, or even severe facial expression; prone to infrequent but severe infections from which recovery is slow.
Behavioral Symptoms: Spends little time with friends and family; avoids social events or remains on their fringes; an observer rather than a joiner; occasional alcohol or drug binges to unwind; only break in life routine is planned holidays and trips.
Typical Examples: The competent worker who believes that "work and friendship don't mix" and so is socially isolated at the office; someone frequently described as being "a very private person" (often mistaken for the "strong, silent type").
Early Warning Signs: Diminishing quality of contact with others; increasing social isolation; relationship problems; abuse of alcohol or drugs.
Long-term Consequences: Complete social isolation.
Commonsense Solution: Learn and practice relationship skills; learn to be more emotionally open and expressive.

Loner behavior was the dominant cause of accelerated aging for only 12.1 percent of the study group, but it turned out to be the second most important stress-energy drain for another 20.4 percent. In addition, Loners often have Drifter traits (30 percent) or Basket Case traits (28 percent).

A Loner is not necessarily someone who lives alone or avoids most social contacts, although this may be true when the type has reached an extreme stage. But he or she is someone who feels alone most of the time, even in a crowd and especially at a social gathering of "friends," and who gets next to no nourishment from relationships. Loners are often very single-minded and successful in their work, but they derive decreasing satisfaction from this source. They fail to form close friendships or truly intimate relationships. Quite often the few friends such people have, perhaps from high school or college days, gradually fade away, and no new ones take their place. Over time, they lose the ability to conduct conversations of a personal nature. Quite often, they become solo drinkers, seeking solace within themselves. They feel increasingly trapped by their lives, even though they may appear to be in control and competent.

The Loner is very uncomfortable revealing his or her true self or true emotions. He is uncomfortable around other people, especially in situations where any kind of intimate interaction is likely. He has trouble giving (or receiving) affection. He feels self-conscious about his social behavior and may feel quite uncomfortable about how he treats other people, or he may have justified his solitariness by persuading himself that there is something wrong with everybody else. Although he may not realize it or admit it, the Loner feels lonely much or all of the time.

It's possible to be a Loner while being married or living with someone. However, the relationship will tend to subside to minimal communication, and that communication will rarely be of a personal or emotional nature.

It takes a lot of energy to hold back or suppress your emotions. And not getting feedback from others about who you are and how you are doing results in stressful uncertainty. This is the main area of vitality drain for the Loner. The key to reducing body age for this type is to learn how to better manage intimacy. This approach entails developing the ability to be more open emotionally, a tough challenge for someone so emotionally buttoned down.

Secondary Stressotypes

Many people have one strongly dominant stressotype. Others score highly in two or more categories. And nobody is all one and none of the others. Thus your secondary stressotypes are also important. Three of the six stressotypes showed up as the second most important vitality drain for almost two-thirds (62.3 percent) of those who entered the program. These were Basket Case (22.8 percent), Loner (20.4 percent), and Drifter (19.1 percent). The chart below shows the frequency of occurrence of secondary stressotypes and suggests the most likely combinations of dom-

SECONDARY STRESSOTYPES

(Percentage of 623 entering subjects)

Dominant Type:	Cliff Walker	Basket Case	Drifter	Speed Freak	Worry Wart	Loner
Speed Freak	18%	32%	24%	NA	8%	18%
Basket Case	12%	NA	20%	8%	22%	38%
Cliff Walker	NA	40%	20%	20%	5%	15%
Drifter	18%	8%	NA	28%	24%	22%
Worry Wart	18%	28%	22%	10%	NA	22%
Loner	18%	28%	30%	4%	20%	NA

inant and secondary stressotypes in a single person. In the next section, you'll meet six people who completed the Body Age Program and will get a better sense of how dominant and secondary types show up in an individual.

SIX STRESSOTYPE CASE HISTORIES

The cases described below are good examples of people who exhibit a strongly dominant stressotype along with a fairly prominent secondary stressotype. As with all the case examples in this book, names, occupations, and other details have been altered to protect confidentiality.

CASE 1: Jim, Personnel Manager
Age 46, Body Age 55, Appearance Age 56
DOMINANT STRESSOTYPE: Speed Freak
SECONDARY STRESSOTYPE: Loner

When Jim entered the program, he was a successful personnel manager for a large food-processing firm. At age 46, he could look back at a long and successful climb up the corporate ladder, but not much of a personal life. His first marriage had ended when he was 38; he was rarely home, and when he was there, he was always catching up on paperwork or entertaining business associates. His second wife, whom he'd married when he was 44, was 20 years younger, and they had a young baby. In the two years since this marriage, he'd been moved from one city to another and had bought a new house but failed to sell the old one; he was carrying two mortgages, as well as starting his new family and paying alimony. Jim told us he'd recently been offered a demanding but enticing new job (with high risk and a high salary), which would have meant moving again. But he simply couldn't make up his mind, wanting to "keep his options open."

He had no hobbies and few interests outside his job (as he put it, he "had no time to relax"), but he found time to free-lance on the side, as a consultant to other companies. His one leisure diversion was racquetball, which he played, in his words, "like it was a matter of life and death." In his case, death or serious injury were distinct possibilities. A growing body of research and clinical experience shows that high-spiking stress reactions, even in someone with no cardiovascular risk factors, can precipitate a sometimes fatal heart attack. This type is sometimes referred to as the "weekend warrior athlete."

Recently Jim had experienced an apparent heart attack, severe tightness and pain across the chest, faintness, severe breathing difficulty, symptoms so bad that he practically collapsed. But when he was rushed to the hospital emergency room, the doctors said he was not suffering from a coronary. Further tests revealed no organic heart problem. Too much stress had led to severe tension in his chest muscles, which had restricted his breathing and simulated a cardiac event.

Jim was a product of what is often called faulty learning. As a child, he had learned that high success requires high effort, but he had also come to believe that only if he gave a 110 percent effort all the time would he be successful. He'd always felt that he "had to do more," had to be better, and—especially—had to be seen to be contributing more. He was a conspicuous performer, terribly concerned not only to do well but to be seen doing well. He gave 110 percent whether he was on the racquetball court, in the office, or driving his car. Not only was it important to appear to be in control, but he always had to appear cool, calm and collected.

This approach left Jim with little sense of priorities, and he was constantly in a state of overstress and in considerable internal, emotional turmoil, which he seldom shared with anyone, lest they think poorly of him. He eventually came to feel at the mercy of "a pyramid of life events that is growing and crumbling at an accelerated rate."

CASE 2: Harriet, Hospital Nursing Director
Age 45, Body Age 59, Appearance Age 56
DOMINANT STRESSOTYPE: Basket Case
SECONDARY STRESSOTYPE: Worry Wart

When Harriet walked in for her initial assessment interview, she was the picture of energy—bright, vivacious, "together"—despite the fact she looked about forty pounds overweight. Within two minutes, she was slumped in her chair, and her face, which had been that of a healthy, happy 45-year-old woman, suddenly seemed 10 years older. She looked exhausted. "I often wonder how I keep going during the day," she confessed.

As Harriet talked, it became clear that she was not getting much sustenance from any part of her life. The pleasure had gone out of her existence. She was having serious problems in her marriage. She had no energy for sex or for home life in general. On weekends, all she wanted to do was sleep or lounge around. Her husband complained she was "no fun anymore," but when she offered to give up her administrative responsibilities as the director of nursing at a large city hospital for a less demanding job as staff education director (at a lower salary), he reminded her of the amount still owing on their new cottage. She was aware that her husband had had several affairs; he had persuaded her that this was the price of her success. He'd never approved of her career in the first place.

She felt guilty about not spending more time with her three children, all in their middle to late teens, but she tired so quickly that she easily became irritable, and family activities soon turned sour.

Lately, on evenings and on weekends, she found she was becoming increasingly depressed or immobile. In the morning before leaving for work, she would sometimes have "crying jags" for no apparent reason. She managed to keep up appearances at the hospital but could "barely crawl" to her car at the end of the day. She got frequent colds and strep infections. She was subject to chronic migraine headaches, typically on Friday and Sunday nights.

At the end of her tether, she'd gone to see her doctor, who'd found no specific disease to explain her condition and had prescribed an anti-depressant. But this only raised her stress level as she attempted to compensate for the side effects, including dry mouth and disturbed sleep.

"I just don't seem to have much to offer anyone," she admitted mournfully. In short, Harriet was a Basket Case on a frightening downward spiral toward a complete mental and physical breakdown.

CASE 3: George, Stockbroker
Age 36, Body Age 44, Appearance Age 45
DOMINANT STRESSOTYPE: Cliff Walker
SECONDARY STRESSOTYPE: Speed Freak

At his first interview, George didn't look well. His face was pale and inexpressive, and there were dark circles under his eyes. He was about thirty pounds overweight, and he'd apparently put on a few of them quite recently, judging from the too-tight fit of his expensive suit. Initially, he described himself as "quite healthy, but just going through a tough time right now." As the interview progressed, however, it became clear that he'd been feeling less than chipper since his college days.

At age 36, George was a physical wreck, with a recent history of serious illness. His first ulcer was diagnosed when he was 30. He'd had a minor heart attack at 34. Lower-back pain was a frequent problem. He seemed to attribute most of these troubles to bad genes: His father, who had died at age 52 of a sudden heart attack, had lived most of his adult life with abnormally high blood pressure.

George seemed to be married to his job, but, unlike a Speed Freak, he needed a constant intake of uppers and downers to get him through the day (he didn't think of these as drugs). He had joined a medium-sized stockbrokerage firm at age 25 and had become a partner by age 30.

He handled a number of large and important corporate and institutional clients, as well as raising equity for new business ventures. It was a demanding job, with high risks and very high financial rewards. It meant a good deal of travel, often at a moment's notice.

A typical day in George's life pretty much told the story. He'd wake after about five hours of sedative- or alcohol-induced sleep. He never ate breakfast, grabbing a couple of coffees and a donut on the run, followed by a couple of antacid pills to quell the chronic queasiness in his stomach. By noon, he would have smoked a pack of cigarettes, downed another four or five cups of coffee, and popped a handful of antacid tablets (he consumed two rolls a day).

Unless there was a boozy business lunch, he'd eat fast food at his desk. As the afternoon wore on, he'd keep pumping himself up with coffee and chocolate bars, or soothing himself with cigarettes and antacid. More often than not, he dined with business associates in a fancy restaurant— a high-fat, high-cholesterol feast accompanied by two or three stiff drinks. At night, he'd often have two or three doubles as a "nightcap," or he'd take a sleeping pill. He needed something to damp down the accumulated effects of his daily intake of stimulants.

This self-destructive lifestyle deteriorated further when he was on the road, where he'd eat even more restaurant meals and rely more on booze and sleeping pills.

George seldom saw his wife, a career woman who sounded from his description like a five-star Speed Freak overinvolved in her work. Their only shared pastime was the rare "vacation," but these escapes were geared to her speedy yet aimlessly self-centered pace, leaving little time for him to relax or regenerate. Vacations were a constant round of scheduled activities: tennis, boating, scuba diving, eating. No lying around for her—or him.

George would occasionally try to do something about his self-destructive lifestyle. He'd tried several fad diets, always losing weight quickly and putting it back on, and then some. He would occasionally go on a brief fitness rampage, which usually lasted no more than a few weeks. Every two or three weeks, he'd play racquetball for a couple of hours, usually with a business associate. Between times, there would be virtually no exercise at all.

In sum, George was ready to fall off the cliff.

CASE 4: John, Lawyer
Age 43, Body Age 49, Appearance Age 49
DOMINANT STRESSOTYPE: Drifter
SECONDARY STRESSOTYPE: Loner

When John walked in for the initial interview, he looked like an ad out of *Gentleman's Quarterly*. From his perfectly cut suit to his expensive Swiss watch, shiny gold pinky ring, and shiny patent leather briefcase, he appeared to be a perfect, and perfectly self-confident, package. He announced glibly that he'd come to have his "psychic interior redecorated by the best in the business."

But the packaging was more than a little misleading and required a great deal of effort to maintain. He visited his barber "religiously once a week" and made a "pilgrimage to London, England," twice a year in order to have his suits and shirts made to measure. None of this disguised the fact that he was somewhat overweight, which became very apparent when he took his clothes off for a physical exam. But his manner and appearance did hide a profound lack of life direction.

"I keep doing more, but I don't feel I'm becoming any more of a success," he explained. "Underneath all this icing there has to be a cake somewhere," he went on. His life was "half over with nothing to show for it," and he was frustrated that all his efforts had "led nowhere." More than once during the interview he wondered why he wasn't happy, given all his outward success. He was resentful and angry that his "life had not fallen into place."

His marriage had broken up when he was 36, because he'd been playing around with younger women. He'd found that he felt alive only when he "broke out of the routine." But he complained of being lonely much of the time, except when he rejoined the "boring" rituals of his job and other responsibilities. His mood swung from "black depression" to "periods of brilliance." His energy level went from total exhaustion to an intense high, involving a big expenditure of energy and money (he was always in debt, despite a big salary). Whatever mood he was in, sleep came with difficulty. He was in the habit of taking sleeping pills despite the potential side effects. He "just needed to turn it all off" at night.

John's law partners were becoming increasingly impatient with the amount of time he spent away from the firm; his vacations were getting longer and more frequent as he sought to combat his periods of depression. In addition to all those fancy clothes, he also comforted himself by buying expensive "decorations and baubles" such as rings and other jewelry.

When he described the pattern of his existence over the past few years, it became clear that John was sailing in a rather costly craft without chart or compass. He had been in psychoanalysis for several years, but dismissed this experience as a waste of time. "All the analyst ever said was: Decide what's really important to you and then live that way.'' (It never occurred to him that this might have been sound advice.) His career was characterized by abrupt changes of direction for no apparent reason. He had switched specialties from corporate law to litigation ''on a whim, a decision made in one weekend.'' Several years later, he'd made another 180-degree turn and gone into family law. At the time of the interview, he was seriously contemplating leaving the legal profession entirely and starting his own real estate and renovations business, but he was losing heart. Another change seemed pointless; it would just mean losing several more years of his life.

John had been referred to the Body Age Program by his physician. During the assessment interview, he joked that he hoped ''we could add ten years'' to his life, although he ''wasn't quite sure why.''

CASE 5: Garry, Chain Store Manager
Age 37, Body Age 48, Appearance Age 45
DOMINANT STRESSOTYPE: Worry Wart
SECONDARY STRESSOTYPE: Drifter

In the entry interview, it quickly became apparent that Garry had led one of the most self-obsessed, self-examined lives imaginable. The Body Age Program was only the latest in a long succession of attempts at ''personal growth,'' none of which had lasted long or gotten him anywhere. He had taken every self-improvement course, read every self-help book on the market, and seen at least a dozen psychotherapists (never for more than a few sessions). But all this had done was to give him more sophisticated and conceptually complex ways of worrying. In truth, Garry preferred worrying to actually changing his life in any concrete way. He lived almost totally in the past or in the future. Anxiety was his middle name.

When he entered the program, Garry's worrying had been formalized into a daily ritual. Each evening, he would spend an hour or two reviewing how (badly) his life was going. He'd put recent events under a microscope and dissect them for trends and lessons, brooding over the black messages they bore. When he had ''an especially difficult or problematic'' subject of worry, he would lengthen the time spent in this ritual day-in-review. It was almost as if he ''had to pay a higher price for a solution to a more difficult situation.'' His ''solutions,'' however, never solved anything.

Nor did setting aside time for worry prevent him from gnawing at himself throughout the day, whether on the job or in social situations. At work, his mind would often wander to his problems. During a casual conversation, he would inevitably start thinking about himself and stop listening to the other person. The most innocent remark might trigger a thought that would launch him into a fresh orgy of self-appraisal, self-doubt, and self-recrimination. His friends stopped asking him how he was feeling, knowing they'd be treated to a litany of moans and groans.

Recently he had concluded that he had too few close friends, so he planned a party to correct this problem. Initially he invited fifty people, but the list grew to seventy-five as he worried about offending or leaving out someone. The planning went on for weeks, and his anguish escalated as the party got nearer. Would there be enough food? Would everyone find at least one other person with whom they had something in common? Would people get too drunk and too rowdy, or not drink enough and eat enough and not have a good time? As he put it, "The logistics and planning that went into that party made D-Day look like a piece of cake." By the night of the actual event, he was in such a keyed-up state that there was no way for him to enjoy the actual event. This planned solution to his friendship worries yielded no new intimacies, but afterward he "had more than enough worry material to fill the next six months, doing postmortems of how it could have gone better."

As Garry talked, it became increasingly obvious that his life had taken on the quality of a self-fulfilling prophecy. One perfect example was what happened whenever he entered into a new relationship. It had hardly begun before he was worrying that it would end. Then he would literally worry it to death. This gave him still more material: his lost love and how to get her back.

He had started a new career at least six times—new job, fresh prospects, rosy future. At the time he entered the program, he'd recently quit his job as a computer salesman and started work as a manager of a small chain of convenience stores. Because Garry was bright and a quick learner, his job beginnings were always full of promise. But inevitably within six months he would develop serious doubts about his new choice and begin to explore half-baked alternatives. His work performance would suffer as the alternatives began to receive more attention than his actual job. He always managed to quit before he got fired, and his employers would inevitably provide him with "less-than-glowing references," mentioning his enormous unfulfilled potential. Then, almost as soon as he'd started his new job, he'd commence worrying that perhaps he'd made a mistake.

CASE 6: Ruth, Social Worker
Age 36, Body Age 50, Appearance Age 48
DOMINANT STRESSOTYPE: Loner
SECONDARY STRESSOTYPE: Drifter

When Ruth entered the Body Age Program, she was 36 years old, overweight, and for a professional woman (a social worker), surprisingly careless about her appearance. Her dark hair was messy, her makeup hastily applied, and her clothes ill fitting. It was almost as if she was sending out the message, "I don't think very highly of myself."

In the opening interview, it quickly became clear that Ruth was used to keeping her distance. Her manner was aggressive and defiant, her speech clipped and no-nonsense. "I hear you've got a pretty good program here," was her gruff explanation of why she wanted help. She turned out to be an agile conversationalist—good at talking about herself while keeping the listener at arm's length emotionally. With her, the personal became impersonal; she gave no hint of weakness even as she described her severely troubled life—she was a very artful dodger. It was only well into the interview, as she began to let down her guard, that a more sensitive and vulnerable person began to emerge. But this real inner self was seldom seen by anyone, including her friends and lovers. Her "tough guy" image was a carefully constructed fiction.

Her mother and father had died in a car accident when she was twelve, and it was then that she had learned the importance of keeping up appearances. Her family had been well to do, but her adoptive family was not. Yet they kept their new daughter in her expensive boarding school, at considerable sacrifice. Ruth learned to hide her parents' poverty and to handle the fact that she was different from her classmates by becoming deliberately eccentric, a mode of behavior she continued into adult life. She soon developed a romanticized image of herself as an outsider, someone on the fringes of society. She thought of herself as having rejected conventionality—a lone wolf in a world of sheep.

She would periodically quit work for eight months or so, living on unemployment insurance and dropping out for a while. In her job as a social worker, she described herself as a kind of Lone Ranger, enjoying the role of riding to the rescue in an emergency and then riding off into the sunset, a situation that left her with minimal contact with her co-workers.

Ruth's long-term relationships with men reinforced this attitude. Like her, they rejected the conventional world, sometimes to the point of living in isolated conditions, often on the fringes of the law. (She'd cohabited with a biker who trafficked in drugs and for whom a good time meant tossing live bullets into a blazing fireplace while his "guests" ducked behind the nearest piece of furniture.) And these relationships were as emotionally barren as they were sparse in creature comforts: Nothing was asked for and little offered.

Ruth was also given to occasional bouts of wild promiscuity in which she would sleep with almost anyone who would have her: a clear sign that beneath her defiant pose was a profound lack of self-esteem.

Her few friends were mostly "little sisters," whom she would take under her wing for a time, advising them on their personal problems. Of course, she never intimated that she could have used a confidant herself. She enjoyed manipulating people and situations, not principally for any advantage it would bring her, but because she liked to feel in control and at a distance. Her one ''good friend'' was someone she'd placed on an impossible pedestal and with whom she seldom spent time, preferring to admire her from afar.

In the last few years, Ruth had been less and less in contact with other people (except at work). As a child of the 1960s, she'd experimented with practically every drug and hung out with a tough crowd. Now her main opiate was bourbon, consumed in generous quantities at home by herself (she didn't want others to see her weakness). At one point in the interview, she confessed that her one best friend was her ''high self.''

At the rate Ruth was going, her Loner lifestyle was going to take over to the point of almost total social isolation.

The foregoing cases only begin to suggest the ways in which individual people can live out the stressotypes in their lives. But they all demonstrate what happens when one stressotype comes to dominate a person's existence. If you want to find out how these six people fared in the Body Age Program, you'll find the rest of their stories in chapter 13, ''Six Success Stories.''

What is your dominant stressotype? Are you a Speed Freak, a Loner, a Basket Case, Cliff Walker, a Worry Wart, or a Drifter? After reading this chapter, you probably have some idea where you fit in. Perhaps one of these case histories sounds familiar. It may resemble you as you are today, or as you have been at some time in the past—and might become again during a distressful period.

To identify your dominant stressotype, along with the other stressotype characteristics that are part of your makeup, turn to the Vitality Quotient Test in the next chapter.

CHAPTER 5

Your Vitality Quotient Test

The Vitality Quotient (V.Q.) Test is a modified version of the Stress Inventory Questionnaire that was an important part of the initial assessment of each of the 623 men and women who entered the Body Age Study. We've eliminated some questions in order to streamline and simplify the test. This more focused version will give you a very good indication of your rate of aging and your stressotype profile.

You may wonder why we aren't using a well-known stress test that measures the number of "stress points" in your life. The test you may be thinking of is the Holmes-Rahe Social Readjustment Rating Scale, often referred to as the Inventory of Life Events. It assigns stress points to a range of stressors, life events that are likely to raise your stress level. The death of a spouse (the worst stressor) gets 100 stress points on the Holmes-Rahe scale; getting married is worth 50 stress points; getting fired is a 47; a new baby rates a 39; trouble with your inlaws is a 29; and getting a speeding ticket merits a lowly 11. Adding up all your stress points is supposed to indicate the probability that you'll have a negative health change over the next two years. If your total is 150 or more, your chance of having health problems is 33 percent; if it's over 300, you have a 90 percent chance.

A limitation of this test is that it rates stressors, not people. For some people, the death of a spouse may really be a 100; for others, it may only be a 50. Stress is what you make of it, or as Dr. Selye was fond of saying, "It's not so much what happens to you that matters, but how you take it." He pointed out that some people can handle or even thrive on higher levels of stress than others; that is, the stress-performance curve is different for each individual.

Many executives we've worked with feel that "their engine is barely turning over" at 500 stress points on the Holmes-Rahe scale, and they're probably right. Others are overheating at 250. By contrast, you probably know someone who gets upset if the paper isn't delivered at the usual time or if a favorite brand is out of stock at the supermarket. Selye called people who perform well at higher stress levels racehorses. He characterized people who can't handle much change or uncertainty as turtles. Racehorses need—and usually can tolerate, unless they are too far gone as Speed Freaks—higher levels of stress than turtles.

While one man's distress may be another man's vitality, major life events are only some of the stressors that can lead to chronic overstress. For most of us most of the time, our responses to dozens of minor hassles and annoyances are at least as important. This gradual accumulation can add up to an unbearable stress burden or can leave us extremely vulnerable to a major stressor when it comes along.

The Holmes-Rahe scale, first published in 1967, remains scientifically sound, but only for a large statistical sample. If you randomly selected a thousand people, gave them the test, and then predicted on its basis how many of them would get sick, you'd be quite close. But if you gave it to ten racehorses, it would have little or no accuracy. And ten turtles would be dead or dying long before their stress points added up to 300. That is why, at the Canadian Institute of Stress, we never use it to provide feedback for individuals.

The Holmes-Rahe scale measures external events. The Vitality Quotient Test you are about to take measures your internal "stress fitness," the combination of your inherited resources, your lifestyle habits, and your learned skills that help or hinder your ability to cope with stressors of whatever intensity. It charts your stress-energy patterns and the ways in which you let stress get the better of you. But just what does the term *Vitality Quotient* mean? A quotient is the mathematical result when you divide one quantity by another quantity. In industry, when you divide output by input, the result is called productivity or efficiency. But we're dealing with human beings, not factories and assembly lines. Your Vitality Quotient is what you are getting back right now in terms of higher vitality and lower body age from how you live your life. It is the result when you divide your personal output—career achievements, peak experiences, feelings of self-esteem, satisfying personal relationships—by your personal input—the amount of stress energy you spend to get these rewards. You can think of this Vitality Quotient as the number of units of satisfaction you purchase with every unit of stress energy you spend. This quotient, or rate of return, is made up of feelings of vitality and well-being, and comes with ample reserves of energy for what you want to achieve. As the Body Age Study suggests, a very high V.Q. is within your reach—very high vitality in an unusually young body—which means a very slow rate of aging. Whatever your score on the following test, you can raise your V.Q. dramatically.

Answer all the questions as honestly as you can, giving the answer that best describes you. The more honest you are, the more accurate your results will be.

YOUR PERSONALIZED VITALITY QUOTIENT TEST

Section A

SCORE

_____ 1. **"Remedies" with Negative Side Effects:** Add up how many of the following you use once or more during a typical week:
- aspirin
- antacids
- laxatives
- antihistamines
- cough syrups
- decongestants
- diuretics (water pills)
- nonprescription sleeping pills
- nonprescription stimulants (such as pep pills) or tranquilizers

Score 0 if one or none
1 if two
2 if three
3 if four
4 if five
5 if six or more

_____ 2. **Alcohol Use on a Typical Day:**
Note: 1.25 ozs. liquor = one beer or one glass of wine.

Score 0 if nondrinker–1 oz./day
1 if 1–2.5 ozs./day
3 if 2.5–4 ozs./day
5 if 4–6 ozs./day
6 if 6–9 ozs./day
8 if 10+ ozs./day

_____ 3. **Exercise Routine Frequency:**
(more than 20 mins. at training heart rate—see p. 285)

Score 0 if three or more times/week
      2 if twice/week
      4 if once/week
      7 if rarely or never

_____ 4. **Sugar Intake:** Count 1 for each food you use more than once per week.
- sugar added to tea/coffee/cocoa
- colas/sodas
- ice cream
- canned or frozen fruits
- baked desserts
- cookies
- doughnuts/cakes
- jam/jelly
- candy/sweets
- chocolate
- sweetened breakfast cereal
- honey
- raw fruits more than twice/day
- dried fruits
- alcohol
- sweet wines/liqueurs
- canned fruit juices

Score 0 if none
      1 If 1–4
      2 if 5–8
      3 if 9+

_____ 5. **Fat Intake:** Count 1 for each food you use at least once per week.
- steak/roast beef/veal
- butter
- hard cheeses
- fried, sautéed foods
- nuts, raw or processed
- canned meats
- bologna/salami
- frankfurters
- fast-food chicken
- bacon/breakfast sausage
- ham
- pork
- avocados
- margarine
- french fries
- pastries/doughnuts
- hamburger

- ice cream
- eggs
- whole milk or 2% milk
- chocolate
- peanut butter
- salmon
- poultry with skin
- tuna/sardines (in oil)
- cream
- processed cheeses
- TV dinners

Score 0 if none
1 if 1–6
2 if 7–12
3 if 13+

_____ 6. **Salt Intake:** Count 1 for each food you eat at least once per week.
- salt in cooking
- salt sprinkled on food during meals
- salt sprinkled on food before tasting
- salty foods
- pickles
- soy sauce
- cheese
- pizza
- bologna/salami/frankfurters
- canned meats
- salted nuts
- potato or corn chips/puffs
- anchovies
- olives
- saltines/crackers
- sauerkraut
- fast-food hamburger
- fast-food chicken
- canned vegetables
- tomato ketchup
- Worcestershire sauce
- powdered soup/gravy mixes
- corned or smoked meat/fish
- pretzels
- TV dinners
- commercial salad dressings
- frozen vegetables
- bacon

Score 0 if none
1 if 1–6

    2 if 7–12
    3 if 13+

_____ 7. **Refined or Processed Foods:** Estimate the proportion (the percentage) of your diet made up of refined foods.

NOTE: Refined foods include ham, bacon, sausage, smoked fish or meat, *all* canned foods and beverages, all white or enriched flours, breads and cookies, dessert pies, candy, ice cream, chocolate, and *all* protein powders, such as soy powder.

    Score 0 if less than 20% refined
            1 if 20–50%
            2 if 50–75%
            3 if 75+%

_____ 8. **Smoking:**

    Score 0 if nonsmoker
            1 if nonsmoker exposed to smokers
            2 if smoke 1–8 cigarettes/day
            4 if smoke 8–20 cigarettes/day
            7 if smoke 20+ cigarettes/day

NOTE: 1 pipe = 2 cigarettes
      1 cigar = 3 cigarettes

_____ 9. **Caffeine:** Add up the cups of coffee, tea, and colas you drink per day:

    Score 0 if none
            1 if 1–3
            2 if 4–7
            3 if 8+

NOTE: For questions 10 and 11, please tick any relative who has or has had these disorders.

_____ 10. **Heart Disease**
         • father _____
         • mother _____
         • siblings _____ _____ _____
         • grandfathers _____ _____
         • grandmothers _____ _____
    Score = total number of ticks, to a maximum of 4

_____ 11. **Hypertension** (high blood pressure)
         • father _____
         • mother _____
         • siblings _____ _____ _____
         • grandfathers _____ _____
         • grandmothers _____ _____
    Score = total number of ticks, to a maximum of 4

Section B

Instructions: Write a number in the blank at the left of each statement below, based on the frequency scale provided.

How frequently has each of the following statements been true about you during the past year? (Use all the numbers. For example, use 1 to express "almost never" and 7 to express a frequency between "occasionally" and "frequently.")

0 = never
1
2 = rarely
3
4 = infrequently
5
6 = occasionally
7
8 = frequently
9
10 = very frequently

Be honest with yourself. As you go through the statements, try to avoid looking like Superman or Superwoman or like a total wreck unless your situation truly warrants it. Use your best judgment. Your honest first thought is usually the most accurate.

Enter one number in the blank to the left of each statement.

_____ 12. I feel used up at the end of the day.
_____ 13. I am callous about a lot of things.
_____ 14. I feel critical of others.
_____ 15. I have a tendency to blame myself for things.
_____ 16. I feel uncomfortable about the way I treat people.
_____ 17. I tire quickly.
_____ 18. I wish I could be as happy as other people seem to be.
_____ 19. I get annoyed and irritated easily.
_____ 20. I can't turn my thoughts off long enough—at nights or on weekends—to feel relaxed and refreshed the next day.
_____ 21. I find that long periods of time around people is a real strain.
_____ 22. I feel low on energy, exhausted, tired, or unable to get things done.
_____ 23. I feel sad, depressed, down in the dumps, or hopeless.
_____ 24. I find myself waking up earlier in the morning than I plan to.
_____ 25. When something difficult or stressful is coming up, I find myself thinking about all the ways things can go poorly for me.
_____ 26. I am not able to give what I would like to the people closest to me.
_____ 27. I seem to get a lot of tension headaches.
_____ 28. I feel blocked in getting things done.
_____ 29. My sleep is restless or disturbed.
_____ 30. I takes me a long time to get over distressful situations.

_____ 31. I don't feel really close to or accepted by the people around me, both family and friends.

_____ 32. Pain in my lower back is a problem for me.

_____ 33. There are a lot of people who would take advantage of me if I let them.

_____ 34. I get into arguments.

_____ 35. My friends would worry about me if I wasn't worrying about something.

_____ 36. I feel lonely.

_____ 37. Allergy problems seem to bother me a lot more than other people.

_____ 38. The ways I organize and use my time aren't a very accurate reflection of my interests.

_____ 39. I sweat easily, even on cool days.

_____ 40. I feel that being upset or worried a lot seems to be part of the price of success.

_____ 41. I feel very self-conscious with others.

_____ 42. I have migraine or tension headaches.

_____ 43. I feel that other people have made a lot more out of their talents than I have.

_____ 44. I tend to anticipate others in conversation (interrupting, finishing sentences for the other person), rather than listening well and letting the other person finish speaking.

_____ 45. Whenever I try to put a worrisome situation out of my mind, it comes right back.

_____ 46. I really don't spend as much time with my friends as I should.

_____ 47. I have aching or tight muscles in my neck and shoulders.

_____ 48. I doubt that the goals I've set for my life are really what will make me happy.

_____ 49. I get uneasy when I'm waiting.

_____ 50. Decisions are hard for me because I spend a lot of time wondering if I've thought of all the alternatives.

_____ 51. I feel I should be spending more time with my family.

_____ 52. I have cold hands or feet.

_____ 53. I feel that many people see me as being a lot more successful than I really feel I have been.

_____ 54. I try to do two or three things at once, rather than taking one thing at a time.

_____ 55. If I could stop worrying so much, I would accomplish a lot more.

_____ 56. I don't handle conflicts or disagreements with people as well as I'd like to.

_____ 57. I get the flu or a cold.

_____ 58. I feel that my leisure time and recreational life don't express the really creative side of me.

_____ 59. I tend to hold my feelings inside, rather than expressing them openly.

_____ 60. I find it hard to take my own advice and to follow through on it.

_____ 61. I don't seem to get the same kind of lasting satisfaction that I used to from the time I spend with friends.

Your Vitality Quotient and Stressotype Score Sheet

Instructions: In the numbered spaces below, enter the numerical scores and answers from the 61-item questionnaire (sections A and B).

Add the numbers across each of the six rows. The total score for each row becomes your score for that stressotype. (Note that the total score on row #1 must be multiplied by 2 to yield your Cliff Walker score.)

Add up your six stressotype scores. Enter this grand total in the space provided. Subtract your grand total from 600. This final number is your personal Vitality Quotient, reflecting *your current rate of aging.* In theory, your V.Q. can range from 0 (are you sure you're not dead?) to a high of 600 (Superman or Superwoman, with no kryptonite in sight).

STRESSOTYPE
SCORE

Cliff Walker

Items ___ ___ ___ ___ ___ ___ ___ ___ ___ ___ ___ ×2 = _____
     1 2 3 4 5 6 7 8 9 10 11 Total

Basket Case

Items ___ ___ ___ ___ ___ ___ ___ ___ ___ ___ = _____
    12 17 22 27 32 37 42 47 52 57

Drifter

Items ___ ___ ___ ___ ___ ___ ___ ___ ___ ___ = _____
    13 18 23 28 33 38 43 48 53 58

Speed Freak

Items ___ ___ ___ ___ ___ ___ ___ ___ ___ ___ = _____
    14 19 24 29 34 39 44 49 54 59

Worry Wart

Items ___ ___ ___ ___ ___ ___ ___ ___ ___ ___ = _____
    15 20 25 30 35 40 45 50 55 60

Loner

Items ___ ___ ___ ___ ___ ___ ___ ___ ___ ___ = _____
    16 21 26 31 36 41 46 51 56 61

GRAND TOTAL = _____

600   minus _____ = _____
             GRAND   VITALITY
             TOTAL   QUOTIENT

Interpreting Your Scores

Your Six Stressotype Scores

Each of the six stressotype scores can range from 0, meaning that you bear no resemblance to that stressotype, to 100, meaning that you are a classic, "textbook" example of that stressotype. For each stressotype, your score will place you in one of three groups:

RANGE OF SCORES	GROUP
0 to 30	Positive: Build on strengths.
31 to 36	Early Warning Signs: Take preventive measures.
37 and up	High Risk: Take corrective action now.

Your Vitality Quotient Score

When you add up your six stressotype scores and subtract that number from 600, the result is your Vitality Quotient. The higher your V.Q., the more slowly your body is aging, and the more energy and vitality you have.

As a first step, your V.Q. can be interpreted as placing you in one of three broad groups:

V.Q. SCORE	V.Q. GROUP
420 +	Positive: Build on strengths.
382 to 419	Early Warning Signs: Take preventive measures.
0 to 381	High Risk: Take corrective action now.

YOUR BODY AGE GAP

You now have three important pieces of information about yourself: your V.Q., your stressotype subscores, and your body age (from chapter 3). The gap between your body age and your calendar age—what we call the body age gap—will shed further light on the meaning of your V.Q. If your body age gap is positive (if your body age score is lower than your calendar age), then most likely your V.Q. score is a high one (420 or higher). If your gap is negative (if your body age score is significantly higher than your calendar age), then you likely have a low V.Q. score (382 or lower). But this correlation isn't always the case. (See the Body Age Gap chart.)

BODY AGE GAP

(in plus or minus years)

	−20	−15	−10	−5	0	+5	+10	+15	+20
V.Q. of 0–381	Much accelerated aging in a much younger body		Much accelerated aging in a younger body			Much accelerated aging in an older body		Much accelerated aging in a much older body	
V.Q. of 382–419	Accelerated aging in a much younger body		Accelerated aging in a younger body			Accelerated aging in an older body		Accelerated aging in a much older body	
V.Q. of 420 and up	Decelerated aging in a much younger body		Decelerated aging in a younger body			Decelerated aging in an older body		Decelerated aging in a much older body	

If your body age is below your calendar age but you also scored a low V.Q., this suggests that fairly recently you've stopped taking good care of yourself or possibly have been going through an intensely demanding experience, such as a marriage breakup or starting a new and demanding job that's giving you trouble. Whatever the reason, your body age hasn't yet caught up with the fact that you are now suffering from accelerated aging. Unless you take corrective action, your positive body age gap will narrow.

If you scored high in body age but also have a high V.Q., this is a very positive sign that you've already started to take the corrective action you need to turn things around. You are probably now experiencing decelerated aging. And the fact that you have slowed down your aging process will soon show up in a lower body age score. You can enhance this process by writing your own prescription in the next chapter—and following through on it.

Whatever your V.Q., look at it positively. It is information you can use to improve the quality of your life. Unlike your intelligence quotient, or I.Q., your V.Q. is highly variable. In small part, it is influenced by the genes you were born with. But mainly it is determined by what you have done, and are doing, with what you've been given. To learn how to use your anti-aging resources more effectively, turn to the next chapter.

CHAPTER 6
Write Your Own Prescription

You are now ready to write your prescription for change. You understand that stress is a powerful energy source that you can use wisely or unwisely. You've seen how the continued misuse of this resource, over months and years, leads to chronic distress and premature aging. You've tested your body age and know whether you are biologically younger or older than your calendar years. And you've taken the V.Q. test, which revealed your current Vitality Quotient (rate of aging), as well as your dominant stressotype and your main secondary stressotypes. As a result, you now have a rather detailed picture of the ways in which your life is out of balance.

PRESCRIBING FOR YOUR STRESSOTYPE

Before we get into the specific anti-aging prescription that's right for you, a few words about understanding the makeup of the stressotypes and evaluating the scores you achieved for each.

The Stressotype Tree

A useful way of thinking about your dominant and secondary stressotypes is as trees whose branches are formed by the questions you answered on the V.Q. test. The two most important questions in defining each stressotype are the two main branches rising from the trunk: These are almost unbreakably attached to the tree; you virtually never have this stressotype unless you scored high on both branches. As you proceed outward along the two main branches of the tree, the connections become less strong. In other words, these less important questions aren't necessary conditions of this stressotype, but they help refine and modify it. You can score high in a stressotype without having a high score on all the questions in the cluster, but the two main branches will almost certainly be present.

The tree illustrations that follow show you this interrelationship for each of the six stressotypes.

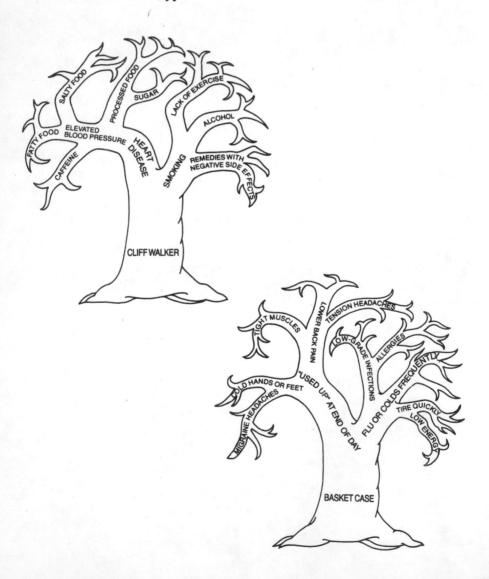

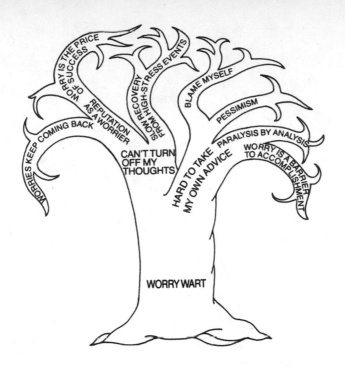

WORRY IS THE PRICE OF SUCCESS
REPUTATION AS A WORRIER
SLOW RECOVERY FROM HIGH-STRESS EVENTS
BLAME MYSELF
PESSIMISM
WORRIES KEEP COMING BACK
PARALYSIS BY ANALYSIS
HARD TO TAKE MY OWN ADVICE
WORRY IS A BARRIER TO ACCOMPLISHMENT
CAN'T TURN OFF MY THOUGHTS

WORRY WART

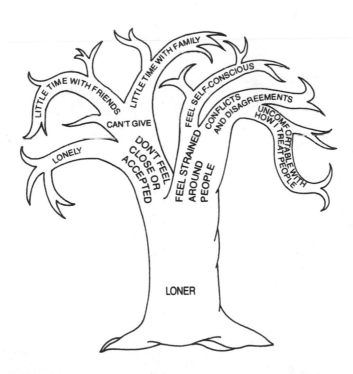

LITTLE TIME WITH FRIENDS
LITTLE TIME WITH FAMILY
FEEL SELF-CONSCIOUS
CONFLICTS AND DISAGREEMENTS
UNCOMFORTABLE WITH HOW I TREAT PEOPLE
CAN'T GIVE
LONELY
DON'T FEEL CLOSE OR ACCEPTED
FEEL STRAINED AROUND PEOPLE

LONER

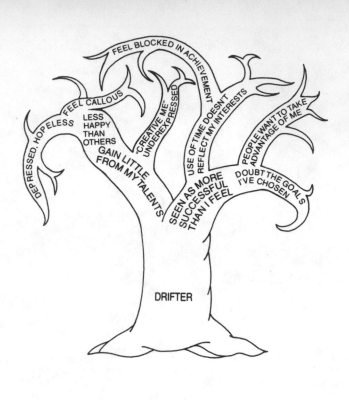

FEEL BLOCKED IN ACHIEVEMENT

FEEL CALLOUS

"CREATIVE ME" UNDEREXPRESSED

DEPRESSED, HOPELESS

LESS HAPPY THAN OTHERS

GAIN LITTLE FROM MY TALENTS

USE OF TIME DOESN'T REFLECT MY INTERESTS

SEEN AS MORE SUCCESSFUL THAN I FEEL

PEOPLE WANT TO TAKE ADVANTAGE OF ME

DOUBT THE GOALS I'VE CHOSEN

DRIFTER

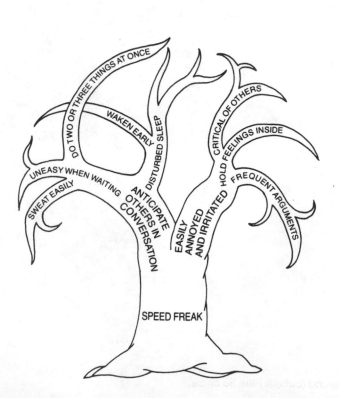

DO TWO OR THREE THINGS AT ONCE

WAKEN EARLY

DISTURBED SLEEP

CRITICAL OF OTHERS

HOLD FEELINGS INSIDE

UNEASY WHEN WAITING

SWEAT EASILY

ANTICIPATE OTHERS IN CONVERSATION

EASILY ANNOYED AND IRRITATED

FREQUENT ARGUMENTS

SPEED FREAK

The Stressotype Wheel

In effect, your V.Q. is a summary statement of your stress-energy efficiency at the moment. Your individual stressotype subscores pinpoint your key areas of inefficiency—your vitality drains. They indicate where you are off kilter in your life. You can get a vivid sense of this by shading in the Stressotype Wheel below. The six segments of the wheel represent the six stressotypes.

STRESSOTYPE WHEEL

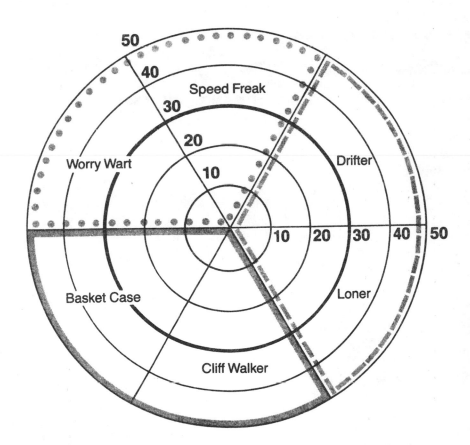

In your Body Age Program, you will concentrate on the stressotypes that you shade beyond (outside) the 30 circle.

Shade in each of the six segments in accordance with your score for that stressotype. Use the numbered rings as a guide: They mark increasing stressotype scores, up to a maximum of 50 (at the rim). The more you resemble a particular stressotype, the more of that segment you'll shade in. If you scored 50 or higher in any stressotype, shade in that segment right to the rim. The result is a visual representation of your stressotype profile: the areas in which you are most susceptible to accelerated aging. Your key stress-energy drains are indicated by the areas outside the third ring (beyond the boldface line), indicating that you scored 30 or higher in that stressotype.

Note that the six stressotypes have been subdivided into three groups of two: Cliff Walker and Basket Case; Speed Freak and Worry Wart; Loner and Drifter. Each pair is made up of related stressotypes, types susceptible to similar vitality drains and having similar prescriptions. If you scored high in one member of a pair, it is likely that you scored high in the other.

The Stressotype Wheel provides you with a stressotype self-portrait that shows you where you need to take immediate action to improve efficiency and restore balance. The more of a segment you've shaded in, the more work you have to do in that behavioral area. You probably have characteristics of all six stressotypes, but your prescription will consist of actions that most directly address your main areas of stress-energy inefficiency.

Rating the Five Interventions

The five interventions, or Vital Life Skills, that you'll learn in Part Two are a compressed version of the ten anti-aging interventions we taught our study participants (see p. 49). The five Vital Life Skills our study showed to be the most potent techniques and approaches for combating aging are:

> Values/Goals Clarification
> Effective Relaxation
> Self-Affirming Communication (For More Rewarding
>   Relationships)
> High Performance Nutrition
> Essential Exercise.

When you read the five chapters on these essential life skills and perform the various tests and exercises they contain, you'll get a distilled version of the training we provided for those who entered the Body Age Study, and you'll be benefiting from their experience.

On the whole, the results were fairly predictable. The most effective interventions for each stressotype generally matched what common sense suggested as the best way to treat a particular vitality drain. For example, the primary intervention for the Cliff Walker was nutrition, and the most effective at lowering body age for Speed Freaks was relaxation.

But some of the results were somewhat unexpected and initially quite surprising. For the Loner, for instance, working on relationships (communication skills) was important, but not the most effective place to start, seemingly because the Loners in our study group found their relationships difficult to deal with right away. To do so would have meant changing habits and challenging attitudes so deeply entrenched as to seem permanent parts of their personalities. Instead, Loners had greatest success concentrating *first* on Values/Goals Clarification. As they felt clearer about what they wanted from life, they began to acknowledge that getting such satisfaction often involved other people and that satisfaction was more deeply felt when accompanied by feedback from others. This clarity enabled them to tackle the thorny area of relationships. In fact, more satisfying relationships almost inevitably turned out to be an important goal for Loners.

Similarly, common sense suggests that a Drifter should sit down and line up his priorities, figure out his life direction, and get moving. But Values/Goals Clarification is often too threatening for someone who's grown accustomed to journeying through life without a compass. Much more effective for Drifters was *first* to more actively affirm and acknowledge the value of the relationships that meant most to them. These relationships invariably held clues to their underlying goals and values.

The Prescription Wheel

The Prescription Wheel below depicts each stressotype, with the five basic interventions ranked according to their effectiveness in reducing body age for that type. The top Vital Life Skill for each type is at the outer rim of the wheel. As you move toward the center, the interventions become less effective for that particular stressotype.

Prescriptions would be simple if an individual were all one stressotype, but in reality, each person is a combination of stressotypes. You may have one clearly dominant stressotype and one that's clearly in second place. Or you may have two or three that are almost equal. As a general rule, any stressotype for which you score higher than 30 is an essential part of your prescription. (If none of your scores are higher than 30, you can still benefit from the program. To lower your body age further and increase your vitality, simply write your prescription based on your three highest stressotype scores.) To refine your prescription to suit your individual stressotype profile, follow these three simple steps:

PRESCRIPTION WHEEL

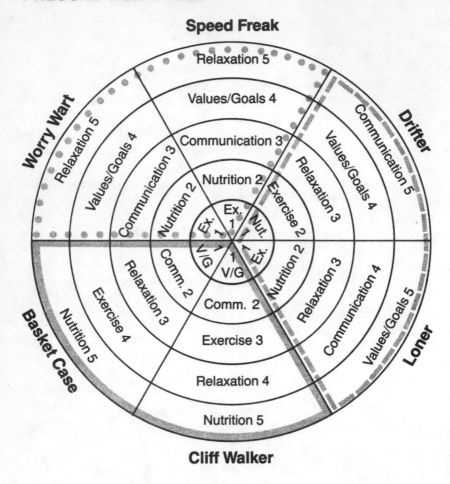

Speed Freak

Relaxation 5
Values/Goals 4
Communication 3
Nutrition 2
Ex. 1

Worry Wart

Relaxation 5
Values/Goals 4
Communication 3
Nutrition 2

Drifter

Communication 5
Values/Goals 4
Relaxation 3
Exercise 2
Nut. 1

V/G 1

V/G

Comm. 2
Relaxation 3
Exercise 4
Nutrition 5

Basket Case

Ex.

Nutrition 2
Relaxation 3
Communication 4
Values/Goals 5

Loner

Comm. 2
Exercise 3
Relaxation 4
Nutrition 5

Cliff Walker

1. *Start with the prescription ranking for your dominant stressotype.* The interventions have been weighted from 5 (most effective) to 1 (least effective). Use the weighting numbers indicated on the Prescription Wheel to calculate your prescription. If you're a Speed Freak, that means Relaxation is 5, Values/Goals is 4, Communication is 3, Nutrition is 2, and Exercise is 1. Simply consult the wheel as you write your prescription.

2. *Look at your secondary stressotypes.* If you have more than one higher than 30, pick only the highest two subsidiary scores. Give each secondary intervention a value half of what it would earn for your dominant stressotype (2.5, 2, 1.5, 1, .5). For example, if your secondary stressotype is Loner, you'd assign values as follows: Values/Goals—2.5,

Communication—2, Relaxation—1.5, Nutrition—1, Exercise—.5. Perform this exercise for up to two subsidiary stressotypes.

3. *Add together the numbers for each intervention to get a total for each.* If your dominant stressotype is Speed Freak and your secondary stressotype is Loner, the result will be this: Values/Goals Clarification —6.5; Relaxation—6.5; Relationships—5; Nutrition—3; Exercise—1.5. Values/Goals and Relaxation are tied. Start with the one that ranked higher for your dominant stressotype: in this case, Relaxation.

The Prescription Pad below makes it easy to calculate your prescription. On it, we've allowed for one dominant and up to two secondary stressotypes. Scores over 30 are your priority.

PRESCRIPTION PAD

Dominant Stressotype: _____

List the interventions in their effectiveness order for this stressotype:

Intervention #1 _____ Value: 5

Intervention #2 _____ Value: 4

Intervention #3 _____ Value: 3

Intervention #4 _____ Value: 2

Intervention #5 _____ Value: 1

Secondary Stressotype #1: _____

List the interventions in their effectiveness order for this stressotype:

Intervention #1 _____ Value: 2.5

Intervention #2 _____ Value: 2

Intervention #3 _____ Value: 1.5

Intervention #4 _____ Value: 1

Intervention #5 _____ Value: .5

Secondary Stressotype #2: _____

List the interventions in their effectiveness order for this stressotype:

Intervention #1 _____ Value: 2.5

Intervention #2 _____ Value: 2

Intervention #3 _____ Value: 1.5

Intervention #4 _____ Value: 1

Intervention #5 _____ Value: .5

Intervention Totals

You've now assigned at least one and possibly three values to each intervention. Add these together to arrive at the total value for each intervention in your personal stressotype profile. Then list the *top three* interventions and corresponding values, in descending order of importance. This is your Vitality Prescription.

Intervention #1 _____ Total Value _____

Intervention #2 _____ Total Value _____

Intervention #3 _____ Total Value _____

Now you know your prescription. If you've answered the questions on the V.Q. test honestly and carefully, it will be an accurate anti-aging prescription—a recipe for reducing your body age. Other interventions may seem more appealing, or easier, to tackle than the first three on your list. But according to your stressotype profile, these are the three you should concentrate on during the Vitality Action Program. For best results, follow your prescription to the letter.

THE VITAL BALANCE

Your vitality prescription is a straightforward recipe for increasing your stress-energy efficiency and moving toward a more balanced way of living. But what do you do once you've achieved the dramatic short-term gains in increased vitality and lower body age that the next few weeks and months will bring? In other words, what is the right prescription for the rest of your life, for honing your vital balance?

Part of the answer is to keep practicing the three interventions that make up your prescription until they become second nature. But that's only the beginning. Think of your prescription as emergency first aid for someone in distress. A longer-term approach to stress mastery and increased vitality is for you to become an expert in all five of the Vital Life Skills described in Part Two.

It is clear from the experience of our study subjects that the interventions gain potency in interaction with each other. If you're a Speed Freak and you learn to relax, you'll feel better and your body age will go down. But the more of your prescription you phase in, the more accelerated your improvement will be. Because success in one area spills over into another, as you increase energy efficiency in one area it will be easier to increase efficiency in others, and your overall efficiency will increase exponentially. This phenomenon is similar to the principle of synergy: The total effect of your actions is equal to more than the mere sum of the actions themselves. Practicing all five Vital Life Skills increases this interactive synergy even more.

If you exercise regularly but eat poorly, you'll never be truly physically fit. Even if you get your values clear, you won't have much energy to act on them unless you learn to relax. If your diet includes a high intake of stress enhancers (such as sugar, nicotine, alcohol, or caffeine), you may not be able to relax, no matter how hard you try. In sum, once you've completed your prescription, start honing the other two Vital Life Skills. If you do, who knows what new plateaus of vitality are possible for you?

To this end, you may be interested in an additional set of rather provocative findings from the Body Age Study. This is the overall ranking of the five interventions for the study group as a whole. The results here were somewhat unexpected and suggest that some approaches to stress regulation and health promotion have a better reputation than they deserve.

The table below shows the relative effectiveness of each of the five interventions in reducing the body age of our entire study group of 602, regardless of stressotype. We determined this effectiveness by means of a rigorous statistical analysis of the study results that carefully correlated each subject's body age improvement with his or her degree of adherence to each of the five interventions. Effectiveness is defined in terms of the percent of change in body age improvement accounted for by the particular intervention.

OVERALL INTERVENTION RANKING

Intervention	Effectiveness
Values/Goals Clarification	24.4%
Effective Relaxation	16.8%
Self-Affirming Communication	14.4%
Essential Exercise	12.3%
High-Performance Nutrition (without vitamin/mineral supplement)	7.9%

NOTE: The above numbers do not add up to 100%. In no study of this type can all of the "variance" be explicitly accounted for. We were, in fact, able to account for an unusually high degree (77.8%). (A further 11.5% was attributable to the vitamin-mineral supplement.)

Values/Goals Clarification, which teaches techniques for figuring out what is important to you and for putting your mental and spiritual houses in order, ranked a suprising first overall, ahead of the physical relaxation techniques that most people emphasize when they teach stress management. There are a couple of possible ways of explaining this. First, Values/ Goals is the intervention that promotes inner harmony, balance, self-acceptance, and self-love. Because positive feelings about yourself are very health-enhancing, it makes sense that this Vital Life Skill would be particularly powerful. Second, it follows that, in order to use stress energy efficiently, you need a clear sense of your priorities, of the direction you want to go and where you want to invest your precious capital of energy and time. Effective time management is simply an example of Values/ Goals Clarification in action. Third, there is growing evidence (for instance, in Aaron Antonovsky's *Health, Stress and Coping*) that people who have survived highly distressful experiences, such as World War II concentration camps, have been those who had a deeply rooted sense of values that could be translated into day-to-day behaviors that helped them achieve a sense of control over their environment. In other words, these were people well equipped to deal with a high degree of uncertainty.

It is really not so suprising that Effective Relaxation ranked second when this intervention is looked at in terms of the concept of stress efficiency. Relaxation helps you gear down, but it doesn't stop you from going right back to the same old grind after your ten minutes of relaxation. It's tough to break ingrained mental and behavioral patterns. Thus the simple ''time out'' use of relaxation has important, though limited, benefits. On the other hand, if you use physical relaxation within the context of getting in touch with your values, or looking after yourself better in your relationships, or making your exercise more effective, then it becomes a very powerful tool for pacing yourself through the day and in your life generally. A core technique involving relaxation—autogenic training—is fundamental to the success of all five interventions.

Another surprise was the fourth-place ranking of Essential Exercise. It seems that exercise, while important, is somewhat overrated by experts in stress and health. This finding echoes a growing theme in studies analyzing the effectiveness of corporate fitness programs. It turns out that the clear benefits of these programs, as measured by such factors as drops in absenteeism, are more attributable to actions other than or in combination with increased exercise, such as greater involvement with and liking of fellow employees (corresponds to our Communication/Relationships intervention); improved self-esteem ("I'm doing something for myself"; "I like myself"; "I'm a good person") and so less depression (corresponds to our Values/Goals intervention); better nutritional habits (corresponds to our High-Performance Nutrition intervention); and more awareness of the importance of taking time out to relax (corresponds to our Effective Relaxation intervention). In short, the Body Age Study confirms what other studies suggest: Exercise by itself has only modest benefits; in interactive combination with other Vital Life Skills, it is very powerful indeed.

In fact, too much exercise may actually be bad for you. At Canada's University of Waterloo, recent research into the effect of exercise on the immune system suggests that there's a point of negative return after which exercise does more harm than good by actually weakening your immune system. In effect, too much exercise becomes a negative stressor. For example, one study of fifteen middle-distance runners had to be abandoned when seven of the subjects were forced to drop out because of illness.

But there is no research that diminishes the importance of regular, moderate exercise. Actually, this intervention might have ranked higher had our study sample been different. The bulk of our study group were middle-class professionals who already did a certain amount of exercise.

Although High-Performance Nutrition ranked last, it would have ranked second if the effects of our vitamin-mineral supplement had been included. This may in part stem from the fact that sound nutritional advice is relatively easy to teach but very difficult for most people to follow. In theory, if our subjects had followed our nutritional guidelines to the letter, they would not need a vitamin-mineral supplement. However, even if they had, their good habits might have been undermined by variations in food quality: Two fresh oranges can have widely differing nutrient contents (from 0 mg. of vitamin C to 180 mg.). Another factor that erodes sound nutrition is the widespread presence of chemical additives in food.

Because of the last-place ranking of nutrition, we concluded that a vitamin-mineral supplement is an essential part of High-Performance Nutrition. But one thing is clear: Proper nutrition has great potential for promoting optimum health and vitality.

You now have all the information you need to begin your personalized Body Age Program.

Part II

The Body Age Program

CHAPTER 7
Taking Action

Part One of *Your Vitality Quotient* provided you with important information about yourself that you can use to put your prescription into action. The only outside support you need, other than the information in the five intervention chapters that follow, is a buddy, or partner, who will go through the program with you (more on this later). This chapter provides a basic roadmap of what lies ahead, and it teaches the one technique you'll be using regardless of your prescription. This technique, autogenic training, enables you to root the change process in your very core until it becomes instinctive.

At this point, you may still be a little skeptical. You may be asking yourself, "Why will this program work for me when others I've tried have failed?" We have three answers. The first is simply that we know our program works. The 602 people who completed the study proved it: They lowered their body ages, and they felt better and looked better. The second answer is that your prescription, the action you will be taking, is geared to you personally. It is based on your behavior type—on the ways in which *you* are most likely to waste stress energy, on *your* typical vitality drains, on *your* susceptibilities to accelerated aging.

The third and most powerful answer is that your prescription will literally *become a part of you*. The specific changes you choose and the steps you take as you learn each Vital Life Skill and put it into action will become second nature. With the powerful aid of autogenic training (self-hypnosis, visualizations, and affirmations) you will alter, under your own direction, your neural pathways and behavioral tendencies. What started out as a small but concrete change will become a self-affirming habit. As this happens, the techniques we teach you for increasing your vitality will stop being a matter of choice and self-discipline ("I must take this medicine because it's good for me") and become instead a natural form of self-expression ("I choose to do this because it expresses who I am and the way I want to be"), as natural as breathing.

Those familiar with the Japanese martial art of Karate will understand what we're talking about. In Karate, as you move up the ranks from white belt to green belt to brown belt, it is primarily a question of learning and perfecting a series of rigorous techniques. But the black belt Karate master has gone beyond this. He is free of techniques: They have become part of his way of being. In a similar fashion, the skills you'll learn in the intervention chapters will free you from techniques. It's true that at first, as you follow your prescription, you will simply "have" more vitality. Yet one morning you will probably wake up, as most of our study participants did, to find that you "are" vitality—that you have become a stress master.

However, before any of this can begin to happen, you must make a serious but manageable commitment. You know what your prescription is, but are you honestly prepared to act on it, to set aside sufficient time each week? Your time commitment need not be great: For the next four weeks you need set aside no more than an average of twenty or thirty minutes a day. Remember, the smallest change makes a big difference. But be honest with yourself and realistic about what you can tackle. You may be tempted, as were some of our study participants, to try to do too much too quickly (a sure recipe for failure).

As you begin the program, most of you will start to feel better very quickly, usually in a few days or at most in the first two or three weeks. And many of the techniques will yield immediate results; for instance, the first time you successfully do a deep relaxation technique, you'll emerge refreshed and energized. But along the way there may be some discomfort, particularly at the very beginning. For instance, if you are starting to exercise after a long layoff, you will probably experience some temporary aches and pains. As you become more assertive in your communication, you may have to deal with some puzzlement or resistance in others who are used to the old you. All our study participants encountered roadblocks and had to deal with shortfalls. When you encounter these, realize that they are signs you are actually doing something new —signs of success.

Your friends and family may find themselves changing, too! In the early stages of the program, the husband of one of our female study participants made the following comment to his wife of sixteen years: "I'm having trouble adjusting to the you who got adjusted to me." In fact, since they both had the courage to communicate more fully and honestly, the program was a big success for both of them. As the wife commented at her eight-month checkup, "For the first time since the early days of our marriage, we both know we're living with a real flesh-and-blood person. But it took a little adjusting."

In sum, it won't always be easy. After all, stress is the body's response to uncertainty, and any change involves introducing some uncertainty into your life. You're bound to experience anxiety—as well as excitement—as you introduce new behaviors and begin to believe that significant change really is possible for you. By concentrating on small, concrete changes that you have designed and chosen for yourself, you keep this uncertainty to a minimum.

THE INTERVENTION TRAINING

Each of the intervention chapters is divided into three sections: "Rate Yourself," "Basic Training," and "Your Four-Week Start-Up Program." In the "Rate Yourself" section, we invite you take stock of your strengths and weaknesses to help you identify specific opportunities for change. Then we help you develop clear images of yourself doing, feeling, and looking better. In the "Basic Training" section, we explain how the intervention works and teach you the specific skills you need to put it into practice. In the "Start-Up" section, we provide you with a structured four-week program to get you off on the right foot. In more detail, here's how the intervention chapters work.

Rate Yourself

You will begin each chapter by taking a personal inventory of what you already are doing and aren't doing to practice a particular Vital Life Skill. This section includes a series of quizzes and other exercises in self-evaluation.

The detailed self-knowledge these self-tests provide allows you to get a clearer fix on what you want to accomplish. If nutrition is at the top of your prescription, perhaps you want to lose weight, or lower your blood pressure, or be less tired at the end of the day. As you become more specific about what you want, you are able to set specific, realistic, short- and long-term goals.

You can think of this process as getting in touch with the person you would really like to be. Your current sense that you aren't living in the way you'd really like to—or up to your potential—is not only a source of day-to-day frustration and nagging dissatisfaction, it is the origin of much of your stress. One of our study participants put this well when he described the difference in his life before and after the Body Age

Program: "Most days I just wished the 'fuller and better me' would go away and leave me alone; then at least I could live my life as a peaceful slob. But it wouldn't. And now I'm glad it stuck with me. Now I don't feel it's gnawing away at me. I feel as though that 'fuller and better me' is waving to me, in a kind of encouraging, understanding way."

The final step in the "Rate Yourself" section is for you to develop the affirmations and visualizations that will help engage your unconscious mind and deepest feelings in the change process. These powerful aids to self-expression are discussed in more detail below.

Basic Training

The second section of each chapter introduces you to the Vital Life Skill. For example, in the chapter "Effective Relaxation," we explain how deep relaxation techniques slow down your metabolism and quiet your brain-wave activity, enabling you to relax at will. Then we teach you various techniques for making this intervention a natural part of your life.

Your Four-Week Start-Up Program

Although many people initially resist structure, our experience with the Body Age Program confirms that the more you are willing to work within a clear framework, the more effective your prescription will be. As a result, we've designed a four-week start-up program for each of the five Vital Life Skills. The basic four weeks are:

> Week 1: Get Ready
> Week 2: Take Your First Step
> Week 3: Build on Your Success
> Week 4: Consolidate Your Gains.

It's up to you whether or not you follow this structure in detail, or merely use it for ideas to get you started.

Spend your first four weeks phasing in only the top-priority intervention on your Prescription Pad. We recommend that you don't start phasing in the second intervention of your prescription until about the eighth week of the program. This provides time for you to get comfortable with your new skills and for the stress of this first series of changes to subside.

THE ACTION DIARY

Our program participants found it particularly helpful to make a formal, written agreement with themselves (sometimes called a self-care contract) detailing the changes they planned to make each week. Other studies have shown that 97 percent of those who make contracts for health improvement actually successfully accomplish change. The self-care contract is a renewable and flexible agreement you make with yourself to achieve a progressive series of clearly targeted behavior changes. It is a way of supporting and focusing yourself as you go through the change process, a blueprint of the new self you are creating. To paraphrase the Zen philosopher D. T. Suzuki, "You are an artist, and your life is your work of art."

Our study participants also found that keeping a daily diary provided them with a regular opportunity to monitor their progress, note opportunities for improvement, and give themselves daily positive feedback.

The Action Diary that we recommend combines both these elements. The Planning Page is the contract you make with yourself each week. The Progress Recording Page is your daily record of how you're doing. A filled-out sample Planning Page and Progress Report Page for week 3 of Effective Relaxation is reproduced below. Blank forms for you to photocopy can be found in appendix A, "Your Action Diary." They can be kept in a loose-leaf notebook.

Before you fill out a Planning Page, we recommend that you give each behavior you're agreeing to undertake the SMART test. (A new behavior is as simple as not interrupting other people or limiting yourself to one glass of alcohol a day.) SMART is an acronym for Specific, Measurable, Acceptable, Realistic, Truthful. For each behavioral goal you set, ask the following series of SMART questions:

> Is it specific? (What? How? Where? When? With whom?
> For how long?)
> Is it measurable? (Will I know when I've done it?)
> Is it acceptable? (Will I feel good about doing this?)
> Is it realistic? (Am I really able to do this?)
> Is it truthful? (Do I really want to make this behavioral
> change?)

As you sit down to fill out your Planning Page, remember not to be too hard on yourself. Set realistic and achievable goals. Don't attempt too much. We've provided space for up to five new behaviors each week, but you may need only one or two until you are simultaneously working on more than one intervention. Also, be prepared to be flexible and to

ACTION DIARY FOR WEEK OF ___8th___ TO ___15th___

Planning Page

Affirmations (My self-themes for this week in key words and phrases)

I _am smooth energy_

I _feel my stress signs and let them go_

(Other) _I flow like a cat_

_____

Opportunity Visualizations (I clearly see myself . . .)

- _breathing away my stress_
- _maintaining a relaxed posture, while others get tense_
- _Keeping my "Stress tachometer" in the green zone until I really need the energy_

_____

_____

I choose to deepen this Vital Life Skill as follows (My specific behavioral objectives this week)

I choose to _Listen to the Autogenic tape and repeat my affirmation for 5 minutes on Monday, Tuesday, Thursday, Saturday & Sunday_

Under the following circumstances: _in the guest bedroom while Jim prepares breakfast with sign on door "Danger Mom Meditating"_

I choose to _practice the Spiral Relaxation for 5 minutes once per day, everyday_

Under the following circumstances: _With my door closed just before I make my "return phone calls" at 2:00 pm_

I choose to _repeat at least one of my favorite affirmations as many times as I feel Comfortable (each workday)_

Under the following circumstances: _As I walk at a slow flowing pace from bus stop to our home (remember it's the Kids house)_

I choose to _____

_____

Under the following circumstances: _____

_____

My other opportunity situations for skill practice are:

- preparing for Friday's staff meeting (spiral)
- responding to boss's question
- dealing with kids questions as I prepare dinner

_____

I have arranged to check in with my partner . . .

When?

Tuesday & Saturday around dinner time

About

My "Stress Tachometer" read out
- her getting religious about going to the gym (she told me to be merciless)

Progress Recording Page

Vital Life Skills Being Mastered: _____Relaxation_____

	Congratulations on Vital Actions	Opportunities for Doing It Better
Monday	- listened to tape - "Spiraled" my way through phone Calls	Wasted energy writing angry memo I didn't send
Tuesday	- ditto plus affirmation - relaxing walk from bus.	felt guilty and tense because I hadn't bought junk food for kids snack
Wednesday	Kept cool when photo copier broke down	

Thursday	- Cancelled a useless meeting - still doing tape	over-reacted to Jimmy's after school snacking
Friday	fielded boss questions with no headache afterwards	one too many (ouch) before dinner drinks
Saturday	- Tape and affirmation are becoming a habit - Kids respect my sign	
Sunday	positive solution to kids argument: I didn't take sides just to end it	I really could have left that brief case at the office

My Summary of Progress at End of Week (Have any patterns emerged? Does my self-care contract require modification?)

modify your contract if it proves too tough to honor or if a more strategic opportunity presents itself. Old habits die hard. And making lots of "mistakes" can be a good sign. Remember that you are changing the mental and behavioral patterns built up over a lifetime. Perfection is one of the most stressful goals you can set for yourself, so don't attempt to become a new person overnight.

On your Progress Recording Page, learn to give yourself credit for things you are already doing well (most of us have a tendency to discount or downplay our successes). Give yourself positive feedback every step of the way.

The daily self-feedback aspect of the Progress Recording Page of your diary is particularly useful for helping you spot opportunities and overcome roadblocks. Even an honest awareness of a shortfall can give you an increased feeling of self-control. The important thing here is that the feedback you give yourself be positive and self-enhancing. Find ways to reinforce your new behavior; don't undermine it.

One Speed Freak who started the program reported that, during the first week, he resisted the feedback part of his self-care contract as "namby-pamby, self-congratulatory back patting." He did it (his wife was his program buddy), but he thought it was a total waste of time. By the third week, however, he reported, "I'm beginning to pace myself in long meetings, saving my energy for the items I'm really responsible for. I realize I've been able to do that from time to time in the past, but I didn't recognize it—how I did it or how good it felt—until I started giving myself feedback in my diary. Now, at least I recognize when I do pace myself well, and what a tremendous skill it can be. I guess my usual feedback to myself was 98 percent critical. Now that I'm celebrating my successes, I firmly expect I'm going to have more of them."

THE BUDDY SYSTEM

Making a weekly contract with yourself and recording your daily progress in your Action Diary doesn't mean you have to, or even should try to, go it alone (especially if you happen to be a Loner). Before you begin your Body Age Program, we recommend that you develop some sort of support system, the simplest of which is the buddy system used by those who participated in the Body Age Study. During the training sessions, we asked everyone to pick a partner. The partners agreed to monitor each other's progress on a regular basis, preferably at least once a week. Monitoring was often as simple as a phone call at a previously agreed time, but in many cases it included regular get-togethers.

Charlie and Tony used the buddy system to particular advantage. Charlie (age 39, body age 48) was a Speed Freak dermatologist who made good progress in the first couple of weeks using his autogenic tape and affirmations. But by the end of week 3, he had gotten almost nowhere in actually building brief "breathing spaces" into his nonstop ten-hour office days. Like most Speed Freaks, he interpreted this as: "None of the relaxation stuff works. I've got to try something else."

He told this tale of woe to his partner, Tony (age 37, body age 44), a dentist and a recovering Loner. Tony saw Charlie's roadblock as an opportunity to be actively helpful (a challenge for his stressotype). The two made a pact to "tell each other the truth," and Tony suggested that Charlie have his nurse schedule at least three fictitious patients sometime in the midafternoon during the next week. Charlie would use this time to do things that had nothing to do with work and would report back to Tony at week's end.

Initially, Charlie admitted that he felt angry with his nurse each time she scheduled blank time and that he had to fight the temptation to see the next patient early. But he resisted—because of his pact with Tony. Soon the fictitious patients became part of Charlie's weekly routine. At their eight-month checkup, Charlie jokingly reported, "Well, at least one of my patients follows the prescription I give him . . . me, although at the beginning it was a case of a doctor following a dentist's orders." (Charlie's body age was down 8 years to 40, virtually the same as his calendar age.)

Tony had also benefited from the partnership (his body age was down 7 years to 36, younger than his chronological age). He commented that Charlie had been a "real sounding board for all the good advice I should have been following." And when he asked himself, "Why should Charlie bother to change, anyway?" he was taken back to one of the basic values that had led to his becoming a health professional in the first place: "To be of value and service to others." It was this awareness that led Tony to realize he wanted to be of *personal* service—not just to be paid to help people. As a result of this value clarification, he joined the local Rotary chapter and reported at his eight-month checkup that he had found "more friendship time" in the past six months than in the previous fifteen years. And it all had started with his buddy Charlie.

In addition to the buddy system, another important means of getting support from your environment is to prepare those around you for some of the changes you'll be making. If you have a family, enlist their cooperation—which could make all the difference. For example, nutritional changes will be much more difficult if the other people at the dinner table aren't willing to cooperate. When you decide to acquire a new behavior that will affect them, find subtle ways to alert your family, friends, and co-workers.

THE SELF-BEHAVIOR CYCLE

In recent years, psychologists have come up with various theories and models to explain the processes people go through when they undergo significant change. They all seem to agree on one point: The simple fact of taking well-chosen action makes you feel different—and better. It literally makes a different you.

This deceptively simple truth is encapsulated in the diagram below: As you change in attitudes (self-concept), your behavior changes; as your behavior changes, your concept of yourself changes. Doing is becoming.

SELF-BEHAVIOR CYCLE

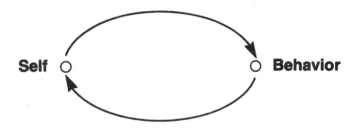

Self ○   ○ Behavior

This diagram gets to the core of why the Body Age Program works so well. To a very great extent, your emotional makeup at any point in time (including how good or bad you feel and how you see yourself in relationship to the world) can be thought of as resulting directly from the way you have experienced yourself in the past. You are the sum of all you have done and felt. If you have typically experienced yourself as successful and in control, you bring this self-image into the present moment and will likely re-create it in reality again and again. If, however, you have usually seen yourself as falling short, failing to live up to your or other people's expectations, you will behave in ways that tend to reinforce this belief.

Hundreds of times during every week, you are presented with opportunities to choose to behave differently. Recognize and seize just one or two of these choice points each day, or each week, and the resulting change in your self-image and self-esteem will surprise and delight you.

For example, you are sitting in your office and the phone rings. The person at the other end (your boss?) has a pressing request for information.

Your instinct is to stand up, salute, and ask how high you should jump in an effort to satisfy the caller and the request. You put the caller on hold while you frantically search through your files for the nugget that will satisfy him or her, all the while worrying about keeping this busy person waiting, occasionally interrupting your search to go back to the phone to apologize for taking so long, dropping the file on the floor as you try to do three things at once, rapidly bringing yourself to a boil. By the time you have found what is wanted, you need a two-week vacation.

The self-affirming alternative to this scenario might be something like the following: When the request comes in, you say, "I'll give it my immediate attention and call you back in fifteen minutes."

The hundred such choice points in your day may now go by largely unnoticed. But each one lets you see yourself as either a driven dog or a person who is in control. At the end of the month or the year, your thousands of specific, chosen behaviors have either led you to feel you've sold out to your job or that you have bought into it. In short, each choice you make is self-creating, and the self you make is up to you.

The positive self-behavior cycle takes about three weeks to transform a new behavior into a self-affirming habit. In effect, your Body Age Program is a series of small, specific, concrete, behavior changes that become habitual—a part of you.

AUTOGENIC TRAINING: ROOTING THE CHANGE PROCESS IN YOUR DEEPEST SELF

One of the ten original interventions we taught our study subjects was something called self-hypnosis and anti-aging imagery. It involved the use of a relaxation technique called autogenic relaxation and two mental techniques: affirmation and visualization. Autogenic relaxation is a technique of self-hypnosis that allows you to root positive affirmations and self-affirming visualizations in your unconscious mind. It brings your mind and feelings into harmony with your body as you take on and adjust to new behaviors.

In chapter 1, we explored some of the mounting scientific evidence of the power of the mind and emotions to affect the body negatively or positively. Autogenic training taps into this extraordinary positive mental power. Those participants in the Body Age Program who consistently used autogenic relaxation combined with affirmation and visualization showed greater and more lasting progress than those who used them little or not at all. We concluded that autogenic training was so important that it ought to be part of all five interventions.

The three techniques that comprise this training are in fact "autogenic,'' which means self-generated. They arise naturally from your deep-est self, and they reflect your care for and faith in yourself. Any one of them can be used effectively on its own. Each can help your prescription take firm root in your personality, so that your new behaviors become as natural as breathing. However, used together they are a much more powerful force in support of positive change.

Autogenic Relaxation

Modern man is primarily a creature of the left brain: the logical, an-alytical, verbal, and time-conscious part of the brain. The right brain, which comes into play during sleep and deep relaxation, is believed to be the center of intuition, inspiration, and imagery—of space rather than time. In a deeply relaxed state, the two halves of your brain are functioning as a synchronous whole, with the potential of greater creativity and mental productivity. Numerous experiments have suggested that increased mental capacity results from deliberate use of relaxation. As described in the book *Super Learning*, by Marilyn Ostrander, foreign language students who alternated periods of relaxation with periods of study took half the time (in some cases much less) to learn language skills.

Autogenic relaxation involves using full, comfortable breathing and mind-focusing techniques to engender what essentially is a form of self-hypnosis. For our study participants, we developed a thirteen- to fourteen-minute autogenic relaxation tape. We gave a version of this tape to everyone who entered the Body Age Program and asked them to use it at least four times a week during the program. (The script for the tape begins on page 127.)

Positive Affirmations

If you're like most people, you conduct a fairly continuous internal dialogue. It can be positive or negative, but for most of us roughly 80 percent of it is self-critical, self-denying stuff, what psychologists refer to as negative self-talk. Negative self-talk—"I can't do this"; "I'm dumb"; "I'm inadequate"; "I'm confused"; "I'm unworthy"—feeds into a weakened sense of self. Very often, this negative chatter comes in a more subtle form of undermining; for example, "I have a feeling I could have done that better"—but "better" is never defined. If you devalue or discount your legitimate accomplishments and qualities, you are guilty of this most insidious form of negative self-talk. Phrases such as "Yes, but . . ." and "Well, this may be so, but . . ." are sure signs of its presence.

You can think of self-talk as the way you communicate with yourself. The more positive your internal communication, the more likely your outward behavior will be positive (self-affirming). This will have an impact in every area of your life, including your relationships with other people. One of the purposes of positive affirmations is to substitute positive for negative self-talk. Self-affirming internal communication reinforces effective external action.

Affirmations can be very powerful tools. One writer has accurately described them as "depth charges of positive energy." An affirmation is a word or a phrase that you choose to express meaningfully a goal you want to achieve or a value you want to express. The emphasis here is on the process—of moving in a satisfying direction, of "being" a satisfying way—rather than the end result. For example, before a competition, a weight lifter might repeat to himself an affirmation such as "I am strength." Or he might choose the cluster "Strength, power, now." A poor example of a weight lifter's affirmation would be the phrase, "I will lift 500 pounds," which emphasizes an end result rather than the process, and which casts the affirmation into the future. Coming up with the right affirmation is like being your own advertising copywriter. It involves finding a slogan that captures very succinctly what this phase of the program is all about for you (that's why your affirmations go at the top of the Planning Page of your Action Diary). A number of people in the program found that lines from favorite songs made powerful affirmations.

There are many ways to use your affirmations, other than as part of an autogenic relaxation session. You may, as some people do, say your affirmation each morning as you face yourself in the mirror and then give yourself a warm and sincere smile or then nod and say, "You bet!" to yourself. Or you may, as one of our study participants did, tape your affirmation to your wristwatch so that each time you check the time you are reminded of your self-theme. Find the method that's right for you. You may feel a little silly when you first try one of these advertising slogans for your better self, but if you persist, you'll find that affirmations work.

Once you get over feeling silly, good things start to happen. A secretary-receptionist named Ann who entered the program at age 27 (body age 35) had particular problems with procrastination: She got so wrapped up in personal problems at work that she let her filing and appointment logging get days behind. One lunch hour she went into one of the office's soundproof interview rooms (she worked at a large mental health center), complete with three videotaping cameras, to do her relaxation and affirmation session. She felt so good saying her affirmation to herself that she said it out loud: "I do what I say. I finish what I start."

Ann didn't realize that throughout her private relaxation session the video cameras had been rolling. The next therapist to use the room rewound the tape only to see Ann looking very relaxed and talking to herself. Although Ann was initially mortified when she found out, the therapist was interested in learning what she was doing. In the end, five professionals from the center joined one of the Institute's stress programs. And with the help of her affirmations, Ann stopped procrastinating.

Effective single-sentence affirmations have key characteristics. For one, they are usually positive, devoid of any negative connotation: "I am strong and confident" is much better than "I am overcoming my weaknesses." They begin with the first-person singular pronoun: "I." Sentences that begin with "I" are more forceful. (You can experience the difference by taking a sentence that begins with "I" and changing it to "we.") The first-person singular pronoun implies that you are taking full responsibility for the statement you are making, that you and the statement are one. Second, the affirmation is a simple declarative sentence in the present tense. The statement "I eat nutritious food" is more powerful than the sentence "I will eat nutritious food." It states your intention as if it were already a fact, emphasizing process rather than result. "I want to become vital" is weaker than "I am vital" or "I am vitality." Also note that comparison words take oomph out of your affirmation. "I get along better with my co-workers" is weaker than "I get along well with my co-workers." In sum, a simple affirmation in the present tense generates a feeling of increased confidence: You *are* what you affirm.

In our training sessions, we gave our students a wide range of possible affirmations that we have found useful in our courses at the Canadian Institute of Stress. Here are some short lists of examples.

Personal and Interpersonal

I am a good person.
[Joe] is a good person.
I understand and appreciate others [name(s) of family member, friend, spouse, colleague] more every day.
I accept myself as I am.
I choose to love and be loved.
I enjoy life fully.
I use the past and the future to enhance the quality of my present.
I contribute to humanity through the joy I bring to my work and social life.
I feel strong and clear, alone and with others.
I can feel critical of others and still accept them.

Work

I am happy and effective in my work.
People enjoy paying me for what I enjoy doing.
I open myself to create solutions.
All mistakes are forgivable.
I forgive myself [and others] for mistakes and unkindnesses.
I now communicate clearly and effectively, with one or with many.
I accept setbacks along the road to success and achievement.
I remain calm and balanced in my work.

Stress Efficiency and Anti-Aging

I feel alive and vital every day.
Health, happiness, and well-being are mine.
I relax at will.
I breathe pain away with every breath.
I sleep easily and soundly.
I am losing weight and gaining beauty.
I eat fresh, healthy foods.
My joints are flexible and comfortable.
My body is quickly cleansing out all congestion and weakness.
I choose to breathe fresh, healthy air. [Good for smokers]
Full breathing relaxes and satisfies me more than alcohol.
I choose actions that express me, now and in the future.
I eat well and eliminate well. [Good for constipation]
I run relaxed and give my all. [This type of affirmation can be used
    with any sport.]

Philosophical/Spiritual

I am becoming more and more aware of the pattern of good in my
    life.
I am happy and blissful just to be alive.
Everything now is as it should be.
I find God in everything I think and sense and do.

You may or may not find some of your personal affirmations in the
list above. We'll be suggesting many other possibilities in the five intervention chapters. The important thing is to find the affirmations that
feel right for you and try them out, even if at first they make you feel
awkward or silly.

Visualization

Visualization means using mental imagery to rehearse for success. It's as simple as picturing yourself doing and experiencing a successful behavior—one that expresses an important self-theme. The potency of visualization has been demonstrated by professional athletes and other high-achievers who employ it as part of their training. Studies have shown that the time athletes spend rehearsing by means of a series of mental images can be even more productive than time spent in physical practice. Because the brain perceives these mental pictures not as imagined events but as though they are actually happening, visualizing the perfect performance can bring your actual performance much closer to perfection.

Figure-skating fans will remember all the press coverage given to the "Battle of the Brians," the race for the 1988 Olympic gold medal between Brian Boitano of the United States and Brian Orser of Canada. Both these superb athletes talked freely about their use of mental imaging techniques to prepare them for the big performance. At one point, Boitano described his technique of visualization as really just a form of daydreaming. Indeed, visualization is a kind of deliberate, creative daydreaming. It certainly worked for Boitano, as anyone who saw his final performance in Calgary will remember.

Even more impressive is the mounting evidence that these mental imaging techniques can help combat disease. Carl and Stephanie Simonton are well known for their use of visualization with cancer patients. In their book *Getting Well Again*, they describe the remarkable recovery of the first patient they worked with, a 61-year-old man with serious throat cancer. He could barely swallow his saliva, breathing had become difficult, and he had dropped from 130 pounds to 98 pounds.

The Simontons' approach was, in their words, "to help this man actively participate in his treatment," radiation therapy. This entailed three five-to-fifteen-minute relaxation sessions each week, followed by a series of visualizations. The patient was to

1. "Picture himself in a pleasant, quiet place" and then "to imagine his cancer vividly in whatever form it seemed to take."
2. Visualize his radiation therapy "as consisting of millions of tiny bullets of energy that would hit all the cells, both normal and cancerous, in their path. Because the cancer cells were weaker and more confused than the normal cells, they would not be able to repair the damage . . . so the normal cells would remain healthy while the cancer cells would die."
3. Picture "his body's white blood cells coming in, swarming over the cancer cells, picking up and carrying off the dead and dying ones,

flushing them out of his body. . . . In his mind's eye, he was to visualize his cancer decreasing in size and his health returning to normal.''

Two months after commencing treatment with the Simontons, the man showed no signs of cancer and at the time their book was published had remained healthy for six years.

None of our study participants were suffering from a serious disease such as cancer, but many discovered the power of mental imagery.

A salesman who entered the Body Age Program found that combining affirmation and visualization helped him be more successful in his job. Previously he had experienced high stress levels and less than ideal results when selling one particular product in his line. He knew it was a good piece of merchandise, but for whatever reason he couldn't seem to get himself to fully believe what he was saying when he made his sales pitch to a new customer.

In the training session on affirmation and visualization, he developed the affirming phrase "Right, tight, and bright," which expressed for him the idea of a tight, facts-focused, optimistic presentation. His visualization started with the scene of him shaking hands to conclude a sale with a client, then moved back two steps to scenes of other clients using the product with a high degree of satisfaction. The final scene in this mind movie was of him listing for the prospective client specific ways in which this product would prove its cost-effectiveness. By the end of the eight-month program, his problem product had become his number-one seller.

The Power of Autogenic Training: Putting the Three Together

A number of studies have attempted to measure the power of autogenic training to improve performance. Some of these have yielded startling results, such as slowing or eliminating the growth of cancerous cells, increasing female breast size by an average of 1.5 inches over a twelve-week period, and accelerating weight loss for dieters.

At the University of Toronto, the Canadian Institute of Stress conducted two studies of the effectiveness of autogenic training for athletes. One study was of thirty-two competitive power lifters; the other was of thirty-six 10-kilometer runners.

In each case, the study subjects were divided into four test groups of equal size. The first test group continued its standard training program in preparation for an upcoming competition. The second group was taught the basics of autogenic relaxation and given a fifteen-minute relaxation tape to be used at least four times per week at home during the training period. The third group used the tape and was taught to use visualizations. And the fourth group used the tape, plus visualizations, plus affirmations.

For example, the weight lifters in the third and fourth groups learned to form clear mental pictures of lifting the winning weight and being congratulated immediately after the lift. They rehearsed these images for at least ten minutes at least four times a week immediately following their use of the autogenic tape. They also used mental images during their training. One image was of blood flowing to the key muscle groups and bringing with it essential muscle-growth nutrients while taking away the tissue being broken down by increased weight demands. During their workouts, this visualization was reinforced by their imagining (mentally "feeling") warm, dampened cloths placed on their shoulders and chests, a sensory highlighting of the key muscle groups they were building.

Weight lifters in the fourth group added affirmations to the visualizing techniques described above. Each athlete developed his own affirmation as the expression of his "personalized maximum strength release" theme. Two examples that were chosen were "Strength, power, now" and "I am power." Both were used as part of the autogenic relaxation and during training.

A similar test-group breakdown was used for the thirty-six long-distance runners. In both cases, the results of autogenic training were impressive. For example, over a mere six weeks the four groups of weight lifters increased the number of pounds they could bench-press as follows: the first group (regular training): 2.2%; the second group (autogenic relaxation only): 4.6%; the third group (autogenic relaxation plus visualization): 7.4%; the fourth group (autogenic relaxation plus visualization and affirmation): 12.1%. Chest size increased in a similar pattern, as did dominant arm size. And the four groups showed increasing stress efficiency as measured by their resting heart rate five minutes before the lift and again three minutes before the lift (when stress is usually on the rise).

In the other study, the runners were able to increase their personal best time over the 10-kilometer distance as follows: the first group, by 8 seconds; the second group, by 1 minute, 12 seconds; the third group, by 3 minutes, 8 seconds; the fourth group, by 3 minutes, 39 seconds. A similar pattern was exhibited in their resting heart rates immediately before and immediately after the race.

You are not training for an athletic competition, but for something even more important—the challenges and opportunities of the rest of your life. The use of autogenic relaxation, combined with affirmations and visualizations, will increase your fitness for the demands of daily living.

It certainly made a big difference for our Body Age Study subjects. Committed and full use of autogenic training more than doubled the effectiveness of the five Vital Life Skills. That is, the more frequently this technique was practiced, the greater the improvement in body age. The chart on page 126 summarizes the effectiveness of autogenic training for 602 of our Body Age subjects after eight months on the program.

AUTOGENIC TRAINING EFFECTIVENESS

Subjects Used Autogenic Training:

Body Age Reversal	Very Frequently	Frequently	Occasionally
10 or more years	188 (59%)	20 (10%)	0 (0%)
7–9 years	127 (40%)	138 (66%)	22 (28%)
6 years or less	1 (1%)	50 (24%)	56 (72%)
	316 (100%)	208 (100%)	78 (100%)

Very Frequently: Used the autogenic tape followed immediately by ten minutes of visualization and affirmation at least five times a week, as well as using affirmations three or more times per day on four or more days each week.

Frequently: Used tape at least three times per week, two or more times followed by five or more minutes of affirmation and visualization, as well as sporadic use of daily affirmations.

Occasionally: Irregular and brief use of tape and affirmation and visualization.

The average body age reversal for those practicing autogenic training "very frequently" amounted to 10.04 years, compared to 4.46 years for those doing so only "occasionally." Fully 59 percent of those who practiced autogenic training "very frequently" achieved a body age reversal of 10 or more years, while less than 1 percent of this frequent practice group were in the "6 years or less" category. By contrast, 72 percent of the "occasional" autogenic practitioners were limited to a body age reversal of 6 or fewer years.

Two things stand out on the chart. The first is that a very high proportion of our study participants used autogenic training to the fullest: Clearly they found it effective and kept with it. The second is that those with high compliance reduced their body age by an average of 10 or more years, regardless of their V.Q. or their stressotype profile.

Autogenic Training: The Technique

No matter which intervention you are working on, you will begin the first day of week 1 of your start-up program with an autogenic relaxation that incorporates one or more positive affirmations and that is followed by a visualization appropriate to the Vital Life Skill in question. The affirmations and visualizations are ones you choose, based on your overall goals for the program and your specific goals for the intervention you are about to tackle.

Relax. Find a place where you can be quiet and uninterrupted for about half an hour. Be sure you can sit or lie comfortably. Now you're ready to begin autogenic relaxation.

Below we have provided the script of the tape we gave to each person who entered the Body Age Program. Ask a friend who has a pleasant reading voice to record the script on an audiocassette. The script, not including the minimum of five minutes of blank tape for affirmation and visualization, should be paced to last about thirteen or fourteen minutes (we've provided time indicators to help the reader monitor his or her speed). If no reader is available, record the script yourself. The script reader should use calm and even tones while recording. (You may find that it helps to partially or completely turn the bass up and the treble down when you play the tape.) If you prefer, you can order from the Canadian Institute of Stress the autogenic tape we used for the study. (See appendix C.)

Use your tape each time you practice the technique of autogenic relaxation.

Autogenic Relaxation: Basic Script

(Reading time: approximately fourteen minutes)

Autogenic relaxation is one of the world's most effective exercises for achieving a physically relaxed and mentally alert state.

By focusing your mind on the instructions, you will be able to experience comfortable feelings of heaviness, warmth, and deep relaxation in every part of your body.

And with each time you practice, it will become easier and easier to relax whenever you choose.

Begin by lying on your back, or by sitting comfortably in a chair.

Become aware of sounds inside the room and outside, and allow yourself to be separate from them.

Allow thoughts to come and go.

[1 minute]

As I count from 5 to 1, picture each number as clearly as you can. By the time I reach 1, you will notice that your thoughts are becoming quieter, more distant, and less distracting.

5 . . . , 4 . . . , 3 . . . , 2 . . . , and . . . 1.

Focus your attention on the tip of your nose. Notice that the air on the inhalation is slightly cooler than the exhalation. And with each exhalation, notice how the tension you don't need continues to leave your body.

Let go of all physical, emotional, and mental tension.

[2 minutes]

Give yourself permission to enjoy this time for your relaxation.

By focusing on the instructions, your mind becomes more and more calm, as your body becomes deeply relaxed.

Inhale now, and bring the air down into your abdomen. Let your abdomen expand, and then the chest. And exhale through your nose.

[3 minutes]

Once again inhaling and filling the abdomen more and more, let your chest expand as you continue inhaling.

Then pause and exhale, releasing tension you don't need on the exhalation.

This time, inhaling slower and deeper, feeling the abdomen expand, and then the chest. And notice the comfortable fullness. Pause, and then exhale slowly.

And continue breathing in this way, consciously allowing the breathing to become slower and deeper.

Once again, inhaling, filling the entire body, and pause, and when you exhale, release all tension from your body.

[4 minutes]

And on the next inhalation, put your awareness on the feelings in the muscles in the abdomen and chest, feeling them expand and tighten. And then, release and relax.

Slowly inhaling, and slowly exhaling.

Breathing in now, and inhaling fresh air. Let the air into the lungs, and let it pass into the bloodstream, bringing nourishing, healing oxygen to every part of your body. And exhale.

[5 minutes]

Now, with a slow, comfortable, deep breath, breathe in light air, and let it spread throughout your entire body. When you exhale, the lightness remains behind.

With your next inhalation, the body becomes even lighter. And on the exhalation, the lightness remains.

This time inhaling, and consciously taking the light air through your nose, into your arms, to the tips of your fingers, and into your head. Now, into your chest, and abdomen, and down your legs to the tips of your toes. And when you exhale, your body feels so light, you feel as if you are almost floating.

[6 minutes]

Now inhale, and breathe in heavy air. Let it spread throughout your body. Feel yourself sinking comfortably into the chair, or the floor.

When you exhale, let the heaviness remain.

With each inhalation, allow your body to be more and more comfortably heavy and relaxed.

Your mind is clear and focused. And it becomes clearer as your body becomes more relaxed.

Feel the pull of gravity now all over. Imagine and feel yourself being drawn comfortably down onto the earth. Feel the pull of gravity across your entire body.

[7 minutes]

Now imagine wearing a heavy suit of clothing. Feel it on your chest and stomach, and abdomen. Feel the heaviness on your back and shoulders.

Imagine and feel a heavy belt around your waist.

Feel the heaviness in your arms, and repeat to yourself: My arms are very heavy. And feel your arms becoming even heavier. Even your hands are wearing heavy gloves.

[8 minutes]

And now, feel the heaviness of your clothing across your hips, thighs, calves, and feet.

Your whole body is very heavy, and very relaxed.

Now, with your awareness on your chest, repeat to yourself: My heartbeat is calm and regular. My breathing is deep and even.

And with your awareness on your stomach, imagine and feel warmth on your stomach. Imagine, perhaps, a comfortable warm heating pad. Imagine and feel warmth, and repeat to yourself: My stomach is relaxed and warm.

[9 minutes]

"I feel warm, and relaxed, and calm."

Your entire body is warm and comfortable.

And as I count from 10 to 1, allow yourself to move into a deeper, and deeper state of relaxation. Picturing the numbers as I count, and when you get to 1, your body will be even more relaxed, and your mind will be even calmer.

[10 minutes]

10 . . . , 9 . . . , 8 . . . , 7 . . . , deeper and deeper, 6 . . . , 5 . . . , 4 . . . , 3 . . . , 2 . . . , and . ... 1.

Become aware of how every part of your body feels, and know that you can return to this state whenever you choose.

Now enjoy this time for your relaxation . . . as you silently repeat your affirmations . . . and rehearse your visualizations.

[*NOTE*: Leave at least five minutes of blank tape at this point, or record five minutes of low-volume, relaxing background music. After this interval, complete the autogenic tape as follows.]

Now, as you begin to come back to an alert and awake state, you will find yourself rising up like a bubble to the surface of a pond as I count from 1 to 20. When you open your eyes, you will feel very relaxed and alert.

[11 minutes]

For the rest of today you will continue to be very alert, and focused. You will notice your body's stress reactions, and let them go.

Tonight you will sleep well, and wake up tomorrow alert and self-confident. And this state of well-being will improve day after day.

Counting up now, 1 . . . , 2 . . . , 3 . . . , 4 . . . , 5 . . . , 6 . . . , 7 . . . , 8 . . . , 9 . . . , 10. . . .

[12 minutes]

. . . more and more awake . . . 11 . . . , 12 . . . , 13 . . . , 14 . . . , 15 . . . coming up to the surface . . . 16 . . . , 17 . . . , 18 . . . , 19 . . . , and . . . 20.

[14 minutes]

Affirm. Note that you introduce your affirmations while you are in your most deeply relaxed and highly suggestible state. If you are working on nutrition, your affirmation might be "I eat for high performance." If you are working on exercise, it might be "I am lean energy." If you are working on Values/Goals Clarification, it might be "I make time to be with my friends and family." The important thing is to choose an affirmation that fits you and what you are doing, one that feels right.

We also recommend that you include at least one general anti-aging affirmation. Here are some possibilities in addition to the affirmations we listed earlier: ''I use stress energy efficiently.'' ''I am energy efficient.'' ''My body renews itself each day.'' ''I am youthful health.'' ''I am vital energy.'' ''I flow smoothly.''

Visualize. As you move on to your visualization, you remain in the relaxed state with your eyes closed. This is your chance to do some creative daydreaming. Now that you have achieved the heaviness and warmth of autogenic relaxation and have thought some very positive, self-affirming thoughts, your mind and body are ready to receive these mental seed images of success.

Visualization is most effective when it is very specific and includes details of all your senses—smell, taste, sight, sound, temperature, texture. The more totally you experience a visualization as if it is really happening, the more powerful and lasting will be its effect. Remember: Your mind makes no distinction between a visualization and a real event.

Here is the basic visualization technique. You can practice it at any time, including during an exercise workout or while taking the bus to work, although it is most effective during or immediately following some form of meditation or deep relaxation.

> Feel the warmth and heaviness of your body while experiencing your mind as calm, clear, and aware. Imagine yourself in a specific situation in which you would like to function more effectively or in which you would like success to be the rule, not the exception (the specific situation will depend on the intervention you are applying). Mentally rehearse how the highly successful ''you'' would ''just naturally'' express yourself in this situation. Visualize it exactly as you want it to be. Throughout, you are calm, relaxed, in control, and deriving great personal satisfaction from your behavior. Repeat the scene in your head until all the details are clear and you have involved as many of your five senses as possible.
>
> Affirm your visualization. Perhaps employ a phrase using the following form: ''In this situation, this is how I am.'' For example, ''When I talk to my father-in-law, I feel calm and confident. I listen to him fully without interrupting.'' If the scene you have been visualizing involves a person who you often feel is negative, you might say something like, ''I see the pluses in this person.'' As a result, you will start to see the positive aspects in this person and spot opportunities you otherwise might have missed.
>
> Feel the satisfaction of having achieved your goal. Savor the feeling.

Continue your visualization until the voice part of the tape begins again. It will bring you back to your normal, awake state. Once the tape is finished, take your time before getting up. Let the feeling of success linger. Feel the power of the affirmations and visualizations flow through your bloodstream and permeate the cells in every part of your body.

The three-part technique we've just described is a powerful tool for planting the seeds of success in your psyche. If you use it faithfully, it will increasingly become a part of you, a natural expression of your inner self, as natural as breathing. It will smooth the road to success.

[Note that on our standard tapescript we allow only five minutes for both affirmation and visualization. Many people find this time too short: At first it may seem more than enough, but later you may want more time. Feel free to give yourself more time, or to make versions of the tape with longer periods for affirmation and visualization. You can also spend some time after the autogenic tape finishes, while your eyes are still closed, continuing your affirmations and visualizations. But it's very important that you complete your tape with the instructions for coming out of your deeply relaxed state.]

THE SUCCESS CYCLE

Regardless of which intervention you tackle first, the self-reinforcing self-behavior success cyle is the same. It consists of a sequence of four basic steps that you will be repeating over and over again during the Body Age Program as your actions re-create your self and as that firmer sense of self (and growing self-esteem) motivates further meaningful action. The four steps or stages are affirm, plan, do, and congratulate yourself.

Affirm. This is the sum of all the positive preparation you do. Define and visualize a more vital "you" as clearly, specifically, and firmly as you can. Affirm how these changes are a natural extension and expression of you. Affirm both your long-term goals for the program and your short-term weekly objectives. Remember the times in your life when you really did make a difference—whether it was losing weight, turning down a tempting job that was wrong for you, or learning a skill you still value. Draw on the memory of past successes to empower the present. Identify your personal affirmations, the high-impact slogans, or the self-themes you will bring to life through concrete action.

Plan. Use visualization to mentally rehearse the specifics of each concrete behavioral change, whether it's going to your first aerobics class or asking a co-worker out to lunch. Recognize in advance—and on the spot as they occur—specific opportunities for greater self-expression. These are your choice points, situations in which you have a chance to introduce new self-affirming behavior. Plan for increasingly challenging behavior changes.

Do. Put your plans into action, and don't be discouraged by setbacks and disappointments. There will be times when, despite your positive affirmations and your careful planning, you will seem to lose your way. The well-meaning but overprotective voices inside your head will start their negative talk: "You'll never be fit—you were meant to be a wimp." "You'll never make any new friends—you're a boring person." "You'll never change what you eat—you're too weak-willed." "You don't deserve success or happiness." At times like these, substitute positive self-talk for negative self-talk. Take the leap of faith. Remember that getting there is half the fun, that doing is becoming. The main thing is to behave consciously and deliberately more like your ideal self (or even to choose on a particular occasion to behave like your old self). Don't be afraid to modify your plan: Adjust your goals as you learn more about yourself.

Last but not least, learn to enjoy the anxiety of change: It's a sign that you are in fact having an impact on you, that you are making a difference. Anxiety may be uncomfortable at times, but it is a vital sign—evidence that you are alive and kicking. One of our study participants, who lost more than forty pounds in her eight months in the program, took pleasure in each hunger pang: These told her, as soon as they began, that she was losing weight.

Congratulate Yourself for Every Success. Mentally and viscerally recreate (visualize/affirm) the successful "you's" that you have been expressing. The importance of this positive self-feedback cannot be overemphasized. You might think of it as affirmation and visualization after the fact. Even if the first week goes by and you have only one tiny success to celebrate, savor it to the fullest. The salesman who used the affirmation "Right, tight, and bright" had this phrase engraved onto a plaque that he hung on the wall of his office, next to several sales citations. The plaque symbolized his power to make a difference in something important to him.

If the week goes by and you have merely noted your missed opportunities for change, congratulate yourself for this deepening awareness. Awareness precedes action; it is the prerequisite to choice and change. Relish each new awareness: These are the first signs of success.

The next five chapters contain a great deal of useful information and many suggestions for effective action. What you do with this resource is entirely up to you. You can follow our program to the letter, or you can ignore it completely and design your own timetable for change. As long as the motivation for change comes from you, you'll succeed. If you make your prescription your own, anything you do that's new will make a difference.

For each of the five Vital Life Skills, we've attempted to give you the essentials as succinctly as possible: the basic information you need to understand the skill and the basic techniques you need to practice it. In fact, we could have written a book instead of a chapter for each one. (If you want more information about any of the interventions, there are all sorts of books you can read and courses you can take. Many of the best books are listed at the back of this book, under "Further Reading.")

For the most part, the next five chapters contain nothing revolutionary, although we have summarized the latest thinking in each area. What's new is the framework we've provided—your personal stressotype profile and the personalized prescription to fit it. What's new is a program that's geared to *you* and rooted in *your* unconscious mind and throughout *your* body by autogenic training. The Body Age Program succeeds because it comes from *you*.

If you remember nothing else about what you've read so far in this book, keep in mind the following three points. They are the Body Age Program in a nutshell.

1. Plan for and make
2. at least one small, concrete, realistic change each week
3. rooted by autogenic training in your deepest self.

It's now time for you to act on your prescription. Read your primary intervention first. Then your secondary intervention. Then your third. Then start your program. The rest is up to you.

CHAPTER 8
Values/Goals Clarification

PRIMARY INTERVENTION FOR: Loner
SECONDARY INTERVENTION FOR: Drifter, Speed Freak, Worry Wart

Core Message

This vital life skill boils down to a simple, four-step process:

1. Get in touch with your basic values.

2. Identify concrete ways in which you can express these values more frequently in your life: These are your "valued experiences," the things you really love to do.

3. Prioritize and plan. Prioritize your valued experiences, identify your opportunities to enjoy some of them more often, then plan for specific action to take advantage of at least one of these opportunities in the coming week.

4. Take concrete action by introducing valued experiences into your life (make small, specific, concrete changes that reflect your core values).

Values/Goals Clarification emphasizes the process, not the end result. Getting there is at least 95 percent of the fun—and delivers 100 percent of the benefits.

The ability to clarify and express one's values and goals turned out to be the most powerful single intervention for participants in the Body Age Study. Values/Goals Clarification proved the most powerful part of the prescription for the Loner stressotype, and was almost as important for the Drifter, the Speed Freak, and the Worry Wart.

This Vital Life Skill is a potent one. The world is full of people who don't seem to know what they want and who expend a lot of energy not getting it—or even worse, getting it. (George Bernard Shaw once said, "There are two tragedies in life. One is not to get your heart's desire. The other is to get it.") How often have you gotten what you thought you wanted (a new car, a new job) only to discover that you still weren't satisfied?

In a very real sense, clarifying your goals and values is fundamental to the Body Age Program as a whole; it is an important part of the "Rate Yourself" process for each of the five interventions. And this life skill gains potency in combination with other interventions, especially Effective Relaxation (an essential part of every Worry Wart and Speed Freak prescription) and Self-Affirming Communication (part of the basic prescription for Loners and Drifters).

The main benefits of Values/Goals Clarification are:

1. *It eliminates many unnecessary vitality drains.* If you spend your stress energy in valued ways that head you in a satisfying life direction, you'll experience less stress-energy drain and a dramatic increase in your stress-energy efficiency. This happens because you narrow the gap between your "real self" (who you are, what you value) and your "ideal self" (who and how you would like to be).

2. *It feels good to act on your core values.* Every time you consciously do something you really want to do (that is, something that expresses a core value), you affirm your self. This not only makes you feel good while you're doing it; it increases your self-esteem and self-confidence (the gap between the real and the ideal narrows).

3. *You find out "what's in it for you."* This intervention is the process that differentiates between those who have "bought into" their job, marriage, or other life situation, and those who have "sold out" to them. For many people, Values/Goals Clarification is the first time they get answers to questions like "Why bother?" and "What's in this for me?"

Many books and courses do a good job of teaching this Vital Life Skill. We have attempted to meld what the experts have to say with our own experience of teaching the skill to our Body Age subjects. In particular we emphasize process (getting there) rather than end result (specific goals). And we have added our powerful technique for *autogenically* rooting the change process, which greatly increases the potency of this and every intervention.

Herb, who entered the program at age 42 (body age 48, appearance age 49), is typical of the kind of progress possible. He was a Loner/ Drifter, a career military man who had risen rapidly to the rank of major. Faced with the possibility of retiring at age 45 on full pension, he'd decided to stay in the army since, "It's literally the only thing I know; I don't see any options."

Herb had never married and had no close friends, although lots of "buddies." Despite regular exercise, he had developed chronic back problems and complained of frequent fatigue. He occasionally went on drinking binges. His greatest pleasure was writing long letters to his brother's kids who lived thousands of miles away. These epistles often contained children's stories based on situations and children he'd observed in his world travels.

As Herb began to look more closely at his core values, he discovered that his priorities were to be creative with his imagination, to have a close family life, and to help children understand their possibilities. None of these values were finding much expression through the army, and he realized he wanted his writing for children to be more than "just a sideline." —

To test the waters, Herb rewrote several of the short stories he'd sent to his brother's kids and submitted them to a small children's magazine. One of them was published. This encouraged him to sign up for a creative writing course, which he loved. At his eighth-month checkup, Herb was still planning to stay in the army, at least until 45 (and full pension). But he felt as though he'd already been "released from my khaki period." His body age was down 10 years to 38, and he looked even younger (appearance age 36). If he was able to get more stories published, he planned to make writing his second career.

As it turned out, Herb resigned from the army two years later and now spends his time writing children's stories and free-lancing as a writer for kids' television shows.

RATE YOURSELF

What are your most fundamental needs and values? What specific goals would you like to achieve using this Vital Life Skill? In what concrete ways could you express these values and move toward the achievement of these goals? The tests and exercises in this section will help you answer these questions as you do the following:

1. Identify your core values and get in touch with your "real self."
2. Focus your image of your "ideal self" (who and how you would realistically like to be).
3. Assess your capabilities and resources (such as your learned skills and inherited resources).
4. Identify specific valued experiences that you can have more frequently and that will move you in an energizing, self-affirming direction.
5. Pinpoint your self-defeating techniques for avoiding positive change.
6. Develop affirmations and visualizations that will empower your determination to change.

Before we go any further, a few key definitions:

Core value: A core value is an aspect of life that is very important to you once such basic needs as food, shelter, and security are taken care of. It can be quite abstract (for example, "to be creative") or it might be relatively concrete (for example, "time with friends" or "being out in nature"). You might think of these fundamental values as the elements of your personal philosophy. They are things you "need" in order to "fulfill yourself" and be really contented.

Valued experience: This is a concrete way in which you express through a specific action one or more of your core values. For example, you might express your creativity by buying a set of oil paints and some canvas and painting a picture. Or, for you, creativity might mean cooking a gourmet meal. Or it might be as seemingly mundane as taking a different route to work in the morning. An experience that expresses the value "time with friends" could be any of the following: going to lunch with a friend, organizing a dinner party, or playing squash with an old chum.

A value is general and often abstract; a valued experience is specific, an action you know will enable you to express that value—and in so doing express a piece of your inner self.

Goal: A goal is a specific short- or long-term objective you set, based on your core values. It is something you want to have or achieve—anything from owning a fancy car to getting a promotion, taking an exotic vacation, or graduating from a carpentry course. Goals are useful distance markers along the path of Values/Goals Clarification. You can think of them as steps or plateaus you reach as you make your journey. Each time you achieve a goal, it's a sign you're more fully expressing the values that make you who you are. But goals are primarily important because they keep you focused and motivated to move in a valued, self-affirming direction. For example, the pleasure of being able to afford a fancy new car is of two kinds: the immediate gratification of getting what you aimed for, and the long-term reminder it provides that you can achieve the goals you set for yourself.

We live in a goal-oriented culture, and many people get goals and values confused. One of the most common confusions is over money and material wealth: Many people write these down on their list of "core values." In fact, making a big salary or having a lot of money to spend is a goal, not a value. And it only becomes a satisfying goal if you know what you really want to use your hard-earned cash for (that is, if making all this money is moving you in a generally satisfying direction). As important and useful as goals can be, values, not goals, are the nub of Values/Goals Clarification.

Given these three definitions, it may seem somewhat silly to talk about categories such as "career" or "family" or "leisure" when discussing values. A value is a value. Values underlie all areas of your existence and flow one into the other. In practice, however, we've discovered that many people have trouble when asked to "write down your deepest values." This is why the exercises in this chapter are divided into two seemingly arbitrary life domains: career and leisure. Our study subjects found these categories helpful in getting a handle on their core values and in identifying the kinds of experiences they valued most. Like them, however, you will undoubtedly discover that your core values are basic to both domains—in fact, to every area of your life.

Complete all four parts of this "Rate Yourself" section. They will give you a more balanced understanding of who you are and how you want to be. If you take the time to do the tests carefully, being as honest as you can, you should emerge with a clearer sense of your basic values as well as an increased awareness of how you miss opportunities to express these values more frequently. You will also be clearer about the specific goals that will have real meaning for you.

Before you plunge into the tests, one final word of preparation. Values/Goals Clarification can be very unsettling in its initial stages. As you begin to see more clearly just how wide the gap is between your real self (who you are now, what you truly value) and your image of your ideal self (who and how you would realistically like to be, based on those values), you will inevitably experience some discomfort. With this in mind, be as honest as you can as you take the tests. If you find yourself rushing through without much thought, slow yourself down.

A number of the exercises that follow were originally designed for use in a classroom setting. If you do them with your partner, they will be even more effective.

Clarify Your Leisure Values

Because leisure values are often neglected, this domain is a powerful place to start. Do the following tests and exercises with care. Take all the time you need.

What Am I Looking for in a Leisure Experience? Read the following list and check off the items most important to you. Add any other important needs or values that you are aware of.

It's Important to Me:

_____to do something meaningful
_____to be self-confident
_____to contribute to my community
_____to continue learning
_____to be physically active
_____to be creative or expressive
_____to explore new ideas or activities
_____to relax and take it easy
_____to do something completely different from work
_____to be entertained
_____to be able to do what I want
_____to be spontaneous
_____to be challenged
_____to do things with my family
_____to do things with close friends
_____to do things my own way
_____to have support from others
_____to feel committed to something
_____to compete with myself to do better
_____to develop more skills
_____to use and improve the skills I have
_____to have something to show for my efforts
_____to keep busy
_____to organize and get things going
_____to get recognition
_____to be a success at what I do
_____to learn more about myself
_____to develop friends
_____to meet a variety of new people
_____to help others
_____to laugh and enjoy
_____to be in attractive surroundings

Draw a line down the center of a sheet of paper. On the left side, list in order of priority the five most important needs or values for you. Leave lots of space between the five items. On the right side, write down beside each of these needs or values how it is currently being met by your leisure activities.

Things I Love to Do. On the left-hand side of the Things I Love To Do chart, list up to fifteen things you love to do. These should be things you actually do or have done, not new ones you'd like to start. Don't restrict yourself. Brainstorm and. let your ideas flow. If you're having trouble, try some general categories such as: indoor/outdoor; active/passive; alone/with others; different seasons, places, or spaces. There are no right or wrong answers. The things you choose need not necessarily be active. Your list might include items as diverse as working, skiing, writing stories, singing, sitting, being alone, or hugging your kids. Don't worry if you can't come up with fifteen things.

Using the symbols provided, code your list.

Finally, on a separate piece of paper, write down several sentences beginning with the phrase, "I learned that. . . ." These sentences reflect what you've learned about your leisure patterns and priorities in doing this and the previous exercise. These are some of your valued leisure experiences. What overall picture do you get as you review your list of choices? Do you see a pattern of choices emerging?

If you are doing these exercises with a partner, explore with him or her the overall pattern of choices and interests that you've discovered. Do you display a balance? What may be an underlying theme (themes) or message (messages)?

Barriers to Enjoyment. According to your personal experience, what are the major barriers preventing you from enjoying leisure? Using the scale provided, rate each of the following barriers as either a 1, 2, or 3.

This is rarely a barrier for me.	1
This is sometimes a barrier for me.	2
This is often/always a barrier for me.	3

_____Often I don't feel like doing anything.

_____I have too many family obligations.

_____Work is the main priority right now.

_____I don't think leisure is important.

_____I don't know what is meaningful for me.

_____I have a great deal of daily stress.

_____I have a bad habit of overcommitting myself.

_____There is not enough money to do what I want.

THINGS I LOVE TO DO

	PL	S	$	Me	Oth	Par	N5	Date
1.								
2.								
3.								
4.								
5.								
6.								
7.								
8.								
9.								
10.								
11.								
12.								
13.								
14.								
15.								

Here is what the symbols stand for.

PL	Requires planning
S	Spontaneous
$	Costs more than $3.00
Me	By yourself
Oth	With others
Par	Would have been on your parents' list?
N5	Would not have been on your list five years ago
Date	Last time you did it: (day, month, year)

————I am unemployed, and I don't think leisure is possible under these circumstances.

————I don't have the physical skills.

————I don't have the artistic or creative skills.

————I am embarrassed about learning something new.

————I don't have enough free time.

————I don't know what is available.

————Sometimes I find it difficult to get started. I procrastinate.

————There is no one to go with.

————Social situations are awkward for me.

————Programs and facilities are not available.

————Family and friends' expectations limit me.

————Making decisions about doing something is difficult.

————I have trouble following through on my intentions.

————I have no outside interests.

————I have little or no energy for leisure pursuits.

————Others [List these on a piece of paper]

If any item on which you scored 3 has repeatedly gotten in the way of a highly valued experience, then don't just hope it will go away. Plan to do something about it when you form your plan of action.

The Someday Game. Even though there is some doubt that we will have a chance to live our lives over again, we still manage to procrastinate and postpone. Your time is precious capital. Like money, it can be spent recklessly or invested wisely.

We've provided "The Someday Game," a form, on which to list your leisure procrastinations: the reasons you give yourself for not spending your leisure time well. In the left-hand column, list five pursuits that you would like to explore but are putting off until the "right" time or circumstance comes along. You may find it helpful to refer back to the first two exercises where you listed your leisure needs and values. Again, don't restrict your thinking. Your list could be as diverse as: slowing down; getting back to exercise; taking up pottery; joining an amateur theater group; reading the classics.

In the middle column, write down your reasons for postponing each desired activity. Sound familiar? How do your reasons for postponing coincide with your barriers to leisure listed in the previous exercise?

Now pick one or more of the valued experiences you are now postponing. In the right-hand column, write down briefly how you can move it up so that you can start acting on it in the next six months—or the next six days.

This is a good time to explore your leisure procrastinations with your

THE SOMEDAY GAME

Things Being Postponed	Reasons for Postponing	Moving Someday Up to Today
1.	1.	1.
2.	2.	2.
3.	3.	3.
4.	4.	4.
5.	5.	5.

partner. Do you impose artifical barriers on yourself? Just what are you avoiding? What are you waiting for?

Pulling It All Together. The following three-part exercise will give you an opportunity to draw conclusions and plan appropriate actions for a more satisfying leisure lifestyle. Take lots of time, and discuss each stage with your partner. In the training sessions, we gave our students a full hour to do this exercise.

Special forms are unnecessary for some of the exercises in this book. When no special forms are provided, we suggest that you write your responses on hole-punched paper and keep these sheets in the loose-leaf binder in which you will collect the pages of your Action Diary.

Reflect on the exercises you've done thus far. Then write down the most important conclusions, understandings, or decisions you have come to about your leisure lifestyle. These might be in any or all of the following categories:

- a value that is especially important to you
- a valued activity or experience that you want to pursue
- a different pace, rhythm, or way of operating
- keeping things more or less the way they are now.

As you write this list, start each entry with a phrase such as one of the following: "I conclude that . . . ," "I understand that . . . ," "I have decided that. . . ."

Once you've pondered and revised this list, determine your three most important goals with respect to your leisure lifestyle. You can think of these as beacons that will help keep you traveling in the direction most in harmony with your core values. Write down your three primary goals.

For each of your three primary intentions, list any specific actions you are willing to take in the next month to move in this valued direction. For example, if one of your primary intentions is to get closer to nature, you might list items like the following: plan a weekend excursion to a park or nature reserve; visit a bookstore that specializes in outdoor books and purchase a field guide; find out about your local naturalist club and attend a meeting; subscribe to a nature magazine.

The simple act of making this kind of list provides you with a repertoire of behavior changes that can form the basis of your Body Age Program.

Clarify Your Career Values

You've probably pondered your career more than once in the past few years, or months. The following tests will help you do this in a way that focuses on your core career values. What is most important to you in the world of work? And what things do you love to do when working? Do the exercises in the order in which they are presented. Don't rush. If you have a partner, discuss each test and what it means.

Career Values Achievement Form. Just how clear are you about what you like and don't like in your working life? In the best of all possible worlds, what values would your career provide you with opportunities to express? Make a Career Values Achievement Form. Look at the example—a form completed by a private-practice psychologist—for the basic format and to get an idea of how to proceed.

CAREER VALUES ACHIEVEMENT FORM

Your Needs and Values: What Are You Looking for in Your Career?

A. Core Values In my career, it's important to me to (be / feel / try to) . . .	B. Valued Experiences In my career, this need or value is now being met by / in . . .	C. Opportunities In my career, I could get more satisfaction by . . .
to help people in real need to solve their problem	• I mostly see patients with real pressing problems	• do one day per week as Consultant at hospitals
to see results of my work	• being little met beyond my reading	• ditto, plus maybe teach an occasional seminar
to have variety in the kinds of problems I deal with	• get sick of this	• become hospital Consultant
to continue to grow intellectually	• only occasionally at Conferences	• a little more satisfaction is possible at hospital
to feel in charge of my hours	• OK	• till my patients will follow-up three month after they leave
to be recognized for what I do ✓	• seeing patients leave in (apparently) better condition	• I'm going to start at 7:00 and finish by 3:00 on Monday - Friday patients want earlier, before work hours
to be with people on an informal give and take basis	• little met; I've kept the same hours for years	

Begin with column A, "It's important to me to. . . ." For each entry you make in column A, make a corresponding entry in columns B and C. This process is one of clarifying your core career values, identifying specific experiences that allow you to express this value in your work, and noting the opportunities for introducing the valued experience more frequently into your working life.

When you have completed your Career Values Achievement Form, take a few minutes to discuss your discoveries with your partner.

Barriers to Accomplishment. This test helps you identify the artifical barriers and self-defeating behaviors you use as excuses for not expressing your values more frequently at work. Once you've done this, you can begin to design solutions. Before you begin, look at the filled-out chart for the basic format to follow and to get a better idea of how this exercise works.

Column 1 (Barriers to Accomplishment): List the five most important obstacles to the achievement of your core career values. (For example, many people write as their number one barrier "Not enough time.") Discuss the specifics of these barriers with your partner. This will help you clarify what you write in column 2.

Column 2 (Reasons): List the reasons that correspond to each of your five major barriers or obstacles. Why don't you have enough time? Are you disorganized? Poor at delegating? Overextended? Busy with a young baby? Fielding too many demands? Why does the company structure prevent you from working independently? Why doesn't your boss allow you to work more independently?

Column 3 (Needed Resources to Solve): Take it as a given that no obstacle is insurmountable. What resources would you need to climb over each of the five barriers you listed in column 1? These can include time, people, money, support services, or other resources.

Pinpoint Your Time Wasters. For most people, the biggest barrier to accomplishing what they really value is time ("I just don't have enough." "I'm being pulled in twenty directions at once.") This quiz helps you pinpoint your favorite ways of wasting time, and to see more clearly all the time you spend on activities you don't value. As we'll discuss in the "Basic Training" section of this chapter, effective time management is an example of Values/Goals Clarification in action.

Rate each of the following possible time wasters, as they apply to your work situation, as L (large), M (medium), S (small), or No (it's not a time waster).

BARRIERS TO ACCOMPLISHMENT

1. Barriers to Accomplishment	2. Reasons	3. Needed Resources to Solve
Not enough time spent with Colleagues... and students	Really - there are few "good reasons" for this - mostly I just wasn't clearly aware of what I value most	Contact local hospital Chief of psychology
Colleagues not aware of new directions in my work and of results I'm achieving		Make a six-month plan for freeing up one day/week for hospital
I'm in a rut - daily habit		Begin plan by changing my monday + thursday hours - small but real progress! Most basically: A couple of decisions and a plan to "Get more satisfaction"

_____Lack of delegation
_____Procrastination
_____Lack of planning, scheduling, organization
_____Trouble getting started in mornings
_____Idle time, talk, daydreaming
_____Sorting and dispensing with mail
_____Searching for files, information
_____Reading magazines, junk mail
_____Shuffling papers
_____Proofreading and signing letters
_____Frequent checking on co-workers or employees
_____Spending time on nonpriority items
_____Interoffice travel
_____Too long on telephone
_____Rewriting memos and letters
_____Lack of written goals
_____Inability to say no
_____Attending unnecessary meetings
_____Poor control of meetings
_____Relying on mental notes
_____Delaying distasteful tasks
_____No "quiet hour"
_____Not using prime time for priority work
_____Not utilizing waiting time and travel time
_____Filing too much, throwing out too little
_____Self-interruptions
_____Indecision
_____Not utilizing forms
_____Utilizing forms
_____Allowing constant interruptions by others
_____Writing instead of phoning
_____Inefficient office or workspace layout
_____Insisting on knowing all and seeing all
_____Not having facts or telephone numbers at hand
_____Unclear communications
_____Not taking advantage of time-saving gadgets
_____Too much attention to detail; perfectionism
_____No daily plan
_____No self-imposed deadlines
_____Leaving tasks unfinished and starting new ones
_____Doing other people's work
_____Co-workers not effectively trained
_____Firefighting: constantly reacting to minor crises
_____Preoccupation with problems

_____No follow-up system
_____Not actively listening
_____Worry, lack of confidence
_____Lack of clear procedures
_____Poor writing skills
_____Absentmindedness
_____Others [List these on a separate piece of paper]

Pulling It All Together. The following three-part exercise will give you an opportunity to draw conclusions and plan appropriate behavior changes for your career life. You can do it alone, but if possible do it with a partner so you can discuss what you discover. Invite your partner to play devil's advocate—first to challenge you and then to make positive suggestions.

> Reflect on the exercises you've done thus far. Then write down the most important conclusions, understandings, discoveries, or decisions you have come to about your career life. These might be any of the following: an activity or experience you want to pursue; a different pace, rhythm, or way of operating; keeping things more or less the same as they are now because you are more satisfied with your life than you realized. Whatever they may be, make a list of your conclusions, understandings, or decisions. You might begin each point with a phrase such as "I conclude that . . . ," "I understand that. . . ," or "I have decided that. . . ."
>
> Contemplate this list and decide which are the three most important goals that you have with respect to your career life. Write them down. Your list might look like this:

> > My goals are:
> > To spend more time working as part of a team
> > To find more outlets for my creativity
> > To make more money

> For each of these goals, list any specific action you could do in the next month to move in that direction. For example, if one of your primary intentions is to take on more responsibility at work, you might list the following: make an appointment to talk to my boss about additional responsibility; check out night-school courses that could enhance my suitability for a more satisfying job (not always one that pays more); sign up for one of these courses; make an appointment to visit a career counselor to find out what sorts of jobs are available for people with my skill level.

The simple act of making this list helps you form a possible plan of action that can become the basis of your four-week start-up program. Discuss the list with your partner. (Note that you can use this basic format, which we've applied to both career and leisure, to clarify other areas of your life such as family and friends.)

Clarify Your Core Values

You have probably become aware by now of imbalances between your working life and your leisure time. The exercise that follows will help you deepen this awareness and give you an even clearer sense of your ideal self—the way you want to live in a whole and balanced way. The clearer and more realistic this image becomes, the more energy you will have to move in a satisfying life direction.

Your Personal Coat of Arms. We have provided you with a shield divided into six segments of roughly equal size. This will become your personal coat of arms—an emblem of what you stand for, what you most value in your working and leisure life. Take your three most important core values for leisure and your three most important core values for career and portray them in the six segments. Perhaps some of them overlap? How does your career complement your leisure?

In each segment, write a word or a short phrase or draw a picture that epitomizes one essential value. If the support of your co-workers is important for you, you might draw a group of people or write the word "harmony" or the word "support." If you value having control over your time, you might draw a clock, or write the phrase "Time is mine." If being physically active is an important aspect of leisure, you could draw an image that suggests your favorite sport or simply write the word "sweat." If you particularly appreciate a clear work structure, you might draw a latticework, or you could write the word "structure." If one of your core leisure values is getting close to nature, you might draw a tree or a bird, or write the word "nature."

Finally, if you want to, give your coat of arms a motto that summarizes the values you've portrayed or that somehow expresses the key value that underlies all the others. Your motto might be a word like "Creativity" or a phrase such as "Self-Affirming Self-Expression."

You are painting a picture of your best self: the person you want to be and know you can be. The values that are most important to you will appear in the top segments. Less important values will appear near the bottom. In which domain—career or leisure—will your most important values most easily find expression? This domain is the place to begin your start-up program.

A SAMPLE COAT OF ARMS

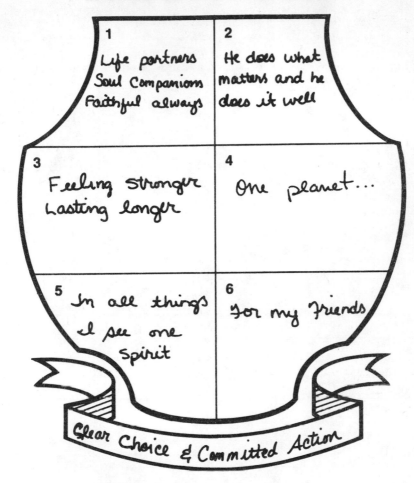

This coat of arms was developed by a Drifter bank manager (age 42, body age 48). The areas on the shield reflect his values as follows:

1. *Family.* He recognized that his wife and children were the most constant sources of value in his life.
2. *Career.* Since he wanted "to be remembered for something," he wrote this one down in the form of an epitaph.
3. *Health.* A line from a favorite popular song.
4. *Recreation.* He had always had a fondness for nature, which he had seldom expressed. (By the end of the program, he'd become very active in an international ecology group.)
5. *Spirituality.* Although not a "practicing religious person," he was strongly interested in clarifying what he believed in.
6. *Friends.* Like so many Drifters, the Body Age Program led him to be aware that "friends are made not once, but continuously through the things I can find to do for them."

When he finished the program, his body age was down 10 years to 38.

MY PERSONAL COAT OF ARMS

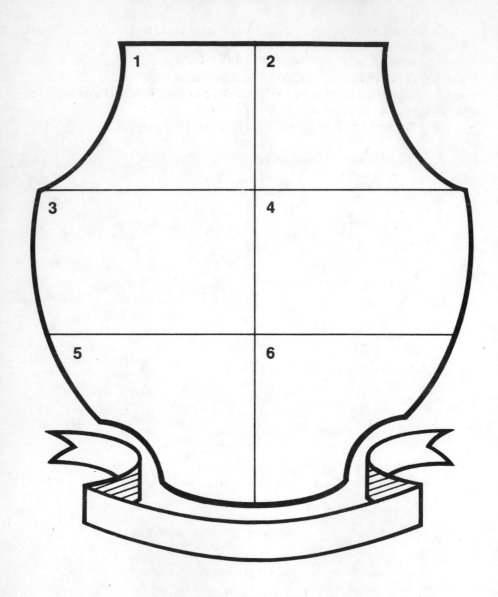

Develop Your Affirmations and Visualizations

As a result of the thorough self-assessment process you've just completed, you've identified some important underlying values that you want to express more fully at work and through leisure. And you have noted some specific valued experiences that are priorities for you. You are now ready to develop the powerful affirmations and visualizations that capture and express these core values.

Here are some typical value-specific work affirmations:

I work to please myself, not others.
I use my time efficiently.
I give and get support from my co-workers.
I discover or give myself satisfaction in my work.
I balance curiosity and results at work.
I seek out the "people" rewards at work.
I challenge my work, and it challenges me.

Here are some possible work visualizations:

A desk with neat stacks of folders indicating levels of priority
A well-ordered briefcase
A friendly lunch with co-workers
Yourself in charge at a meeting
Yourself, cool and articulate on the phone
Yourself being congratulated by a colleague for a job well done.

Here are some typical leisure affirmations:

I use my leisure time to practice relaxation techniques.
I value, above all, the leisure time I spend with my family.
I give myself time for recreation.
I spend time expressing my creative side.
I have a strong affinity for the world of nature.

Here are some possible leisure visualizations:

Walking in the woods on a lovely day with the birds singing
Gathered with friends in an enjoyable social setting
Serving a dinner you've cooked to an appreciative gathering
Admiring a picture you've just painted.

One company vice-president discovered opportunities to use visualization to express his "flair for drama" in leading his troops. He would not only plan his key lines but also conjure up mental images of the costume appropriate for the meeting (for example, Viking warrior, quizzical professor, laid-back salesman). Initially, he felt silly and dishonest doing this mental rehearsal. Then he realized how powerful these visualizations were in improving his performance.

BASIC TRAINING

Mary was an attractive and successful television talk-show host, age 41 (body age 51, appearance age 45). She seemed to have it all—a glamorous job, a big salary, famous and fascinating friends. However, during the course of her entry interview for the Body Age Program, she revealed that her life was in fact a kind of solitary confinement. (Subsequent testing confirmed that her dominant stressotype was Loner.) She was perfectly coiffed. Her movements were stilted, almost calculated, leaving the impression that the interview was the rerun of an earlier ''live'' performance.

Her working day followed a strict, unvarying routine. She arrived at the television studio at 5 A.M. to prepare for a 7 A.M. airtime. After the show ended at 9, she would review the roster of guests and topics for the following day, go home and read the daily newspapers, then sleep until 2 in the afternoon. After that, it was back to the office, where she worked until early evening, digesting the research for the next day. She was home by 8 P.M. and in bed by 9:30 or 10. Her weekends were spent reading books and magazines related to work. She felt she had no time for ''casual'' socializing and got no regular exercise. Worse, for the past fifteen years, as she steadily climbed the ladder of media success, she had made no intimate friends and maintained no long-term relationships. Her life was virtually one dimensional: work.

At the time she entered the program, Mary had been thinking very seriously about leaving the television station, not for a bigger job with a network show (something she had been offered) but for something ''less demanding.'' But since her job was the only area of her life in which she felt successful, she was afraid to leave. She felt that even a relatively small ''90-degree change'' would spring her loose from this prison. She wasn't clear why she wanted the change or what the change would be like, but the feeling kept growing.

The Four-Step Process of Values/Goals Clarification

Mary was badly in need of some self-examination and redirection. Here are the four steps we led her through.

Step 1: Get in Touch with Your Core Values. During the training sessions, Mary took stock of her job skills and experiences as a highly skilled television journalist. Then she made the following list that reflected her core career values:

Conversation with interesting and accomplished people

Discovering new things and new perspectives

Helping others through deepening their understanding of the world

Being in the limelight, but equal pleasure in creating and orchestrating "behind the scenes"

Making a contribution "to the world" on specific, important issues

Traveling to new places, experiencing new environments

Being a "big sister" to younger women working their way up through the media jungle

Flexibility in setting hours

During the training, Mary's entire focus was on her career, which made up her whole life. Any change would have to start here.

This first step is sometimes referred to as getting in touch with your current "real self," seeing yourself more clearly as you are, now. First, you must confront your weaknesses as well as your strengths, honestly assessing both your capabilities (including what you were born with and the skills and experiences you've picked up along the way) and identifying your deepest values. Of these two components of your real self, your values are by far the more important. Given your capabilities, any number of directions are possible (including continuing along your present path, but with a renewed sense of purpose). How much satisfaction you'll find in the direction you choose depends on the degree to which it reflects what is most important to you.

Step 2: Identify Concrete Ways You Can Express These Values More Frequently in Your Life (Identify Your Valued Experiences). Having identified her most important work values, Mary then took step 2. She used them to paint a mental portrait of her "more inner self"—her term for her ideal self. She then had the courage to ask herself the risky question "What would this person look like in real life, acknowledging that she has the skills and experience I have as resources?" The picture she painted was not of a radically different career, but of the same basic job with important differences—experiences that would allow her to express the values she had identified as being important.

Here are some of the significant brush strokes in Mary's ideal self-portrait: wearing blue jeans and a sweat shirt (instead of an impeccably tailored suit); occasionally phoning the office to say she had decided to work at home; teaching a graduate-school course to a small group of radio and television arts students; lounging in her apartment in deep discussion with several of the world's best minds; encouraging her producer to try some risky experiments with their program format; "simply having the time to feel content with what I've built in my career."

As Mary contemplated this picture, the keys seemed to be "less of a time burden" and "more contact with other people." So she set out to move toward these goals.

As you get clearer about the concrete experiences you really value (and want more of) and as your ideal self comes more and more into realistic focus, the stressful gap between your real self and your ideal self automatically begins to narrow. When a tyrannically elevated ideal comes down a notch or two, or an "embarrassed slob" comes up a few notches in his own esteem, the gap gets smaller, uncertainty is reduced, and stress levels go down. After months or years of stalemate, action suddenly seems possible.

Now you can begin to set goals. Goals are useful signposts along your self-affirming path; they are not ends in themselves. It is primarily the process of moving in a valued direction that brings satisfaction and increases self-esteem.

Step 3: Prioritize and Plan. Mary now had to decide which of these valued experiences to work on first, and which specific goals to aim for. The goals and experiences she gave priority to were: persuading her bosses to hire an understudy who could eventually take over aspects of her job she wanted to downplay, and who could at the same time be someone to whom she could be a "big sister," passing on her knowledge and skills; getting approval to begin making documentaries and traveling to other parts of the world on assignment; and doing more stories about worthy organizations that are often neglected in gloom-and-doom news coverage.

The priorites you developed in the "Rate Yourself" section are specific experiences you want to enjoy more often (or for the first time). These are the basis for forming a plan of action. There are literally hundreds of opportunities each week for you to introduce a new valued experience. Plan to capitalize each week on just one or two of them and you will have completed step 3.

Step 4: Take Concrete Action. Now that Mary had a clearer idea of the direction in which she wanted to move, she was ready to take meaningful (valued) action. She set up a meeting with her boss to discuss hiring an assistant. He agreed. Her choice was a recent graduate from journalism school, someone who'd admired Mary's work for years. At first the "understudy" did occasional interviews on the show, then a regular lifestyle spot. By the end of the year, she became junior cohost, giving Mary much more time to devote to doing more of her own research, and more "up close and personal," in-depth interviews. Mary also had more time to search out stories about people and organizations who were making a difference, and had the clout to showcase these on the air.

In her next contract, she negotiated six yearly specials that would allow her to travel to "exotic and innovative" settings to do more in-depth treatments of more diverse subjects "behind the news." This exploration of new territory led to her becoming a founding member of an important international think tank on world issues, which led to the first close friendships of her adult life.

At Mary's eight-month checkup, her body age was down to 40, and her appearance age was 37.

The sum total of these four steps is a narrowing of the gap between the ideal and the real, and a growing sense of freedom. Of course, the gap between the real and the ideal will never disappear—and if it did, life would be rather boring, with nothing to strive for. But the narrower the gap, the less it is a crippling obstacle to change and the more your ideal self becomes a motivator of further action. To paraphrase Dr. Selye, it motivates you to strive for your highest attainable aim.

Mary continued to act on her core values after she graduated from the program. Soon the job she had wanted to abandon had evolved in new and satisfying ways. Mary helped create a successful new format that gave her cohost even more exposure. When the next job offer from the network came along, Mary turned it down because she was "having too good a time" right where she was.

But Mary never did directly address the leisure deficit in her life—during the training sessions, she never could make much of the leisure values tests—in truth, she didn't put that much value on leisure. She continued to live an existence that was mostly work and little play (a long weekend in New York twice a year was one of her few leisure pleasures). But instead of becoming an increasing drag, her work had turned into her pleasure (and a source of rewarding relationships). This change was accompanied by renewed vitality and a sharply enhanced sense of self-worth. Today Mary is less of a Loner, but despite the strong progress she has made, she will probably always be a somewhat solitary figure.

There is an important lesson here: Perfectionism—or always striving for the perfectly balanced life—is in itself very stressful. The key is to acknowledge and accept, as Mary did, that you may not be "everyone's ideal of a well-rounded person," but that, for you, your life works well.

The Process Is the Reward

Mary had learned that the process of getting there is the real reward of Values/Goals Clarification. This concept had a powerful impact on many other participants in the Body Age Study. A successful entrepreneur who had founded a real estate company with offices across the country commented that this idea helped him feel "finally free." It had enabled him to realize that, no matter how big his annual sales volume became, he would "never have made it" or "arrived." He now saw that success was an endless process, not a destination—that it was the ongoing daily expression, acceptance, and appreciation of his self. Each time he achieved a goal, he felt good—his self-esteem went up—but he derived much more satisfaction from his awareness that he was on the right path, one that he had chosen.

Many of our study subjects felt liberated by this radical shift away from the achievement of specific goals or results to an emphasis on life process. In our training sessions, we told them to invest 95 percent of their stress energy in valued experiences—things they perceived as heading them in the right direction—and only 5 percent into immediate or long-term measurable goals. Getting there is 95 percent of the fun and 100 percent of the reward.

This emphasis on process over end result is quite different from traditional types of goal selection, for example, the old-fashioned career aptitude test that reveals you should be a wildlife biologist or an accountant. Like the Zen archer, you are not so much aiming at a target as becoming at one with the process of drawing the bow and releasing the arrow. You *are* the flight of the arrow. And when the process is honored in this fashion, the arrow almost inevitably hits the bull's-eye.

Investing Your Time Capital

Time management was one of the original ten interventions we tested in the Body Age Study. But the experience of our study subjects made clear that how you spend your time says more than anything else about your self-concept (your values and how much you value yourself). In other words, choosing to use your time in valued ways is the essence of time management. And the reason we included it as a technique is that how efficiently (self-servingly) we use our time is a litmus test of how efficiently we use our even more basic resources, for example, our stress energy.

If you prioritize your life on the basis of the experiences you value most, all those excuses for getting things done, or changing the way you do things, will simply evaporate. Nonetheless, many of our study participants found specific time-management skills useful in overcoming the most common barrier to change: "I just don't have enough time."

You'll find a number of the best books on time management listed in "Further Reading" at the back of this book. But most of the suggestions these books contain can be boiled down to the following three basic principles (closely related to the four-step process described in this chapter).

> Set clear priorities based on clearly defined values. (Based on your short- and long-term goals, what is the best use of your time?
> Form a plan of action.
> Be flexible and creative in solving time problems.

Here is a list of tips for mastering this essential life skill.

Prioritize

1. Identify some long and short-range goals to help in identifying your top-priority work or leisure activities (you have already done this in the "Rate Yourself" section).

2. Keep an activity diary for a few days to help you find out where your time is going now. Take a good look at how well your time usage jibes with your overall goals.

3. Make a reasonable list of what you'd like to accomplish at work and at leisure. Then go back and rate the activities you've listed according to their importance. Try the A B C system: A for high-priority activities, B for medium-important activities, and C for lowest priority activities. Follow the 80/20 rule: Spend 80 percent of your time on the A activities and only 20 percent on B and C activities.

4. During the course of the day, frequently stop and ask yourself: "What is the most valuable use of my time right now?"

5. Do your most demanding work during your hours of peak energy and alertness. But don't relegate leisure to the low-energy back burner. For example, it's best to exercise when you have some pep, not at your lowest energy ebb.

6. Identify activities that you'd like to delegate, and discuss them with family members and co-workers. Whenever possible, make specific agreements with people about dividing up tasks.

7. Focus your attention on one activity at a time.

8. Learn to say no (or to negotiate a satisfactory middle ground between yes and no), including no to leisure activities that don't really reflect your interests. Because your time is valuable, be choosy about where you spend it. This may be the most important time-management skill of all.

Plan

1. Plan your day and your week. Make specific contracts with yourself to use your time more efficiently, for example, to tackle priority activities first or to take shortcuts.

2. When you have a busy day ahead, get up a little early and spend a few minutes organizing your time. Better yet, do it before 9 P.M. the night before. You will sleep better if tomorrow is laid out on a piece of paper, not nagging away in the back of your head.

Be Flexible and Creative

1. Use waiting time productively and creatively: to do relaxation exercises, to read, to do stretching or strengthening exercises, or to complete some other work. Or treat it as flexible leisure time, an opportunity to do something valuable.

2. Do things in quantity; for instance, make several batches of a dish and freeze the extras for future meals.

3. Compartmentalize your work. If telephone interruptions are a problem, you might make and return calls at a designated time or times during the day.

4. Try adjusting your schedule if you see a way to use time more efficiently or in ways that suit you better. If possible, change your schedule to avoid rush-hour traffic. Occasionally give yourself a "sabbatical" day at work, on which, to the extent possible, you deliberately do things in a different sequence than is your habit.

5. Continually look for shortcuts and time-savers. For example, you might be able to find a shorter route to work or to organize a car pool for driving your kids to school. Consider purchasing time-saving devices, anything from a tape recorder for making notes while away from your office to a slow cooker, microwave, or bigger freezer.

When doing all of the above, appreciate your accomplishments. A sense of self-appreciation is a good way of increasing your productivity at work and your satisfaction with leisure. For example, as you leave the office in the evening, replay the day's accomplishments with a colleague, or review your To Do list and take pleasure in the items you can check off. After a leisure outing, make a point of telling a friend what a great time you had and offer to include him or her next time.

Time isn't money, but it is precious capital to be invested wisely. The clearer you become about what you value, and the concrete ways in which you can express these values more frequently, the more time management will become second nature.

The Domains of Leisure and Career

There are many ways of subdividing your life into different spheres of activity, but for the participants in the Body Age Study we chose the categories of career and leisure. Our experience suggests that these work well in helping you to organize your priorities and plan for fruitful action.

The career domain requires little further comment beyond the obvious fact that many people mistakenly assume that their work provides them with few opportunities to express their deepest values. Leisure is another story. Many people give short shrift to their leisure time. They define it in negative terms—as the absence of work—instead of as something positive, active, and restorative.

Rewarding leisure activities can be summarized by the word "re-creation," or creative leisure: the positive, active, self-affirming, self-restoring use of your free time. It means filling this time with valued experiences. Doing nothing—really relaxing—can be extremely "re-creative" and should be a component of everyone's leisure. In fact, actively choosing to "rot" occasionally in front of the television set is great, especially if you resist guilty urges to "do something productive" while you're glued to the tube. (Many Speed Freaks and Worry Warts can't tolerate unplanned or unscheduled time, and schedule activities that don't really give them much satisfaction just so they can be doing "something." Practicing relaxation techniques is a very good way for them to schedule leisure time productively.) Truly restorative leisure is usually either physically or mentally active, or both. But it will re-create the self only if it speaks to some of your deeper needs and underlying values. In sum, successful leisure means re-creation of the self through self-affirming (valued) behaviors.

Many of our study participants were deeply dissatisfied with the way they spent their leisure time. One woman in the program reported that one day, as she was watching a sitcom rerun for the fifth time, she suddenly became aware of what "killing time" really meant. A male program participant reported that he felt so trapped by his weekly bridge night that, on several occasions, he had an almost irresistible urge to jump up in the middle of a hand and scream. He didn't, however, consoling himself with the thought that "maybe next week" he would skip bridge and find something better to do. (He hadn't found anything better in twenty years.)

Dissatisfaction with leisure time is often much closer to the surface than a person's disappointment with his or her work. Since most of us must work to earn a living, we tend to take for granted an imperfect job and its dissatisfactions. But our leisure time should by definition be fun and rewarding, even if our work is not. We expect a lot out of leisure and are very disappointed when it doesn't deliver, usually because we approach leisure passively instead of actively.

Taking a hard look at leisure proved a very powerful experience for many of our study participants. One company president remarked at the end of a training session that this had been "the second most impactful experience" of his life. (The first had been his conversion to "born again" Christianity.) A partner in a management consultant firm who had always thought that his recurring fantasy of taking up hot-air ballooning was only that—a fantasy—suddenly realized that it was "only a matter of choice and action." (Shortly thereafter, he joined a ballooning club.) And a university professor, who felt trapped in the expected academic role (faculty-club outings to the opera and playing the role of a cultivated Renaissance man), finally indulged his secret, lifelong passion for country and western music. Previously he'd been embarrassed to buy country records or go to country concerts. Now he not only openly catered to his repressed interest, he actually "liberated" several of his colleagues with similar "deviant preferences."

Work and leisure are most satisfying and energizing when they are in balance. Of course, the right balance is different for different people (Mary, for instance, found some of the rewards of leisure in the context of work.) The key to balance, however, is active, self-affirming leisure rather than empty time that is little more than the absence of work. For many participants in the Body Age Program, turning leisure time into re-creation seemed to cause other parts of their lives to fall into place—they enjoyed their work more and found they had more energy for their families.

In sum, aiming for a healthy balance between work and "re-creative" leisure will make this Vital Life Skill even more effective. You'll become more productive, and your life will be considerably more fun.

YOUR FOUR-WEEK START-UP PROGRAM

Week 1: Get Ready. Refine your priority list of specific valued experiences that you want to introduce into your life. Plan for concrete action in week 2.

Week 2: Take Your First Step. Begin implementing your plan by choosing one recurring opportunity to turn a core value into a valued experience—and doing it. If you are working on the career domain, this might be something that happens every working day. If you are working on leisure, it may mean making room for just one prescheduled leisure activity this week.

Week 3: Build on Your Success. This week you can either continue doing what you did last week (but do it better) or take advantage of a second recurring opportunity to act on your core values.

Week 4: Consolidate Your Gains. The change that began in week 2 as a novelty is becoming a habit.

Your four-week start-up program for Values/Goals Clarification is divided into two parts: leisure and career. It's up to you which one you start with and whether you work on one or both domains. The key is to get started. If you follow the program, over the next four weeks you will experience a significant change in the way you behave and how you feel about yourself.

The following program for action is only a guide. Some of you may wish to move more quickly, some may want to take more time (you're sure you're not just procrastinating?). Adopt the approach that is right for you. But if you find you want to speed up, make certain it is because you are ready to move and are not just impatient with the process (Speed Freaks, take note).

LEISURE ACTION

Follow this format if leisure is the life domain you wish to tackle first. If you feel ready, you can turn your attention to career action at the end of week 4. If you want to start with career, turn to page 173.

Week 1: Get Ready

The purpose of week 1 is to deepen your awareness of what you really want out of your leisure time (including simply more of it) and to refine your priority values and valued experiences. In essence, this week you'll be repeating the first three steps of the four-step Values/Goals Clarification process: identifying your core values; identifying your most valued experiences; and prioritizing and planning for action.

Fill out your Action Diary Planning Page. Agree to do the following things in the coming week:

1. *Begin with autogenic relaxation plus affirmations and visualizations.* Before you do anything else this week, find a quiet time to listen to your autogenic tape and introduce your leisure affirmations. Follow this with a leisure visualization: See yourself in a satisfying and fulfilling leisure situation. Use your affirmations daily, ideally at least three times each day.

2. *Dream about the great times.* While you are still in a relaxed and receptive state, do the following exercise. It is a kind of guided visualization that will help you deepen your awareness of your leisure needs and values.

> Read each of the following questions. Think about your dreams by closing your eyes for a few moments and visualizing. Take as much time as you want. Let your thoughts flow.
>
> If you won $ _____ in a lottery, would your lifestyle change? If so, how? (Fill in your own dollar amount.) List the main elements of your new lifestyle on a piece of paper.
>
> Project yourself into the future, immediate or long-term. Imagine two days (forty-eight hours) that would be ideal for you. Fantasize whatever you want—skill, money, location, and resources are not a problem. Write on a piece of paper about your two perfect days—use point form or, if you like, write a short story. Talk about where you would be, what you would be doing, and with whom. Would this experience be something isolated or part of your ideal ongoing lifestyle? Go into as much detail as you can, including sights, sounds, and specific events. Have fun as you imagine this ideal forty-eight hours of perfect re-creation.

This exercise will be especially effective if you discuss what you've written with your partner.

3. *Refine and prioritize your list of leisure values.* Looking back over what you've written, jot down a list of the key values expressed in the scenes and situations you've just described. The more fundamental the value, the more important. For example, if you described forty-eight hours at a resort in the tropics, an underlying value might be the company of good friends or being close to nature. A warm climate, on the other hand, wouldn't qualify. (Note the difference here between valued internal experiences that make you feel better about yourself and external conditions, such as weather, that are not subject to your short-term control.) Check back over the leisure exercises in the "Rate Yourself" section to see if your new list lacks any essentials. Add them.

When you've made your list, reduce it to no more than eight items. You may find that you can combine some things that overlap. Go down the list and beside each item write either A (essential) or B (merely important). The A items are your priority leisure values. These form the key to your directional self. Each time you perform an activity that expresses one or more of these values, you are following the compass heading toward your realistically realizable ideal self.

4. *Keep a leisure diary.* Keep a daily diary in which you note both basic categories of leisure activities—flexible time, or "flex time," and scheduled activities, such as a game of squash with a friend or a trip to the zoo with your kids.

Many people find it much easier to plan a two-week vacation or an overnight excursion than to deal with flexible time. "Flex" time is unpredictable. It occurs every day, such as when you arrive early for an appointment or your guest arrives late. It comprises all that unscheduled time, especially when you're at home "relaxing," when many people feel "at loose ends," faced with time "to kill." (Speed Freaks generally fill their flex time with any activity, however pointless, that keeps them busy. Either that, or they start to boil with impatience. A first step for them is often to do a relaxation technique instead of stewing or keeping themselves busy just for the sake of movement.)

The key to planning for flex time is to have a repertoire of self-contained experiences you can draw on when empty minutes catch you unawares, and to make sure that any materials you need for these experiences are readily available, whether they are a book, a tape recorder, or wool and some knitting needles. Relaxation techniques are an especially satisfying way to spend some of your flex time, and most require no equipment or planning beyond the simple realization that they are available to you. (You can even use some of your flex time to keep your diary up to date!)

Beside each diary entry indicate whether the activity was satisfying or not, whether it reflected one of your essential leisure values (the A's on your list).

At the end of the week, make a rough estimate of how many hours of leisure time you spent—that means time when you were neither working nor attending to other responsibilities. How much of it was flex time? How much of it was prescheduled? What aspects were most satisfying? Is there a reasonable balance in your life between work and play? There is no ideal ratio of flex time to prescheduled leisure, but increasing your prescheduled, re-creative leisure is a more important basis for rewarding leisure action. Flex time is at least partly a product of the kind of life you lead, and it may diminish somewhat as you learn to invest your total time capital in more valued ways.

You now have a much better idea of the valued ways you already use your leisure and of your many opportunities every day for getting more true re-creation.

5. *Prioritize and plan for action.* Prioritize your list of valued leisure experiences, and set your objective for the next three weeks. Plan the concrete actions you will take in week 2.

6. *Check in with your partner.* Make an appointment to call or be called. Discuss any problems and get the support you need to continue the process.

7. *Record your progress in the Action Diary.* Each day, note the leisure experiences that express your underlying values. Identify the obstacles you place in the path of satisfying leisure and the opportunities you missed because you were poorly organized, too busy, or had your priorities skewed.

Week 2: Take Your First Step

Fill out your Action Diary Planning Page. Agree to do the following in the coming week:

1. *Continue autogenic relaxation with affirmations and visualizations.* Continue the affirmations you've been using, or modify them to reflect your deepening awareness of your core values. This is the mental training that will make action easier and more satisfying. Use your affirmations at least once daily, ideally three or more times each day.

2. *Either introduce new flexible time behaviors . . .* Every morning (or the evening before), plan one or two self-contained activities you can use during your flex time each day. If your flex time happens when you're away from home, be sure to carry with you whatever equipment you might need. In the evening, take stock of how you've done, and note opportunities you've missed.

For nearly twenty years before entering the program, one Loner had enjoyed composing short, humorous songs and limericks while driving to work. In week 2, he began taking his tape recorder in the car so that he could record new inspirations, as well as hundreds of half-forgotten old favorites, for his colleagues at work.

A psychiatrist Speed Freak who was often called as an expert witness in court cases typically had to wait several hours before testifying. In week 2, he tried filling this flex time by tying new salmon-fishing flies (a recently rediscovered passion).

3. *. . . Or plan for prescheduled leisure.* At the beginning of this week, plan at least one rewarding leisure activity that requires a fair chunk of your time (at least an hour or two) and that has to be scheduled in advance. If you come up blank, consult the exercise ''The Someday Game,'' earlier in this chapter, to refresh your memory about specific activities you might schedule. Perhaps it is a squash game with a buddy or a visit to the art museum. Maybe it's a trip to the country just to walk in the woods, or a photography excursion in the city, or simply finding out where you could take a photography course.

4. *Check in with your partner.* You're making a concrete change this week. Your partner can give you support and feedback.

5. *Continue to record your progress in the Action Diary.* Your record will reflect the addition of new or more frequent self-affirming (valued) leisure activities in either flex time or prescheduled time. At the end of the week, pause to take stock. What leisure values are you still failing to express adequately? What obstacles are still giving you trouble? Congratulate yourself for your increased awareness and for each time you've expressed yourself more fully, faithfully, or frequently.

Here is a sample Action Diary Planning Page for week 2 of Values/Goals Clarification. Your contract will reflect the specific valued experiences you use this week to express and affirm some of your core leisure values. Find ways to incorporate each specific behavior into your lifestyle without major dislocations. Don't overdo. Remember: Change is stressful, so take it one step at a time. Above all, remember to give each behavior you undertake on this self-care contract the SMART test. Ask yourself whether it is Specific, Measurable, Acceptable, Realistic, and Truthful.

ACTION DIARY FOR WEEK OF June 12th TO June 18th

Planning Page

Affirmations (My self-themes for this week in key words and phrases)

I _find the natural me in nature_

I _am open to all positive energy_

(Other) _____

_____

Opportunity Visualizations (I clearly see myself . . .)

I clearly see myself walking in a sun-dappled woods, studded with gorgeous wildflowers and filled with the scents and perfumes of the forest

I choose to deepen this Vital Life Skill as Skill as follows (My specific behavioral objectives this week)

I choose to _Repeat my leisure affirmations once each day this week_

Under the following circumstances: _On first waking up in the morning, before getting out of bed_

I choose to _buy a wildflower guide this week_

Under the following circumstances: _At lunch hour Wednesday, I'll go to the nature bookstore that's a few blocks from my office_

I choose to _take a walk in the woods this weekend_

Under the following circumstances: _After breakfast on Sunday I'll drive to the Conservation area near my home & spend a couple of hours walking in the woods and looking for Wild flowers_

I choose to _____

Under the following circumstances: _____

My other opportunity situations for skill practice are:

1. *To plan something on weekends (usually I just sit around and watch sports on T.V.)*

2. *I have three evenings free a week*

3. *I could also arrange to play squash with a friend at lunch hour once in a while*

I have arranged to check in with my partner . . .

When?	About
- *On Sunday evening after my hike*	*I'll tell her about the walk, how it felt, and promise to bring my sketch book or developed photos to Wednesday lunch.*
- *Wednesday lunch*	

Week 3: Build on Your Success

Fill out your Action Diary Planning Page. Agree to do the following this week:

1. *Continue to use autogenic relaxation with affirmations and visualizations.* Repeat your affirmations daily, ideally three or more times each day.

2. *Increase the value of your flex time or prescheduled leisure time.* Continue in the priority area you concentrated on last week. If you increased the quality of your flex time, continue to explore how you can use these previously empty minutes in ways that you value. If more prescheduled leisure was your goal, plan another self-affirming activity for this week, or perhaps even more than one. (Do you dare to pig out on satisfying leisure?)

A Drifter whose pattern was to "devour" her occasional vacations when they were happening, now planned ahead, picking up books (the more obscure the better) in order to steep herself in the history and culture of the place she planned to visit. Now her vacations were with her all the time. (Her first vacation after entering the program was "the best of my life.")

One Speed Freak executive began taking his camera along with him on busy business trips, pausing to photograph unusual nature and city scenes. He later joked, "I may not be stopping to smell the flowers as much as I should, but at least now I'm pausing to notice them."

3. *Check in with your partner.* How is it going? Are you starting to have fun? If not, why not? What are the options?

4. *Record your progress in your Action Diary.* At the end of the week, pause to reflect on your accomplishment. Plan the concrete actions you'll take next week to increase your leisure pleasure.

Week 4: Consolidate Your Gains

Fill out your Action Diary Planning Page. Agree to do the following for the coming week:

1. *Continue autogenic relaxation with affirmations and visualizations.* Enjoy the sense of control and self-nurture these techniques give you. And remember to use your affirmations daily, ideally three or more times each day.

2. *Consolidate your new leisure style.* This is the third consecutive week you've been expressing your core values more fully through your use of leisure time. Where and how can you deepen this process still further? Continue to work in the area you've chosen—either flex time or prescheduled leisure, finding new ways to increase the number and quality of your valued leisure experiences.

One Speed Freak had always felt too pressured by time to take up any hobby requiring new skills and patience. He discovered intense satisfaction in learning to repair antique clocks, later commenting, ''I never knew 'time' could be so entertaining, especially when you can make it stop and go to please yourself.''

3. *Check in with your partner.*

4. *Record your progress in your Action Diary.* At the end of this week, look back with a sense of real accomplishment at the concrete changes you've made. You really are using your leisure time differently. Congratulate yourself for every success.

Take stock of how far you've come. Do you feel more self-confident, more energetic? Do you find that work is less onerous and overwhelming? Do you feel that you're living a more balanced life? Do you choose to continue to move in this self-affirming direction?

After these first four weeks, you may feel confident enough to turn your attention to the domain of career, while you continue to make changes in your leisure time.

CAREER ACTION

Week 1: Get Ready

The main purpose of this first week is to deepen your awareness of what you really value and want in terms of your work and working environment. This week you'll be repeating the first three steps of the four-step Values/Goals Clarification process: identifying your core values; identifying your most valued experiences; and prioritizing and planning for action.

Fill out your Action Diary Planning Page. Before you do anything else, make a contract with yourself to introduce the following behaviors in the coming week:

1. *Autogenic relaxation plus affirmation and visualization.* Begin this week with a fifteen-minute autogenic relaxation using your autogenic tape, after which you introduce your career affirmations and visualizations. Plan at least three more autogenic sessions this week. Use your affirmations daily, ideally at least three times each day. This is especially important on work days. It will keep you in touch with the values you tend to lose sight of while at work.

2. *Visualize your ideal job.* Immediately following your initial autogenic relaxation session, spend a half hour or so visualizing your perfect job. Here's how to do it.

> Read the following questions and suggestions with care. Then think about your ideal job by closing your eyes for a few moments and letting your thoughts flow.
>
> If money were no object, and if any job in the world could be yours if you asked for it, what would it be? If you don't have a specific "dream job," make one up. Imagine the sorts of things you'd be doing and the kinds of people you'd be associating with. How would your overall lifestyle change if you had this job? How would it affect other parts of your life?
>
> Close your eyes and project yourself into the future, immediate or long-term. Imagine that you've landed your ideal job. Fantasize all the things you'd be doing and the experiences you'd be having in this job.
>
> After you've spent a few minutes enjoying this visualization, write down the details. Where would this job be located? What exactly would you be doing? With whom? What sort of hours

would you be working? How far would you be commuting? Go into as much detail as you can. Then write down in point form what you would do during a day at your ideal job.

3. *Refine and prioritize your list of career values.* As you look back over what you've written, jot down a list of the key values expressed in the scenes and situations you've just described. The more fundamental the value, the more important. For example, if you described a job located in a bustling metropolitan area, an underlying value might be coming into contact with interesting and accomplished people. If you described a job that involved lots of traveling, an underlying value might be experiencing new people and places. If your ideal job was one with few interruptions, an underlying value might be working alone or independently of others. (Note the difference between an external circumstance and an inner value.) Finally look back over the list of core career values you came up with in the "Rate Yourself" section of this chapter. Are all those values reflected on this new list? If not, should any of them be added?

Once you've got a comprehensive list, reduce it to no more than eight items. (You may find that you can combine some things.) Go down the list and beside each item write either an A (essential) or a B (merely important). The A items are your priority career values. These form the key to your directional self. Each time you perform an activity that expresses one or more of these values, you are following the compass heading toward your realistically realizable ideal self.

4. *Keep a work diary.* Carry a notebook to work with you this week, and in it note key experiences that correspond to one of your priority values (the ones you marked with an A). Also note any opportunities for self-expression and chances to experience these values more fully, but do nothing to act on them. At the same time, notice and record any obstacles and any particular low points, experiences that epitomize unsatisfying work experiences or situations. Become aware of how these experiences fail to express your values or get you closer to your goals. You now have a much better sense of the parts of your job you really value and the opportunities you have every day to experience these values more often.

5. *Prioritize and plan for action.* Identify the specific valued experiences you would like to introduce into your working life over the next three weeks. Prioritize this list on the basis of what seems doable and important to do. Decide on your first concrete step. Now plan at least one concrete valued behavior you will introduce next week.

6. *Check in with your partner.* Knowing that you've got a date to talk to your partner will give you a sense of support and responsibility as you embark on this important period of change.

7. *Record your progress in your Action Diary.* Your progress this week is simply in deepening your awareness of what you value, your opportunities for change, and the obstacles in the way of change. Congratulate yourself as you get more in tune with your career needs and goals.

Week 2: Take Your First Step

Fill out your Action Diary Planning Page. Agree to do the following during the coming week:

1. *Continue using autogenic relaxation with affirmations and visualization.* At least four times each week, modify your affirmations or replace them with new ones, as seems appropriate. Repeat your affirmations daily, ideally at least three times a day.

2. *Begin implementing your plan.* You have probably identified one recurring opportunity for expressing one of your priority work values. Do it each time it occurs this week. As you do, make modifications as necessary (be flexible). Each evening after work, take stock of all the valued activities you've done, especially congratulating yourself for meeting your daily goal. If you feel ambitious this week, feel free to add additional valued activities, experimenting with more than one self-affirming change.

If you will introduce just one valued experience this week—and repeat it every working day the opportunity occurs, so that it really takes root —you will take a major step. This one new behavior need not be big or dramatic. This is definitely not the stage to hand in your resignation or confront your boss over a long-simmering resentment. Your aim is to make one small and concrete change and to really enjoy the way it makes you feel.

Our study participants found all sorts of ways to take a first step. One Loner took the initiative to organize an office farewell lunch for a departing colleague. A Speed Freak decided to make all his nonpressing phone calls during two half-hour periods he set aside at 10 A.M. and 2 P.M. And one Drifter resolved to make his boss aware of the several types of experiences he had most enjoyed during a recent project, thereby increasing the likelihood he would have opportunities for more such experiences in the future. (Remember Charlie, the Speed Freak dermatologist who scheduled three fictitious patients into his weekly office routine? This is a creative idea for any professional who sees many clients each day and feels overwhelmed by his or her packed schedule.)

3. *Check in with your partner*. Let your partner know about your success in introducing a new self-affirming (valued) behavior this week. Discuss any roadblocks you are encountering, and brainstorm solutions.

4. *Record your progress in your Action Diary*. In addition to noting opportunities and obstacles, your progress now includes at least one actual new valued behavior. Congratulate yourself for your success and for every awareness of an opportunity.

On day 7 of this week, pause to jot down in point form how you've done and to plan for the next week.

Here is a sample Action Diary Planning Page for week 2 of Values/Goals Clarification. Your particular planning page will reflect the specific valued experiences you use this week to express and affirm your core career values. Find ways to incorporate each specific behavior into your lifestyle without major dislocations. Don't overdo. Remember: Change is stressful, so take it one step at a time. Above all, remember to give each behavior you undertake on this self-care contract the SMART test. Ask yourself whether it is Specific, Measurable, Acceptable, Realistic, and Truthful.

ACTION DIARY FOR WEEK OF Jan 20th TO Jan 26th

Planning Page

Affirmations (My self-themes for this week in key words and phrases)

I *am organized and efficient*

I *respect myself and my co-workers respect me*

(Other) _____

_____

Opportunity Visualizations (I clearly see myself . . .)

I clearly see a stack of finished work on my desk
I clearly see myself handing the completed
report to my boss

I choose to deepen this Vital Life Skill as follows (My specific behavioral objectives this week)

I choose to _do a fifteen minute autogenic relaxation followed_
by affirmation and visualization at least 4x's during coming
week

Under the following circumstances: _Monday, Wednesday and_
Friday before dinner in the den with the door closed.
Saturday morning before breakfast

I choose to _repeat my career affirmations once each_
day this week

Under the following circumstances: _on first waking up in_
the morning before getting out of bed.

I choose to _organize and plan my entire work day_
every day this week

Under the following circumstances: _I will get to the office_
fifteen minutes earlier than usual, close my
door, hold my calls and lay out the coming day

I choose to _____

Under the following circumstances: _____

My other opportunity situations for skill practice are:

—Whenever my work gets too much. I can always close the door and have my secretary hold my calls.

— I will make a point of congratulating anyone who goes the extra mile

— I will take compliments with a simple "Thank you, I'm pleased you feel that way."

I have arranged to check in with my partner . . .

When?

On Wednesday evening

About

How my better scheduled week is going

Week 3: Build On Your Success

Fill out your Action Diary Planning Page. Agree to do the following during the coming week:

1. *Continue practicing autogenic relaxation*. Do this at least four times this week, along with the appropriate affirmations and visualizations. Use your affirmations at least once a day, ideally two or three times each day.

2. *Build on your new valued career behavior*. Last week, you took your first concrete step. This week, you are ready to take another step along the path of your directional self. Make sure it is something you are confident you can do. It may mean doing more of what you started last week, or finding a second recurring opportunity that complements your first changed behavior. Remember that each step, however small, is an important act of self-affirmation. These small acts add up, especially now that you have your career values clear and your priorities for action lined up.

In week 2, a Cliff Walker who was trying to cut back to smoking only after meals saw a golden opportunity for self-affirmation: He volunteered to join his company's committee for a smoke-free workplace and helped them plan the no-smoking policy to be phased in over the coming year.

A Speed Freak who always took his briefcase home with him, although he didn't always do work once he got there, began setting aside at least two evenings per week when he would go home without his "ball and chain." He also promised himself that if he did take the briefcase home, he was committed to doing at least an hour's work.

3. *Check in with your partner*. How is it going for you? Do the obstacles still seem immense? Are you trying to move too fast? Are you missing small opportunities that could add up?

4. *Record your progress in your Action Diary*. Congratulate yourself for every success and every new awareness. On day 7, look back over your progress during the previous week. Then chart your course for week 4.

Week 4: Consolidate Your Gains

Fill out your Action Diary Planning Page. Agree to do the following during the coming week:

1. *Continue using autogenic relaxation with affirmations and visualizations*. Use your affirmations daily, ideally three or more times each day.

2. *Consolidate your new career behavior*. Find ways to deepen (do better) the one or two new behaviors you've introduced in weeks 2 and 3. Consolidate.

An office administrator with advanced Basket Case symptoms was positively ecstatic when in week 4 he finally began to "work smarter, not harder" by requesting his staff to submit requests for supplies on a form. Formerly he had spent much of his day chasing orders and responding individually to dozens of verbal "emergency requests" from subordinates who'd gotten comfortable with him as their gofer.

3. *Check in with your partner*.

4. *Record your progress in your Action Diary*. At the end of this fourth week, pause to look back at your progress in expressing your core values at work. How have you done? How are you feeling about yourself? If you have followed the four-week plan, you are now feeling less anxiety and considerably more self-confidence. You know you can make a difference in your life.

If you began with career, you may feel confident enough to turn your attention to the domain of leisure, while you continue to make changes at work.

Continuing Your Prescription

Now that you've completed your four-week program for leisure or career action, it's up to you what you do next. You can continue to explore either leisure or career, or you can add the second domain while continuing with the first. Or you can begin to phase in the next intervention in your prescription as you continue to practice Values/Goals Clarification. The sooner you do, the sooner your whole vitality prescription can start to work for you. However, we recommend that you work on this intervention for a total of eight weeks before turning to the next item on your prescription pad.

Think of your start-up program as a module or prototype of change. As you continue to work on this Vital Life Skill, it's up to you whether you stay within this formal structure. But we strongly recommend that you keep up your diary and continue to use autogenically rooted affirmations and visualizations.

Many of our study subjects showed inspiring progress as they continued the process of Values/Goals Clarification over the full eight months of the study—and beyond. One of these was Jonathan, a Loner and a highly successful vice-president of a large communications company who entered the program at age 51 (body age 57). He was eligible for full retirement in three years, and for the previous five years, his life had been dominated by the questions ''What will I do then? Who have I been, up until now, other than someone very good at what he does? All I do is my work, and I know that work isn't enough.''

As Jonathan got in touch with his core values—especially the ways he liked to spend his leisure—he could finally see (by putting it down on paper) that all his life he had wanted to be an actor. This bolt of new awareness initially depressed him: ''How can I start a stage career when I'm 51? It's too late. And I'd be embarrassed to start while I'm still with the company.'' This is a good example of the real/ideal gap seeming impossibly large when it is first perceived but vaguely defined.

Then Jonathan came to a crucial realization: A big part of his job every day involved acting. His corporate performances included motivating his employees, being a strong leader, and inspiring his troops. He began to see (and to write down) all sorts of opportunities for effective ''stage management'' of meetings and internal communications. He began to identify his opportunities to ''play leading roles'' and then to rehearse for them. This process began to release the buried actor who had, as he put it, ''been in the dungeon for over thirty years.''

Over the eight months of the study, Jonathan changed dramatically (to use a very apt word). He began picking up on all sorts of little opportunities to make the impression he wanted to make. ''After some meetings,'' he told us, ''I could almost hear the applause—which I was giving myself.'' At his final checkup, he looked, felt, and tested ten years younger (his body age was down 10 years to 47). By having the courage to define his ideal self honestly, he narrowed the gap. (Two years later, we heard that he had joined an amateur theater company and was playing minor parts as if they were starring roles.)

CHAPTER 9
Effective Relaxation

PRIMARY INTERVENTION FOR: Speed Freak, Worry Wart
SECONDARY INTERVENTION FOR: Cliff Walker

Core Message

In this chapter, we teach a range of conscious relaxation techniques that you can use to relax at will and to perform better, both in difficult, high-stress situations and over the long haul. As you lower your day-to-day stress level and reduce your tendency to go into the danger zone of overstress, your performance will improve, and you'll experience less fatigue.

Relaxation is the primary intervention for Speed Freaks and Worry Warts, and the second most potent intervention for Cliff Walkers. In addition, deliberate relaxation techniques will enhance the effectiveness of the other interventions, many of which contain specific suggestions on how to combine them with relaxation. For instance, the exercise chapter includes instructions on how to use relaxation breathing while doing stretching exercises. And your practice of all five of the Vital Life Skills is more powerful when you root the change process in autogenic relaxation with affirmation and visualization.

Relaxation skills directly address the area in which Worry Warts and Speed Freaks are most inefficient in dealing with stress and so most susceptible to accelerated aging. These are people who continue to expend stress energy long after a threat, challenge, or opportunity has passed. They neither fight nor flee: They just tough it out. Typically, they are prone to overdosing on stress, to shooting over the top of the stress-performance curve, to operating in almost continual overdrive.

Regardless of your stressotype, however, you'll benefit from incorporating conscious relaxation techniques into your lifestyle. They will enhance your effectiveness—your ability to concentrate, solve problems, and summon up the energy you need to get things done. Many extraordinarily productive people have incorporated relaxation habits into their workstyles. Hans Selye had a special chair constructed in which he could do certain kinds of work while reclining. And Winston Churchill reportedly handled affairs of state while lounging in a dressing gown or soaking in a hot bath (he had the reputation of being able to do two days' work in one). By learning and practicing relaxation skills and applying them in demanding situations, you too can perform more effectively.

Here in summary are the main benefits of Effective Relaxation:

> The bodily restoration during deep relaxation yields an immediate payoff in extra energy.
>
> The ability to relax at will allows you to regulate on demand your expenditure of stress energy through the day, resulting in more energy when you need it and energy to spare for leisure.
>
> The lowering of your stress thermostat—the overall stress level at which you normally operate—conserves your overall expenditure of stress energy.
>
> The quieting of negative inner chatter or self-talk—Worry Warts take special note—makes these thoughts less distracting and less fatiguing, and you will more easily hear the positive alternatives. (Positive affirmations are powerful aids to this process.)
>
> Increased awareness of your body and your emotions will help you get clearer about what's really important to you. Also, you will gain a sharper awareness of physical and emotional pain that has previously been disguised by the beta endorphins released during a stress reaction—this pain is information essential to your health and well-being.

Your relaxation potential is enormous. By learning and practicing only a few techniques, you can get immediate pleasure and refreshment. In the long term, you can increase your self-control and self-esteem. Learning to relax will increase your sense of control over your environment and your feelings of personal power.

Speed Freaks often show very quick and dramatic results with the relaxation part of their prescription. One such was Jack (age 41, body age 48), a senior account executive with a large advertising firm. Jack lived for ever-increasing speed and pressure. He finally admitted that without such constant stress he was deeply afraid that ''nothing has any meaning, my whole life might just disappear.'' (This is a good example of an irrational negative belief that can be very difficult to get rid of.) Nonetheless, he knew something had to give since he regularly ''just collapsed on weekends.'' Except when he was out cold, however, he was ''so high on stress'' he could no longer feel the ups and downs.

In the first few weeks of the program, Jack began practicing the spiral relaxation technique you'll learn in this chapter. First he did it on weekends (when he wasn't so high). Then he used it several times during the work week. He was amazed: ''For the first time, I could actually physically feel which parts of my day made me feel satisfied and which ones churned my stomach and gave me headaches.'' A few days later, a saying of his father's flashed into his mind for the first time in years (and it came back again and again): ''Life is like sex. If it doesn't feel good, you're probably doing it wrong.'' Now Jack could see and, more important, feel what he was doing right and what he was doing wrong.

As he became more adept at a whole range of deliberate relaxation skills, Jack described his newfound ability as being ''like the seek-and-scan function on my car stereo. It lets me tune in to the messages I've needed to hear for a long time.''

At the end of the program, Jack's body age was down 10 years to 37, below his calendar age by 4 years. And he'd done this without abandoning his fast-track advertising career. He'd learned that, in his business, you ''can't afford to go flat out all the time. The environment changes minute by minute because our clients' worlds are so turbulent. You have to be able to gear back to avoid going into a skid on the curve that lies just ahead. And you have to keep some gas in the reserve tank for opportunities that suddenly appear with no advance notice.''

Like Jack, you can discover your relaxation potential.

RATE YOURSELF

Use the self-tests in this section to:

> Take an inventory of your existing relaxation skills (you may not realize how many you already have).
> Identify your stress hierarchy—recurring day-to-day opportunities for you to deliberately relax.
> Develop your relaxation self-themes: your personal affirmations and visualizations for this Vital Life Skill.

Relaxation Skill Inventory

Everyone has relaxation skills, things they do deliberately in order to lower their stress levels. But you probably don't recognize all the things you are now doing as skills. You may even think of some of them as negative escapes rather than positive ways of taking care of yourself. The purpose of the Relaxation Skill Inventory is to give you an opportunity to take stock of what you already are doing to look after your relaxation needs, including any formal relaxation skills you've learned. Thus your list might include a martial art such as Tai Chi, a meditation technique such as TM, any of the relaxation skills taught in stress-management courses, as well as soaking in a hot tub, going to the club for a workout, or taking a catnap.

On the list below, check off the relaxation activities you regularly use to lower your stress level. We've left space at the end for you to add others we haven't thought of. We recommend that you brainstorm with your program partner.

_____ Getting a massage	_____ Giving a massage	_____ Tranquility tank or hot tub
		_____ Sex
_____ Taking a shower	_____ Hot bath	
_____ Dancing	_____ Dinner out	_____ Listening to music
		_____ Reading a book
_____ Cooking	_____ Doing a hobby	_____ Sports
_____ Watching TV	_____ Meditate	_____ Daydreaming
_____ Socializing	_____ Doing Tai Chi	_____ Gossiping
_____ Gardening	_____ Hot drink	_____ Playing with the kids
_____ Sitting by the fire		
	_____ Singing in the shower	_____ Taking a nap
_____ Listening to music	_____ Bird-watching	_____ Taking a walk
_____ Going to a movie	_____ Painting	_____ Doing odd jobs
_____ Shopping	_____ Exercise	
_____ Going fishing	_____ Yoga	
_____	_____	_____
_____	_____	_____
_____	_____	_____

While smoking and drinking alcohol are both common ways of relaxing—as is the use of tranquilizers—they have negative side effects and so are not on our list. This is not to say that there's anything wrong with the occasional glass of wine at the end of a high-stress day. Drinking moderately in social situations may well enhance your relaxation, but five minutes of deep relaxation will relax you better and leave you energized and refreshed.

How large is your relaxation skill inventory? Are there skills you have but haven't used for a while? If you can't check off at least five on this list and add three more of your own, you need more relaxation resources.

As you start to put Effective Relaxation into practice, be sure to build on your existing relaxation skills. Choose ways to relax that seem enjoyable and that fit into your schedule with relative ease. Although the specific relaxation techniques we teach you are important, a walk in the park at lunchtime is also a good way to relax. And if you combine your walk with a simple relaxation meditation that quiets your thoughts, it will be even more effective.

Your Personal Stress Hierarchy: Identifying and Prioritizing Your Relaxation Opportunities

We recommend that you use this exercise as part of week 1 of your four-week start-up program (see the final section of this chapter). The purpose of the stress hierarchy is: to increase your awareness of when and how you suffer from too much stress (and how you feel when you are under stress); to identify your priority relaxation opportunities, those recurring high-stress situations you want to change (our experience has shown that, on average, 95 percent of these events are predictable); and to prioritize these high-stress relaxation opportunities as a basis for taking action.

For the next week, keep a daily stress diary. (Use a notebook, your daybook, whatever.) You can either carry it with you throughout the day, noting in it everything you experience as stressful, or you can sit down at the end of the day and look back over the stress peaks and valleys of the previous twenty-four hours. Feel free to spend time practicing new relaxation techniques during the week, but do nothing to change your behavior in high-stress situations. Simply observe yourself as you continue your normal life.

The diary can be an important awareness tool because most of us develop emotional calluses: We become so accustomed to feeling distressed in certain situations, or of operating at a hyped-up level much of the time, that we have lost touch with our bodies. Only unusual or acute overstress situations stand out. The diary is a technique for bringing into your awareness all the high-stress events you experience. As you do this, you will notice that the great majority of these events are part of a recurring pattern.

Each time you note a physical or emotional symptom of distress (to refresh your memory of these, see the Personal Distress Checklist on p. 28), rate the intensity of the event according to the following scale: 1 = no distress; 2 = minor distress; 3 = moderate distress; 4 = severe distress.

The entries in your stress diary will look something like this:

> "Morning staff meeting—2"
>
> "Argument with spouse—4"
>
> "Caught in stop-and-go traffic—3"

At the end of each day, go over your stress diary. Observe which situations cause you more distress, which less. Then take the average stress level of these "situational stress points" by adding them together and dividing the total by the number of situations. Using the example of the three situations above, the total would be 9, divided by 3, yielding an average stress level of 3. This is your situational average—the average intensity of those occasions you noted in your diary as distressful. Using your situational average as a guide, subjectively assign a stress-intensity level to your whole day. When you do this, factor in the ups and downs, the times you are tense and the periods when you are more relaxed. Overall, would you give your day a 2? a 4?

Take a moment at this stage to ask yourself how you feel about your overall daily stress level. How does this number compare with the average of your situational stress points? Is your whole day a 2 or 3, occasionally spiking up to a 4? As you ask yourself these questions, you are beginning to get a much clearer picture of your daily stress pattern.

Now analyze your day more deeply by recording any behavioral patterns you observe in relation to recurring or high-stress events. For example, does your stress level hit 3 just before you arrive at work each morning? Is there a weekly meeting that drives you round the bend? Do you grit your teeth when you hear the baby bawl? Do you start to tense up as the weekend ends and you start to think about Monday?

These obstructive patterns interfere with your comfort and effectiveness in every sphere of your existence. They repeatedly and therefore predictably drain your stress energy. Use the Stress Patterns Record we've provided to perform this stress self-analysis. You can either reproduce this form for your Action Diary notebook or use it as is. Make an entry for each significantly distressful situation during the day just past. (Feel free to record your positive stressful experiences as well. Such information

STRESS PATTERNS RECORD

Situation, date, and time	Stress symptoms (tense, upset, hands sweating, heart pounding, can't concentrate)	What I did and thought	How I felt (anger, sadness, joy, fear)	What I would like to have done	Level of stress (1–4)	Outcome (1–4)

will give you more insight into when you master stress and when it masters you.)

In the appropriate columns, briefly describe the situation, your behavior and feelings, and what you might like to have done differently in the situation.

In the last two columns, enter a number, as follows:

In the column "Level of Stress," enter the appropriate distress level score from 1 to 4.

In the final column, "Outcome," pick the number that best describes how you rate your effectiveness in coping with the situation: 1 = very effective; 2 = effective; 3 = somewhat effective; 4 = not effective.

You will use these weighting numbers when you prioritize your relaxation opportunities into your personal stress hierarchy.

At the end of the week, plot your week-long pattern of stress expenditure on a Stress Level Scale and Graph. (Use the sample from one of our study subjects as a model.) Indicate under Day 1 which day of the week you began. Then take the overall stress-level number (the average) you assigned to that day and mark an X on the graph at the correct level

STRESS LEVEL SCALE AND GRAPH

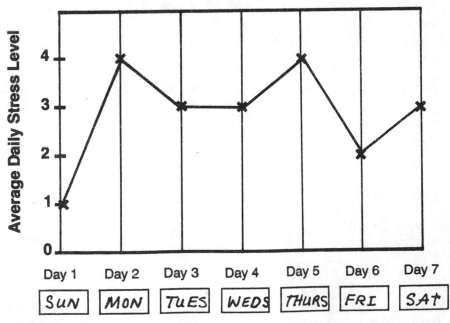

This is a sample graph for a Speed Freak office manager whose staff required very little supervision Friday but whose son had a baseball practice at 6 A.M. on Saturday.

and day. Do this for each day of the week. Now join the seven Xs with a continuous line. This is your week-long stress pattern. How does your week look? Does your stress level go higher as the week progresses, and then drop suddenly at the weekend? When you combine this graphic picture with the information in your week-long Stress Patterns Record, you have a detailed stress self-portrait.

You now have a seven-day stress diary, a seven-day Stress Patterns Record, and a seven-day Stress Level Scale and Graph. This is all the information you need to create your personal stress hierarchy and prioritize your relaxation opportunities; in other words, the recurring situations that you want to handle differently. In our training sessions, we sometimes referred to these counterproductive situations and behaviors as "stress vampires": a very vivid way of saying that they are vitality drains that needlessly sap your reserves of stress energy.

Follow this sequence of steps:

1. Look at your Stress Level Scale and Graph.

2. Read over your week-long Stress Patterns Record.

3. Pick approximately five important recurring situations in which you experience some level of distress: situations and behaviors you'd like to change. Look especially for situations that occur more than once each week or that recur regularly from week to week.

4. Rank these situations in their order of importance (the weighting numbers you assigned in your Stress Patterns Record can help you with this). The more frequently a situation occurs or the higher the stress level you experience during that situation, the more important it is.

5. Prioritize your important relaxation opportunities—your opportunities to break longtime patterns—according to their doability: How willing are you to change these situations? How difficult do they seem? Thus, your top priority is a situation that occurs frequently but that seems relatively easy for you to tackle. Your lowest priority is a situation that occurs only occasionally but that gives you a lot of distress. This is your personal stress hierarchy.

Many study participants found that keeping a stress diary led to some surprising self-discoveries. A good example is Jennifer, a Worry Wart aged 45 (body age 56) who had been appointed a criminal court judge the year before entering the program. As she started to look at her stress patterns, she expected to find that her major sources of stress were the work load and responsibilities of her position, with raising two teenagers also making a strong contribution. So the results of her stress diary "came like a bolt out of the blue." The stresses of sitting on the bench and of dealing with her two teenage daughters rarely rated over a 2 (except for the occasional exceptional day). But she hit 3s and 4s every day on the drive to and from work.

Jennifer pondered these ratings, at first doubting their validity. Finally she concluded that they were true. What gave her the most distress was "making the transition from a flesh-and-blood wife and mother, who sometimes burns the toast and is a pushover for a sob story, to someone who must put intuition and gut feelings on hold, listen only to the legal merits of a case, and then make the tough, right decision."

As Jennifer began to take action, she reported that the counting-breaths and the mind-focusing techniques allowed her to "close the house door emotionally in the morning and the office door emotionally at night." No longer did she feel as though there were "two Jennifers," but rather one person living in two different countries. Her new relaxation skills were the passport she needed to travel less distressfully between the two.

Develop Your Relaxation Affirmations and Visualizations

You now have identified your priorities for action. These will form the basis of your four-week start-up program. But what are your bottom-line relaxation goals? Can you picture yourself and hear yourself behaving in a more relaxed and self-confident way in difficult situations? What affirmative word or phrase would best express this underlying self-theme? Here are some sample relaxation affirmations:

> I am relaxed and calm in stressful situations.
> I relax at will.
> I am calm energy.
> I flow.
> I control my foot on the stress accelerator.
> I shift gears effortlessly.
> No fuss . . . No muss.
> I flow like a cat.
> I bring peace to stressful situations.
> I breathe stress away.
> I am centered.
> Relaxation is my birthright.
> I am harmony.
> I step beyond stress.

Can you visualize yourself performing well in one or more of your relaxation opportunity situations? Here are some sample visualizations used by participants in the Body Age Study:

From a Cliff Walker police officer: A sleek cat striding effortlessly, silently, confidently.

From a Loner hotel chef: As I sit relaxed, I see my released "green aura" extending outward, gradually soothing important people.

From a Worry Wart high school teacher: I am in my garden at the time just before nightfall when there is no wind and only gentle sounds. [Any other healing place works: a waterfall, a woods, a seashore.]

From a Speed Freak politician: I see myself standing at the podium, with minimum muscle tension in my body, smiling warmly at the audience as I prepare to give a speech.

From a Loner production manager: I see my boss becoming more and more emotional at our staff meeting, and for every notch his tension level goes up, mine goes down a notch—and this is reflected in my breathing rate.

From a Speed Freak lawyer: I see myself driving to work in the morning during rush hour: sitting in a relaxed posture, making as few lane changes as possible, and keeping my distance from the car in front. I am enjoying the opportunity to listen to tapes of my favorite music.

From a Worry Wart flight attendant: I feel, see, and hear myself handling an angry passenger calmly and effectively, and then sharing how I did it with other flight crew members.

From a Drifter physician: I see myself at the end of the day, after the last patient, putting my feet up on the desk to make a few notes in my diary about those patients I was really able to help.

From a Basket Case salesman: I see myself putting my heavy sample cases down beside me as I ride up in an elevator while using the "unburdened time" to do the counting-breaths technique.

BASIC TRAINING

In this section, we provide you with your basic training for relaxing at will. You will learn the following:

> A series of simple, enjoyable techniques for achieving the deeply relaxed state known as the relaxation response, in which your mind is calm and focused but awake, and your body is relaxed
> The technique of cognitive reappraisal for rethinking and reevaluating especially difficult situations
> Where and when to use your chosen techniques.

We've selected the particular techniques we'll be teaching you, from among the literally hundreds of relaxation methods that are available, because we find them particularly effective in our stress-management course. But we've listed references to other good sources of relaxation techniques in "Further Reading" at the back of this book. No one has a monopoly on relaxation, and whichever techniques you choose to learn and use, build them on top of your existing relaxation skills as summarized in your Relaxation Skill Inventory.

The Relaxation Response

The *relaxation response* is a term coined by Dr. Herbert Benson of the Harvard Medical School to describe the physiology of deep relaxation. It is a natural process during which your body's level of mobilization is sharply reduced and very little energy is expended. (By contrast, the *stress reaction* is a process of heightened mobilization and high energy expenditure.) Benson's understanding of the relaxation response grew out of laboratory studies he conducted in the late 1960s on individuals practicing transcendental meditation. He discovered some striking things. For one, the deep relaxation engendered by meditation, though definitely a restorative process, is quite different from the relaxation you get during sleep.

The relaxation response lowers the metabolic rate of the body: Your heart rate and breathing slow, your blood pressure often goes down, and your muscles relax. But unlike when you fall asleep, these things happen almost immediately, and the decrease is greater. During a typical night's sleep, it takes four or five hours for the metabolic rate to reach its lowest point, and it typically decreases no more than 8 percent. With the relaxation response, however, the decrease takes place in the first three minutes and ranges from 10 to 20 percent below the normal metabolic rate. In addition, during the relaxation response, you relax much more deeply than during normal sleep. This explains why people practiced in relaxation techniques can emerge reenergized from as few as five minutes in a relaxed state. Indian yogis, for example, can function on virtually no sleep.

During deep relaxation, your brain is much more awake than it is during sleep. Scientists have identified four basic states of electrical activity in the brain, each coinciding with different degrees of wakefulness. In descending order from most alert to least wakeful, these are beta (fully awake), alpha, theta, and delta (asleep). During deep relaxation, your brain is in the alpha state, a condition of keen mental awareness in which it is highly receptive to creative ideas and positive suggestions. The relaxation response is a state in which your mind is fully awake and focused (but calm), yet your body is more deeply relaxed than during even the most restful deep sleep. In addition, the lower metabolic and brain wave levels give your cells and tissues a chance to rest and restore themselves more quickly. Your thoughts are still active, but they become less distracting—quieter and more distant.

The awake but relaxed alpha brain state is highly receptive to positive suggestion (hence the effectiveness of autogenic training). This may be because during the relaxation response the left brain (logic, reasoning) and right brain (feelings, intuition, creativity) function in harmonic balance.

Experiments in biofeedback (a method of bringing involuntary functions into your awareness) have shown that even the body's involuntary systems (for example, blood circulation, the nervous system, and even the immune system) can be "trained" over time to respond to conscious stimuli. By learning to trigger a restorative relaxation response whenever you want to, you can train one of your most important involuntary systems, the parasympathetic branch of the autonomic nervous system, to work for you.

There are many routes to deep relaxation, but all effective relaxation techniques capable of triggering the relaxation response incorporate one or all of the following elements:

> Slow, full, relaxed breathing
> Conscious relaxing of the muscles
> Deliberate focusing of the mind on one specific thing so
> that thoughts and emotions become quieter and less
> distracting, and troubling emotions subside.

Some techniques begin with the breath; others concentrate initially on relaxing the muscles or helping to focus the mind. But all ultimately lead to a state in which your body, mind, and emotions are deeply relaxed.

In the pages that follow, we'll teach you a variety of proven techniques for achieving the relaxation response. Pick your favorites, and practice them until they become easy. Most of those who entered the Body Age Program found relaxation fun, once they got over their initial resistance to setting aside time to relax. And they reported that, when they used one of the methods we describe below, they could feel the difference after even a few minutes.

Before you begin, here is a simple four-step method for beginning any relaxation:

1. Get comfortable.
2. Become aware of the sounds in the room and far away.
3. Say the following affirmation: "I choose this time for my focused relaxation."
4. Consciously slow your breathing (many people like to focus on the tip of their nose).

If you are like many of our program participants, you may be feeling some resistance to trying these techniques. Perhaps the experience of one class of program trainees will inspire you.

The evening this group of twelve had their first relaxation class, the room's thermostat was working poorly and the temperature was a chilly 64 degrees. People had been politely complaining and putting on their coats while listening to the instructor's introductory presentation. They remained bundled up as they were led through the first fifteen minutes of guided relaxation. Afterward, eleven of the twelve reported that they actually felt warm, although the room temperature hadn't changed. And the twelfth, who had been been "very tense all week"—his neck muscles were so tight he couldn't look sideways without pain—could now move his head freely and comfortably. ·

In fifteen minutes, we had twelve believers.

Basic Relaxation Breathing

There can be no deep relaxation without slow, full breathing that fills the lungs fully from belly to chest. Yet most adults are chronically unable to breathe deeply. Ironic as it may seem, they have to "learn" to breathe. Men and women are taught that it's a virtue to "suck in that gut," to keep a flat stomach at any price. The price, however, is that after a few years you can no longer fully expand your diaphragm when you breathe. Your abdominal muscles become chronically tight.

Pay attention to your breathing right now. (At first, you may find it helpful to put your hand on your belly to monitor its rise and fall.) Is it slow and full, or short and shallow? Your breathing is involuntary except when you consciously breathe differently. When you're excited or in the midst of physical exertion, it automatically speeds up. When you're tense, it becomes restricted and shallow. And when you're sleeping, it is usually slower and somewhat deeper.

When you deliberately slow down your breathing, your body's exchange of oxygen and carbon dioxide becomes more efficient, biochemically triggering the relaxation response. Thus the key to successful relaxation breathing is the long, slow inhalation and the long, slow exhalation, especially the outbreath. With each long outbreath, you can literally feel yourself relaxing more deeply.

As a first step to successful relaxation breathing, it helps to become aware of how you breathe normally. To do so, follow this simple exercise, which in itself is an effective relaxation technique, and one you can use in any situation to lower your stress level.

Exercise: How Do You Breathe? For this exercise, you can be sitting or lying in a comfortable position. Make sure your clothes are loose enough that they don't constrict your breathing; in particular, make sure the clothing around your waist is loose.

Close your eyes and place one hand on your chest and one on your belly. As your two hands rise and fall, notice how you are breathing. Do you breathe through your nose or your mouth or both? How fast or slowly? How deeply? Does the hand on your belly move at all?

Now, with your eyes still closed, experiment with deliberately breathing through your nose and down into your belly. Don't force it; just gently inhale as fully as is comfortable. Exhale slowly so that your lungs empty and your belly falls. Let your breath be easy and natural, like the ebb and flow of the tide. Continue breathing this way until it feels comfortable and normal.

Many of us have developed habits that inhibit this kind of breathing. We wear tight clothes or hold in our stomachs unconsciously because we think it makes us look better. Relaxation breathing is an opportunity to let down your hair and "let down" your body, a chance to be yourself.

Now that you know more about breathing, you may enjoy keeping track of how you breathe at different times during the day. Do occasional "breathing checks" when you think you're relaxed and when you know you're not. This is a simple technique for increasing your awareness and your readiness for change.

Exercise: Basic Breathing. It comes down to these three simple steps:

Fully empty your lungs (don't forget to collapse your belly).
Make a deep, slow inhalation (filling first your belly and then your chest.)
Make a long, slow exhalation (emptying first your chest and then your belly).
[Repeat.]

You'll discover that the more you breathe, the longer your inhalation and exhalations can become. Experiment with this. In classes, we regularly had students who could easily take a full minute for one, long, slow out-breath.

Techniques That Combine Breathing with Mind-Focusing

A number of breathing exercises also involve deliberate mind-focusing techniques that help quiet internal chatter (self-talk). You focus your mind by concentrating on a word, an image, or a phrase while doing relaxation breathing. It works so well because you must keep your mind focused on the word or image; in so doing, you allow busy and distracting thoughts to become quieter and less burdensome.

The combination of relaxation breathing and mind-focusing is the basis of all meditation techniques, including transcendental meditation. Your mantra—your focusing word, image, or phrase—can be as simple as the number "one" repeated over and over again in your head, or the word "calm." Your autogenic relaxation tape is just one of many possible mind-focusing techniques. (Autogenic relaxation is one of the two most-used relaxation techniques in the world. The other is progressive relaxation, described below.)

All the exercises in this section use mind-focusing techniques combined with relaxation breathing.

Exercise: Abdominal Breathing. (Note: While most techniques in this chapter are optional, this one is recommended as a basic core technique for all readers.) Abdominal breathing can be practiced lying, sitting, standing, or walking, and so can be utilized in many situations, from walking through the park to sitting in your office or in meetings, or after vigorous sex. In other words, relaxation breathing doesn't mean you have to be sitting cross-legged chanting a mantra. The following instructions are for lying down.

> **1.** Lie on your back, feet parallel and slightly parted, hands at your sides. Remove your glasses or contact lenses, and loosen your belt or the clothing around your waist. If you wish, close your eyes.
>
> Breathe normally a few times through your nose to get comfortable.
>
> Now inhale slowly and visualize the air as it passes through your nose, goes down into your lungs, and starts to fill the bottom of your lungs. Notice how your belly rises. As you exhale, let your belly fall.
>
> For the next few breaths, just feel your belly rise and fall. Put all your attention on your breathing. Each time you exhale, feel yourself relax, letting go of tension. Give yourself permission to enjoy the relaxation as you continue to breathe fully, in and out. Use the affirming words "I choose to enjoy this time for my focused relaxation."
>
> **2.** This time, as you inhale through your nose and take the air down into your belly, let your belly expand as far as it wants to go. (By focusing on the abdominal area, you can let go of more and more unneeded muscle tension.)
>
> Continue to inhale, allowing your ribs and chest to expand

until your chest is comfortably full. Imagine that you are being filled with air, effortlessly.

Begin to exhale slowly through your nose, emptying the air first from your chest, then from your torso, and finally from your belly, letting your stomach fall. With each exhalation, feel your body releasing and relaxing more and more.

If you like, visualize your breath as a wave moving back and forth between the bottom of your abdomen (your belly) and the top of your lungs (your chest fully expanded). As you inhale, first your belly rises and then your chest fills with air. As you exhale, the process is reversed: First your chest falls, then your lower chest, and finally your belly. In and out, in and out, the wave washes back and forth in your body.

Do this for three to five minutes, slowly and with awareness. When you are comfortable with this stage, go on to stage 3.

3. Slowly inhale to a count of 4. Hold your breath for a count of 4. Exhale for a count of 4. Keep up this breathing, increasing the count to 5, then 6, and so on, as it feels comfortable, but always trying to make sure that the inhalation, the hold, and the exhalation are equal in length (for example, 8–8–8).

Each time you exhale, let all the tension flow out of your body as you permit yourself to relax more and more deeply.

(An alternative method for stage 3, which many of our students preferred, is to make the holding stage shorter; a long, slow in-breath, a brief hold, and an equally long, slow out-breath. For example: 10–1–10.

As you become accomplished at abdominal breathing, you'll be amazed at how long you can take for a single breath.

Exercise: Counting Breaths. This exercise seems simple but is usually quite challenging at first. Your mind will tend to wander. Think of this as the beginning of your increased awareness of how self-talk works. When a stray thought breaks your concentration, notice the thought, then "wave good-bye" to it as it passes through. Some people even like to tell the thought they'll see it later. When your thoughts are very stubborn, it is often helpful to briefly half-open your eyes. Keep steering your attention back to your breathing and then your counting. If you get frustrated, recognize what's happening as an overprotective response to an as-yet unfamiliar situation (uncertainty causes stress)—your body tightens and your mind calculates.

Don't overdo it. Never stretch your limits of comfort. As they become more comfortable and fun, gradually increase the length of time you practice this and other techniques.

Sit on a chair or cushion with your back and neck straight and your eyes closed, or open, if you prefer. Although if you sit you may be less likely to fall asleep, you can also lie in a comfortable position. Breathe slowly and deeply through your nose. Scan the body from head to toe for tension areas, and put your focused awareness on each tense part of the body with the positive intention of relaxing it. (For example, you could say to yourself the affirming phrase, "I now let go of the tension in my legs.")

Notice where you feel your breath entering and leaving your nose (it could be the upper lip, the tip of the nose, or inside the nostrils). Experience the breath as it passes back and forth over this point. Notice that the breath is slightly cooler on the inhalation than on the exhalation. Continue for about a minute.

Now start counting your breaths. Inhale fully. As you exhale, count 1 to yourself and visualize the number 1. Inhale fully. As you exhale, count 1, 2 and visualize the number 2. Continue up to the number 4, then start at 1 again.

Continue counting your breaths from 1 to 4 for five minutes or more. After a week or two, you can gradually increase the duration of this exercise. Some people do it for as many as ten or twenty minutes. Whenever your concentration wavers, re-focus on the counting. When you've finished, sit still briefly and become aware of how you feel in every part of your body. Then bring yourself up to a more awake state, by counting 4, 3, 2, 1. Slowly open your eyes and have a good stretch.

As your concentration improves with practice, you can try counting your breaths up to the number 10 and lengthening the time you spend doing this exercise. Find the version of this exercise that's right for you.

There are all sorts of variations to this technique that you can experiment with. For instance, you can simply repeat and visualize a single number. Or you can discover how it feels to count down instead of up, although for one of our students, this had the completely wrong effect: He felt like he was a rocket about to blast off. Or you could use a very brief affirmation (for example, "I am a good person," "I like myself," or "I am vital energy"). Some people like to repeat one word or syllable on each in-breath and one on each out-breath. Find a system that feels good.

Exercise: Repeating a Phrase. Pick a short, suggestive word or phrase that you will repeat over and over. Phrases with multiple "m" sounds are especially effective. They seem to produce the maximum calming and mind-clearing effect. One phrase we like to use is "I am calm."

> Sit comfortably with your eyes closed. Breathe slowly and
>   deeply through your nose.
> Repeat aloud the words, "I am calm."
> Repeat softly, "I am calm."
> Whisper, "I am calm." ·
> Think, "I am calm," so that this is the only thought in your
>   mind.
> Continue this exercise for five minutes.

A number of variations are possible. For example, simply repeat the word or phrase silently on each out-breath or each inhalation. Many people find that repeating the word "calm" is the most effective version of this exercise.

Exercise: Spiral Relaxation. Like most mind-focusing exercises, this one can be done in many different circumstances, from commuting to work to a quiet evening at home. With practice, it can become a technique for almost instant relaxation.

> Lie, sit, or stand comfortably. Breathe deeply and fully. Imagine a point of light, or the sensation of it, at the tip or your nose. Let the light travel up the bridge of your nose to your forehead.
> *Face*: Let the light circle clockwise around the left eye, then up and around the forehead, then down and around the right eye, then down and around the right cheek, then around the left cheek, then around the lips.
> *Neck*: Circle counterclockwise, forming three spirals down the neck.
> *Left Arm*: Make three sprials as you travel from the shoulder down your left arm to your elbow. Continue to the wrist with another three spirals. Trace your thumb to your small fingers, outlining them in white light. Spiral six times back up the arm to the shoulder, through the armpit, across your back, to the right armpit.
> *Right Arm*: Spiral three times down your right arm to the elbow, then three more times to your right wrist. Trace every finger from the little finger to the thumb. Then spiral six times back up your right arm.

Chest: Make seven slow spirals down your chest to your hips, to a point between the legs and under your left thigh.

Left Leg: Spiral six times down your left leg, as you travel down the thigh, past the knee, down the calf to your left ankle. Trace the big to little toes of your left foot, outlining each one in white light.

Allow the light to hop over to the big toe of your right foot.

Right Leg: Trace your big to your little toes and then make six spirals as you travel up the right leg to your inner thigh.

End with an extra turn around your right thigh and up to the base of your spine behind the waist.

You can do this exercise at any speed. You may enjoy experimenting with doing it very slowly or much faster than your normal speed.

Many program participants found breathing and mind-focusing techniques very effective. A telephone operator found she was able to "keep her cool" when an obscene phone call came in by doing several slow, full exhalations. "But I had to be careful," she joked, "not to let the caller think I was into 'heavy breathing,' too."

Speed Freaks find counting breaths very helpful when they are tempted by one of their most characteristic behaviors: interrupting in the middle of a sentence. Counting breaths not only relaxes them, it gives them "something to do." For Worry Warts, counting breaths for several minutes, then getting up and doing something is invariably helpful.

Muscle-Relaxation Techniques

Since elevated stress levels lead to chronic muscle tension, muscle-relaxation exercises are often an excellent place to start your relaxation session. You may want to use them in combination with other techniques or on their own. You are probably quite unaware of many places in your body where you habitually hold on to muscular tension. Among the more common areas in which people hold tension are in tight shoulders, tight jaws, clenched fists, and tensed forehead muscles (which cause tension headaches). Muscle-relaxation exercises will help you become more aware of these holding places, teach you how to relax them, and help you train yourself not to "tense up" so easily. These techniques work wonderfully to break chronic tension patterns.

Your body contains three types of muscles: skeletal (or voluntary), smooth, and cardiac. Skeletal muscles, as the name applies, are attached to your bone structure and are what enable you to move around. Smooth muscles, mostly found in the walls of your internal organs and in the blood vessels, keep food and waste moving through the digestive tract, as well as being responsible for such things as the dilation of the pupil in response to light. The cardiac muscle is the muscle that lines the heart, causing it to pump the blood through your veins and arteries.

Unlike the other two types of muscles, skeletal muscles are responsive to conscious control (although they also respond involuntarily as, for example, when your shoulders tense up during a stress reaction). Since you have some conscious control over skeletal muscles, it is possible to learn to relax them "voluntarily."

Relaxing the skeletal muscles will often also initiate some relaxation of the involuntary smooth muscles. It also decreases the level of blood lactate, the most commonly measured fatigue acid, thus contributing to a decrease in feelings of fatigue.

Relaxation breathing enhances the muscle relaxation exercises we'll be describing. Slowing and deepening your breathing makes it easier to let go of muscle tension, although muscular relaxation alone is sufficient to trigger the relaxation response. In fact, breathing techniques principally achieve their effects by reducing muscle tension.

The first step in muscular relaxation is to become aware of those muscles that are chronically tense. Body scanning is the simplest method of getting to know where in your body you are holding on to tension and then releasing some of it.

Exercise: Body Scanning. Sit or lie in a relaxed position. Become aware of your breathing. Allow it to become slow and regular. Use an affirming statement such as "My body is relaxed and becoming more relaxed with each exhalation."

> Starting at your head, scan your body for tense areas. These include locked knees, hunched shoulders, and a held-in stomach that may be preventing you from breathing from the diaphragm. Go very slowly, stopping at each body part where you detect tightness or holding; discover how you can relax that part simply by putting your focused attention there. To release tension even more effectively, imagine breathing fresh, healing air into that part of the body. On the exhalation, breathe out any tension you don't need.
>
> Place your awareness in your forehead. Allow your forehead to relax; imagine it is smooth and serene.
>
> Focus on your eyelids. Let your eyelids relax.
>
> Place your awareness in your jaw. Feel the tension and let it go.
>
> Focus in succession on each part of your body: lips, tongue, neck, shoulders, upper arms, forearms, hands, chest, stomach,

hips, thighs, knees, calves, and feet. If you like, become even more specific, for instance, paying attention to each finger. Alternatively, perform the body-scanning exercise as if your mind was a kind of roving tension sensor, pausing only at the centers of tightness and giving them permission to relax.

Focused awareness and intention effectively releases muscle tension. Remember that you are probably unaware of many of the places you habitually hold tension and that tension often exists in unexpected places.

The first time you do this exercise, take a few minutes to scan your body. Spend only as long as feels comfortable. Gradually increase the amount of time, until you are able to give your entire body a thorough scan. As you become more skilled at locating tension, you should be able to perform an effective body scan in as little as two or three minutes. As you practice this technique, you will become better and better at knowing where your tension is and relaxing it quickly.

Since tense muscles are contracted muscles, it often helps to deliberately elongate or distend these muscles. This involves various stretching exercises. One of the areas where most of us carry a lot of tension is the neck and shoulders. The following three exercises address this area particularly. (Stretching exercises for other muscles are described in detail in chapter 11, ''Essential Exercise.'')

Exercise: Shoulder Rolls. Stand with your feet parallel at a width of 2 feet apart, and with your knees unlocked. Relax your shoulders. Clasp your left wrist with your right hand behind your back.

Rotate your shoulders slowly forward, up, back, and around—a complete rotation—while inhaling very slowly. Do a second shoulder roll while continuing the same inhalation. Still on the same inhalation, do another half-rotation (forward, up).

Relax your shoulders, letting them fall forward and down as you exhale sharply.

(Throughout this technique, your hands remain clasped behind your back.)

Repeat the exercise at least six times. Then reverse direction and repeat the exercise in its entirety.

Exercise: Head Half-Circles. This exercise helps relax the neck muscles, improving blood circulation to the brain. Remember not to force your head around. If you have chronic neck pain, you should consult a physician before attempting this exercise.

Sit comfortably in a chair or stand with knees unlocked, feet parallel and 2 feet apart. Let your shoulders and arms hang relaxed at your sides.

Lower your head forward until it is hanging in a relaxed position. Now slowly rotate it in a half-circle toward the left shoulder, then across toward the right shoulder, while inhaling through the nose. (Don't circle your head back of a vertical position, as this can harm your neck.)

Exhale slowly through the mouth as you continue the circle down to your right shoulder and then slowly back to your chest.

Repeat the half-circle six times to the left. Then reverse direction and do six half-circles to the right.

Do the exercise slowly, and continue it as you feel your neck muscles relax.

The foregoing exercises involved the gentle stretching of tight muscles. The two exercises that follow involve the deliberate contraction of muscles, followed by their release.

Exercise: Stomach Lifts. This exercise works on the skeletal muscles of the abdomen and thus involves the smooth muscles of the colon and reproductive organs. It can help relieve constipation and stimulate bowel function by relaxing chronically tense abdominal muscles (both skeletal and smooth). It will also relieve tension or stiffness in the lower back.

Stand with your feel parallel and about 3 feet apart. Bend your knees, and then bend your whole body forward from the hips, keeping your spine and neck straight. Your back—from your sternum to the top of your head—should form a nice straight line. Place your hands on your thighs just above the knees with the fingers pointing inward. (Keep your shoulders, hands, and arms relaxed.) Look at a spot on the floor 3 feet in front of your toes.

Exhale sharply, emptying your lungs and pushing your stomach out. Holding your breath out, rapidly contract and release your abdominal muscles three to five times. Make each contraction as deep as possible, but perform the sequence at a comfortable rate and level.

Inhale, taking a moment to catch your breath.

Remaining in the same position, exhale sharply and repeat the sequence again. Do the whole exercise three or four times.

As your skill improves, increase the number of stomach lifts performed during each sequence to fifteen or twenty.

Exercise: Progressive Muscle Relaxation. This exercise was developed more than fifty years ago by Dr. Edmund Jacobson, a physiologist-physician. Along with autogenic relaxation, it is one of the two most-used relaxation techniques in the world. It is simply the contraction (tightening) and release in sequence of all the skeletal muscles in your body. This technique trains you to recognize tension when it appears and accustoms you to the sensation of letting go of tight muscles. Until you've experienced the contrast, you don't know what it feels like to be relaxed.

Once you have practiced this technique, you will become adept at noticing tension when it occurs in your body and learn to substitute relaxation immediately.

Lie comfortably on the floor or on a couch or bed. If you prefer, put a cushion under your knees. Except for the part of the body you are tensing deliberately, keep the rest of your body relaxed. Breathe fully and easily throughout the exercise.

1. Begin by slowly bending your fingers and tightening them into fists, squeezing them tighter and tighter. Now hold this and focus your attention on the tightness. Be aware of how it feels. Then release and let the fingers unfold. Notice the difference. Then allow your fingers to become even more relaxed by simply putting your attention on them.

Repeat this segment, this time selectively tensing only the muscles that tighten the fingers. Release.

2. Clench both your fingers and your biceps. Start by tightening your fingers into fists, then bend your arms at the elbows to create tension in your biceps and upper arms. Tighten as much as is comfortably possible (pain is not the purpose). Hold this tension. (Only the muscles of your hands and arms are tight; the rest of your body is as relaxed as possible.) Now release and feel the difference.

Now release even more as you repeat to yourself, "My arms and hands are becoming more and more relaxed."

3. Breathe into your chest as fully and completely as you can. Hold this deep breath. Feel the tension in your chest muscles while the rest of your body remains completely relaxed. Now release and exhale. Feel the difference.

4. On your next inhalation, take the air fully into your belly and abdomen. Hold this abdominal breath. Feel the tightness of your abdominal muscles. As you breathe out and release, let go of all the tension you don't need.

After an easy in-breath, exhale fully, pulling your abdomen in and tightening it as much as you can. Hold. Then selectively tighten the muscles in your abdomen while the rest of your body (including your jaw and your spine muscles) are as relaxed as possible. Now release and resume breathing in a relaxed and even fashion. Feel the tension continue to drain from your body as relaxation spreads throughout your torso.

Your whole body is becoming more and more relaxed.

5. Focus on your shoulders. Without involving any arm muscles, selectively tighten your shoulder muscles as you shrug your shoulders up toward your ears. Hold this position, while the rest of your body, including your face and jaw, is completely relaxed. Keep your breathing slow and easy. Now release your shoulders and feel the difference.

6. Gently arch the small of your back, hold, and release.

7. Tense your legs by flexing your toes toward your face and then pointing them away. Hold. Release.

8. Tighten your face and scalp by frowning while you clench your jaw. Hold. Release.

9. As you continue progressive relaxation, your body is becoming more and more relaxed as your mind becomes more and more focused and awake. Allow this feeling to deepen even more as you silently count down from 10 to 1. By the time you reach 1, you are even more relaxed and calm.

Be aware of how you feel now in every part of your body. You can return to this state whenever you wish. With practice, it becomes easier and easier.

Focus on repeating some simple affirmations. Examples: "I am a good person." "I like myself as I am." "I trust and value others." "I choose health, happiness and well-being." "I love myself and I love others." "I choose success and find satisfying ways of reaching my goals." "I seek the goodness and wisdom within."

10. Enjoy a minute or two of quiet relaxation while your attention is focused on the slow, steady intake of breath at the tip of your nose. When you come back to a more wakeful state, you will possess a sense of well-being and energy that will stay with you throughout the day.

11. Rise up now, like a bubble rising to the surface of a pond, as you count from 1 to 20. By the time you reach 20, you will feel balanced, refreshed, and ready to continue your day.

Exercise: The Shakeout. One of the most delightful of all muscle-relaxation exercises is called the shakeout. It's a wonderful way to start the day or to relax any time you want to "shake out" tension. It simply consists of five to ten minutes of free-form movement to lively music with a strong beat.

Pick some music you like, put it on, and start to move. The more imagination you use and the more parts of your body you involve, the more effective your shakeout will be. It also makes a wonderful loosening-up exercise as preparation for a physical workout.

A good way to start your shakeout is with your feet planted firmly in place while you begin to move other parts of your body in time to the music. Let the notes and the rhythms inspire you. Be sure to get your hips and arms into the act. Wiggle and sway. Twist and shout. Dip and dive. Pretend you're waving to a friend (or to a crowd), swimming up a waterfall, climbing a rope, taking a bow—whatever images pop into your mind.

After a few minutes of moving in place, let your feet start to move you—dance in place or start boogying around the room. Continue to use your whole body, including your head, arms, and hips, as you shake out all tension and stiffness.

Continue your shakeout for five to ten minutes.

Many of our participants found useful ways to incorporate muscle-relaxation techniques in their lives. A nurse who teaches prenatal classes reported that, once she learned that muscular relaxation was good for more than reducing a woman's pain during birthing, she began teaching the same skills to expectant fathers to help them get through the emotional drain of waiting.

A pro-football player (a 280-pound lineman) credited the shakeout technique with allowing him to go back to 20 m.p.h. stress from 90 m.p.h. when he was sitting on the bench. On the sidelines, he'd shake out instead of tensing up. "So by the fourth quarter I just had a lot more energy left for the trenches, to dominate the other guys who had stayed tense for the whole game."

A commodities broker reported that his muscle tension (clenched fists, hunched shoulders as he talked on the phone) was such a sound reverse indicator of the quality of his judgment (that is, when he was tense, he was most likely making a bad decision), that he began taking his tenseness into account in making "intuitive judgment calls." And he started taking a minute to deliberately release muscle tension (he did shoulder rolls with breathing) before making an important decision.

A Technique for Re-evaluating Difficult Situations

No matter how good you become at your chosen relaxation techniques, there will remain certain situations in which you will find it difficult to relax. These situations constitute your leading edge of learning—your most challenging (and potentially rewarding) relaxation opportunities. If you have started your stress diary, you will already have begun to identify a number of them. You get tense thinking about these situations, you overdose on stress during them, and you take hours (or even days) to come down after them. All sorts of recurring situations fall into this difficult category: a worrisome meeting with the boss; a phone call from someone you are afraid of; a speech you've got to give; a problem class you can't seem to get control of; a long-delayed confrontation with your spouse over a long-standing point of conflict.

Exercise: Cognitive Reappraisal. Cognitive reappraisal means rethinking a difficult situation. The technique can be used to confront an immediate crisis, or as an effective method of reappraising the ongoing stressful patterns in any part of your life, with a view to handling them in a less stress-elevating way. It is based on the simple truth that you won't take action to improve your situation unless you clearly and practically recognize the need and the options available.

As we've refined it, this technique involves four simple steps: recognize that you are under stress and identify the cause (that is, the pattern or situation); stop the upward escalation of your stress reaction, use a simple deep-breathing technique; take a second look at the situation and form a plan of action; listen to your own advice—and follow it. You can use this technique to plan for a recurring event, to deal better with an event when it is happening, and to lower your stress level after a distressing experience. Here it is in detail.

Recognize the early warning signs. Once you have identified your stress hierarchy, you will have a pretty clear idea of the peaks in your daily and weekly stress curve and of the kinds of situations to which you react poorly—that get you "upset" or "drive you crazy." Ideally, step 1 means recognizing the signs of stress before you go over the top, before you get so upset that you become ineffective. But even if you have just overdosed on stress, simply recognizing the symptoms, physical and mental, means you can take action to get yourself down quickly and, more important, to defuse such a strong overreaction the next time the situation happens. (Remember: At least 95 percent of your distress comes from situations that happen over and over again.)

Stop the upward escalation of your stress level. Do this by taking an immediate breather: We recommend a quick and effective relaxation breathing technique we call the *Sigh of Relief*. As with all breathing-relaxation techniques, the key to success is the long, slow exhalation of breath, preferably through your nose.

1. Comfortably exhale all the air from your lungs.
2. Slowly fill your lungs with air, right down into your belly and up into your chest.
3. Hold your breath for several seconds, but don't force yourself to hold it longer than feels comfortable.
4. Slowly and comfortably empty all the air from your lungs, breathing out through the nose and allowing any sound—from a sigh to a groan —to come.
5. As you begin the long, slow exhalation, let your shoulders drop into a more relaxed, slumped position. Repeat this several times until you feel more relaxed and clearheaded. Continue relaxation breathing as you do steps 3 and 4.

The above may sound simple, but it can be a real challenge in the midst of an apparent crisis. If you have practiced the basic breathing exercises we described earlier, you will find it much easier to successfully practice the Sigh of Relief in a high-stress situation.

Look at your situation. With your heart beating a bit more slowly and your head somewhat clearer, you are now in a position to take a second look. The more distressed you are, the more likely you are to see your plight in bleak and threatening tones, and to exaggerate its seriousness. Now that you've calmed down a bit, ask yourself the following three basic questions. If you are honest, your answers will further reduce your stress level and put you in better control of the situation. If you have time, write the answers on a piece of paper. (One idea is to carry in your wallet a slip of paper with the questions on them.)

1. *What really is at stake here for me? (What is the worst that could possibly happen?)* This step entails asking yourself questions such as: What do I really stand to lose here? How may I be hurt in this situation? What are the consequences if I do badly here? Above all, be as specific and realistic with yourself as possible about the worst-case scenario. As you do this, you reduce your general nonspecific anxiety to a manageable-sized fear that you can begin to work with. (Since uncertainty is the root cause of most distress, the best antidote is gut-felt information—in this case, about realistic consequences. And this principle holds for all three questions.)

2. *Is there anything I can realistically do to change the situation?* Notice the word "realistic." If you can identify a practical, immediate change that will alter the situation for the better, then make it. Theoretically, any situation can be changed. But this often requires dramatic or extreme measures (jumping up in the middle of a meeting and running out of the room, or walking out on your spouse). If you are not prepared to take such drastic action, then your answer to this question is no. Now you can move on to improving the existing situation in a less radical way. (Some people, notably Worry Warts, believe that if they worry enough, the problem will magically go away. In fact, this approach only makes matters worse by keeping the worry machine going and stress levels wastefully high.)

3. *If this situation does not go the optimal way, what's my plan? Or, How will I deal with that? (Be as specific as possible.)* Lay out your plan—the steps you will take and how they will help you. It's a good idea to write the steps down on a piece of paper, being as clear and specific as possible. (If you are practicing cognitive reappraisal right after a stressful event, step 3 turns into an opportunity to plan for the next similar event.)

Asking yourself these three questions and answering them concretely is the heart of cognitive reappraisal, enabling you to take a second look at a distressful situation—whether it's in the future, happening right now, or in the past. It can help you in an immediate crisis or with a recurring source of stress, because the questions go straight to the cause of most of our stress: uncertainty, not knowing where we stand or how we are going to handle a new or difficult situation. The questions are designed to reduce the level of your uncertainty. When you answer them honestly, they will. When you succeed at this even once, you teach yourself that you can "feel" in control, even in difficult circumstances in which you used to feel powerless. And your unconscious mind learns to look for the positive solution when an involuntary stress reaction begins.

Listen to your own advice about how you are going to deal with the situation. And act on it. (In a developing "crisis," this advice might be as rudimentary as telling yourself to "keep breathing as slowly and fully as possible.")

This is the basic technique of cognitive reappraisal. Many of the people who entered the Body Age Study found it particularly powerful since they had to deal with many "difficult situations" every day.

Here's a typical situation in which cognitive reappraisal can work wonders.

You're on your way to the airport, and you've cut the timing pretty fine. However, you're moving along nicely—there's not too much traffic. Then you run into an unexpected slowdown caused by an accident. Cars are moving at a snail's pace. You're afraid you're going to miss the flight—and a very important meeting. You start to feel aggravated and impatient, feelings which get worse when you change lanes only to fall further behind. Now that self-critical little voice in the back of your head begins to berate you for being so dumb and incompetent to have left so late. Your stress thermostat goes higher. Here's what you do:

Recognize. Yes, it's true. It's very likely that I'll miss the plane, and my stress level sure is up. At this point, catching the plane will be an unexpected bonus.

Stop. Okay, whether or not I make the flight, I'm going to be a wreck (and I may cause one) if I keep on like this. Sigh of Relief. That's better. I'm beginning to see things a little more clearly now.

Look. Ask yourself the three questions:
What is the worst realistic consequence of missing that plane? People may regret being unable to deal with my part of the agenda, but it's not so urgent that it can't be postponed to next month's meeting, or to a conference call later this week. I'll lose a few brownie points with my boss, but the worst realistic consequence is that I'll miss what happens at the meeting and have to arrange for everyone to get a copy of my report. Not such a big deal after all.
Can I change the situation? Well, I could pull off onto the shoulder, lock my car, and run to the airport (it's four miles away). But realistically, there's not much I can do.
What's my plan? Now I can calmly plan my moves on reaching the airport and, if I miss the plane, take steps to inform people I won't be at the meeting.

Listen. How does my plan sound? I think I'm handling this quite well. Am I prepared to act on my advice? Yes.

What, Where and When: A Thumbnail Guide to Relaxation Skills

What Skills to Acquire. Choose at least one technique or a combination of techniques suitable for an *extended period of deep relaxation*—ten or fifteen minutes of relaxation response. These include autogenic relaxation, abdominal breathing, spiral relaxation, counting breaths, repeating the word "calm," and progressive muscle relaxation. If you enjoy using the autogenic relaxation tape, this is really all you need. But if you have at least one other technique, such as abdominal breathing, that you can use when you don't have your tape recorder handy, this will greatly increase your flexibility.

Choose at least one technique you can use to achieve *deep relaxation in a short time*. Once you've practiced for two or three weeks, you will be able to trigger the relaxation response in several minutes. The more familiar you become with a technique, the easier it will be to activate your innate relaxation mechanism. These techniques include abdominal breathing and spiral relaxation.

Choose at least one technique suitable for a *quick relaxation*—no more than sixty seconds. The quickest relaxation of all is the Sigh of Relief we taught as part of cognitive reappraisal. Or you may prefer to design your own quick-relax technique that's a modification of one of your favorite longer techniques. For instance, if you simply slow your breathing and repeat the word "calm" for a minute, you can become much more relaxed right away.

Where and When to Practice Relaxation. The best times for an extended relaxation session are before breakfast, lunch, or dinner. Don't relax right after eating—unless you want to fall asleep—because it's harder to keep your mind awake when you're using energy for digestion.

Use your shorter relaxation skills almost anywhere, anytime. In fact, simply becoming aware of your breathing and slowing it consciously can lower your stress level throughout the day and let you regulate your foot on the stress accelerator.

Caution: While there's nothing wrong with a few relaxation breaths while stopped at a traffic light, don't do a deep relaxation while driving—you could have an accident.

Relax as preparation for sleep, but don't do more than five minutes of relaxation before bed. It will leave you wide awake and full of energy, rather than ready for sleep. If you want to do a relaxation as preparation for sleep, choose a short technique, such as a brief spiral relaxation or a few minutes of abdominal breathing while repeating a word or phrase, such as "I'm ready to fall asleep" or the word "calm."

If you wake up in the middle of the night and can't get back to sleep, change your physical position, and use a short relaxation technique similar to your preparation for sleep. The idea is to focus your mind and slow down your metabolism. Most important, don't fuss and fume because you can't sleep—Speed Freaks and Worry Warts, take note. Accept the possibility that you may be awake another hour, or even until morning. Lie back comfortably and continue doing your favorite relaxation technique. You may well fall asleep, but even if you don't, just staying in a deeply relaxed state will give you almost the same amount of restoration as sleep. Our study participants estimated that they had 80 to 90 percent of their normal energy the day after using this strategy. And sleep-deprivation research indicates that unless you miss a good night's sleep three days running, you won't suffer if you can compensate by using the high level of metabolic efficiency engendered by deep relaxation.

Your relaxation ability will increase as you fit your new skills to appropriate circumstances.

YOUR FOUR-WEEK START-UP PROGRAM

Week 1: Get Ready. Keep a stress diary for a week and identify your priority opportunities for relaxation. Meanwhile, find quiet time to practice one or two relaxation techniques.
Week 2: Take Your First Step. Use your new skills to relax after three distressful events.
Week 3: Build on Your Success. Practice relaxation following three additional events.
Week 4: Consolidate Your Gains. The distressful situations that used to leave you keyed up no longer seem so difficult.

The four-week start-up program for Effective Relaxation is designed to make you an expert at basic relaxation skills and to give you a taste of the immediate difference they can make. If you follow the program, by week 4 you will be able to trigger the relaxation response after only several minutes of deliberate relaxation. And immediately after a high-stress experience, you will be able to "cool down" more quickly than you could in the past. All in all, you will notice the difference your relaxation sessions are making in the way you feel during the day and in how much energy you have.

At the end of this start-up program, you will be ready to add cognitive reappraisal to your basic relaxation repertoire. You will have become adept at lowering your stress levels before, during, and after the most difficult, high-stress situations.

Week 1: Get Ready

Fill out your Action Diary Planning Page. Agree that during the coming week you will introduce the following new behaviors into your life:

1. *Autogenic relaxation plus affirmation and visualization.* Begin this week by setting aside some quiet time to listen to your autogenic tape, at the end of which you will repeat one or two powerful affirmations that express and reinforce your relaxation goals. Follow this by visualizing yourself behaving in a more relaxed way in a high-stress situation. Practice autogenic relaxation at least four times this week. Keep using your affirmations and your visualizations each time you practice autogenic relaxation. Repeat your affirmations daily, preferably two or three times each day.

2. *Begin practicing your relaxation skills.* On at least four different days this first week, spend fifteen to twenty minutes practicing a mix of physical-relaxation skills that appeal to you. If possible, do this during a "quiet time" when you can practice undisturbed and when your stress level is already fairly low. Include among your training techniques at least one that is appropriate for a brief relaxation (no more than five minutes) during a busy or stressful time, and one technique or a combination of techniques that gives you ten to fifteen minutes of deep relaxation.

Although it may on occasion be necessary to "make" the time for your relaxation practice, most of our study participants reported that, when they looked at their schedule, it was more a matter of "finding" the time. There are naturally occurring periods of down time in the course of a week: times when you are waiting, or have "time to kill." These recur four or five times a week quite predictably. For instance, many people use commuting time to relax.

One woman (a Basket Case real estate agent) told us that more often than not her commuter train was at least ten minutes late. So she planned to use this down time to do a spiral relaxation while sitting in the waiting room.

A Speed Freak dentist reported that, depending on his schedule for the day, there were at least three five-minute periods (which he could forecast) when he just killed time (this really bugged him). So he made little ticks on his daily schedule to indicate when he could practice his counting-breaths exercise.

And a busy Drifter executive who traveled a great deal had complained about the stress of "rushing to wait" every time he went to the airport. Then the "light of opportunity went on," as he put it, and he started using these dead half-hours to listen to his autogenic tape on a portable tape player.

3. *Start or continue your stress diary.* For instructions on how to keep a stress diary and a Stress Patterns Record, and how to plot your daily stress level on the Stress Level Scale and Graph, see pages 186–190. Even if you've already kept a seven-day stress diary, continue it this week to refine your personal stress hierarchy further. If you haven't started your diary, start it now.

4. *Check in with your partner.* At some point during the week, arrange to have your partner check with you to see how it's going. He or she may be able to help if you're having some trouble with one of the techniques or be able to recommend a technique that you haven't tried.

5. *Record your progress in your Action Diary.* Each day this week, take the time to keep track of your progress in your Action Diary. Note every time you practice a relaxation skill and when you use your affirmations and visualizations. This week, as your awareness of your stress patterns increases, you will undoubtedly note numerous opportunities for relaxation. If you write these down in the Action Diary, they will help you plan for action in the coming weeks.

Finally, don't forget to give yourself positive feedback for each new bit of relaxation you do and each relaxation opportunity you notice.

Week 2: Take Your First Step

Fill out your Action Diary Planning Page. Agree to do the following during the coming week:

1. *Continue to practice autogenic relaxation with affirmations and visualizations.* Do autogenic relaxation with affirmations and visualizations four times this week, modifying your affirmations and visualizations to reflect your increasing awareness of your relaxation opportunities and goals. In addition, use your affirmations daily, preferably three or more times each day.

2. *Continue to practice relaxation skills.* Keep up your daily practice of your favorite relaxation techniques. This week, add at least one technique appropriate for a very brief relaxation—something you can do in as little as a minute, such as the Sigh of Relief.

3. *Relax after three distressful events.* In week 1, using your stress diary, you identified the situations that repeatedly elevated your stress level. Some of them drive you crazy (overstress), others are tolerable though unpleasant. You organized these into a personal stress hierarchy.

Pick three events in the coming week that you can predict will be moderately distressful. (Your stress hierarchy should have made these clear to you.) Preview them mentally or use paper and pencil. As soon as possible after each of these events, find an opportunity to practice at least five minutes of physical relaxation, using whatever technique or techniques you like.

This may mean shutting the door to your office and holding your calls, or using your coffee break for some calm instead of some caffeine. If you are a salesman who dreads one of your weekly calls on a customer, after the visit take five minutes to relax in your car before you start driving to the next appointment. Or take some relaxation minutes after any of the following: sitting through another meeting you really didn't need to be at, after all; cleaning up something spilled by your four-year-old; finding you've agreed to a request that, if you'd thought about it, you probably would have turned down or negotiated to modify. What you choose depends on the events that are unpleasant, high-stress events for you.

4. *Check in with your partner.* Communicate at least once this week, although more often is better. Perhaps you might even schedule a dinner with your partner so that the two of you can compare notes and congratulate each other on your progress so far. Are you encountering any roadblocks? How did you feel when you relaxed right after a high-stress event?

5. *Record your progress in your Action Diary.*

Here is a sample Action Diary Planning Page for week 2 of Effective Relaxation. Your own planning page should suit your lifestyle and schedule. Find ways to incorporate each specific behavior without major dislocations—and if your self-care contract turns out to be too ambitious, modify it to lower the stress of change. Remember to give each behavior you undertake on this self-care contract the SMART test. Ask yourself whether it is Specific, Measurable, Acceptable, Realistic, and Truthful.

ACTION DIARY FOR WEEK OF March 1st TO March 6th

Planning Page

Affirmations (My self-themes for this week in key words and phrases)

I _am becoming more and more relaxed every day._

I _feel calm and in control, alone and with others_

(Other) _I breathe away stress_

Opportunity Visualizations (I clearly see myself . . .)

I clearly see myself going into the weekly planning meeting calm, cool, and in control. I listen atten- tively to what others have to say, and when I speak, I use a firm, relaxed voice. I can see that people are listening to what I say. All the time I'm aware that my breathing is slow and regular, and that I feel good.

I choose to deepen this Vital Life Skill as follows (My specific behavioral objectives this week)

I choose to _do a fifteen-minute autogenic relaxation followed by affirmation and visualization at least 4 x's during coming week_

Under the following circumstances; _Monday, Wednesday and Friday before dinner (5:30 pm) in the den with the door closed. Sunday before supper_

I choose to _spend fifteen minutes each day this week practicing physical relaxation techniques_

Under the following circumstances; _Monday through Friday on the train commuting to work each morning. Saturday and Sunday before breakfast_

I choose to _relax immediately after three predictable high-stress events this week_

Under the following circumstances: _Wednesday immediately after the morning staff meeting; Friday after driving_ home in rush-hour traffic; Sunday after the morning phone call from my mother.

I choose to *repeat my relaxation affirmations at least once each day this week*

Under the following circumstances: *As soon as I wake up in the morning, before getting out of bed; as soon as I return to my desk after lunch; as soon as I get into bed at night*

My other opportunity situations for skill practice are:

1. *The weekly planning meeting at the office*
2. *When my son comes home late for dinner*
3. *During rush-hour traffic*

I have arranged to check in with my partner . . .

When?	About
On Sunday morning	*How I've done this week and what patterns I've noted in my stress diary*

Week 3: Build on Your Success

Fill out your Action Diary Planning Page. Agree with yourself to do the following during the coming week:

1. *Continue to practice autogenic relaxation with affirmations and visualizations.* Use autogenic relaxation with affirmations and visualizations four times this week. Continue to use your affirmations daily, preferably two or three times a day.

2. *Continue practicing relaxation techniques.* As you practice your favorite techniques, they will become easier and more pleasurable, and you will be able to trigger a deeply relaxed state more quickly.

3. *Relax after three high-stress events*. These can be the same events as in week 2 or different ones. (Consult your personal stress hierarchy of five top-priority, recurring behaviors or situations.)

4. *Check in with your partner*.

5. *Record your progress in your Action Diary*.

Week 4: Consolidate Your Gains.

Fill out your Action Diary Planning Page. Agree to do the following during the coming week:

1. *Continue to use autogenic relaxation with affirmations and visualizations*.

2. *Continue to practice your relaxation techniques*. Keep it simple, successful, and fun. If you want, add a new technique to your repertoire. But the main thing is to refine your ability to relax at will.

3. *Relax after three high-stress events*. If you've been working on the same three recurring events, you've probably noticed that you can relax more quickly now than you could at the start. The events themselves may even seem less stressful, since you know that relief is just around the corner.

4. *Keep in touch with your partner*.

5. *Continue recording your progress in your Action Diary*. As you come to the end of your four-week start-up program, look back over your diary and take pleasure in the progress you've made.

Continuing Your Prescription

You may have noticed that in the four-week start-up program we made no mention of the cognitive reappraisal technique. The purpose of the first four weeks is to get you started, to give you firm grounding in relaxation. With four weeks of practice under your belt, you should be ready to try cognitive reappraisal to change the way you experience a high stress event *while it is happening*.

In the coming weeks, gradually increase the intensity of the situations you are willing to tackle. If you stick with it, eventually there will be no difficult experience you are afraid to "do differently."

As soon as you're ready (the sooner the better), begin phasing in the next intervention in your prescription. We recommend that you wait until week 8, by which time some of your new relaxation skills will have become relaxation habits.

You'll find that your relaxation skills enhance the effectiveness of the other Vital Life Skills. All our study subjects who learned to relax found that this skill spilled over into other areas and interventions. In Terry's case, relaxation was the linchpin that made his whole prescription work. As a Speed Freak (age 39, body age 46) who'd done "nothing but my job since I was 18," he'd felt quite threatened when his Values/Goals Clarification caused him to face the fact that he was doing almost nothing to look after his leisure interests. (Terry's job managing his successful service station kept him working long hours, including nights and week-ends.) After this self-discovery, he experienced several sleepless nights. "It was as if my whole life was nothing more than the numbers adding up on the gas pump," he later commented.

Thanks to the autogenic relaxation tape, Terry was soon able to sleep again. And he was willing to work toward his primary leisure goal: to be assistant coach of a local boys' soccer team he had helped sponsor for five years (he'd been "quite a soccer star" in high school). But to coach would take him away from the station two evenings a week and part of the day on Saturday, a thought that threw him into a panic.

Back to relaxation, this time cognitive reappraisal. Terry rethought his situation and came up with a compromise plan: He would sign up as assistant coach on a month-by-month basis (this gave him an escape clause); he would hire a part-time assistant manager (a semiretired truck driver he'd known for years, not one of the young "rip-off artists" he feared would "take over the station"); and he arranged a way for his stand-in to reach him at the soccer field in an emergency.

Even with all this preparation, it took Terry six months to "get comfortable enough to leave the station at 6 P.M." When he finally did make the move, he found that the breath-counting technique (five minutes prior to leaving) helped him "wash off the job worries along with the grease." He also found strength in his affirmations ("I run a tight ship" and "The station works for me") and his visualizations (seeing a kid's face after making a great play and shaking hands with proud parents). In sum, Terry reported that "the ability to relax was the key that unchained me from the pumps. I knew there was more to life, but couldn't get free to do anything about it."

At his eight-month checkup, Terry tested 10 years younger, with a body age of 36—below his calendar age by 3 years. And he asked us to help him design a relaxation program for young athletes. He'd noticed that his best players were "those who can keep their cool on and off the field." Meanwhile, he was preparing for next season.

CHAPTER 10
Self-Affirming Communication (For More Rewarding Relationships)

PRIMARY INTERVENTION FOR: Drifter
SECONDARY INTERVENTION FOR: Loner

Core Message

When boiled down to its essence, self-affirming communication means having the courage to reveal to others who you are and what you want.

Effective communication is an essential interpersonal skill that is at the root of all satisfying relationships.

Communication is a two-way street: It means both expressing yourself assertively and listening actively.

Most of us have many self-defeating communication behaviors or styles. These can be replaced by self-affirming communication skills.

Most stress-energy inefficiency stems from feelings of uncertainty, powerlessness, and lack of control. And nowhere (except in internal self-talk) are these feelings more acutely felt than in the realm of interpersonal relationships, whether with the members of your immediate family or with co-workers or strangers. It is hardly surprising that among our study subjects, relationship malnutrition was a major contributor to accelerated aging, and a particularly significant strain for the Loner and the Drifter.

As we pointed out in chapter 6, "Write Your Own Prescription," common sense suggests that working on relationships would be the most effective place for the Loner prescription to start. In fact, Loners usually don't see "any reason for bothering" to work in this area. These are people who say things like, "I don't need people anymore: I have my cat (my dog?), my books (my drugs?)." Becoming clearer about the valued experiences that can only be achieved with others motivates them to take action. For the Drifter—for whom Values/Goals Clarification would seem to be a first priority—taking action to improve relationships turned out to be a necessary prelude to effectively getting in touch with his or her underlying goals and values. This is because core values become more immediate and gut-felt in the context of close relationships. In other words, the Drifter must first be caught up in more involving relationships that lead to greater clarity about what he wants and values. For both these types, Self-Affirming Communication is a very important intervention that will work potently to reduce body age and increase vitality.

Self-Affirming Communication gains effectiveness in combination with other interventions in your prescription. Both the Drifter and Loner prescriptions include Effective Relaxation, as well as Values/Goals Clarification. The latter is almost symbiotically related to this Vital Life Skill. Closing the values gap between the real self and the ideal self makes honest communication easier because you feel you have less to hide. Equally important, Self-Affirming Communication is possibly the most powerful concrete expression of your values and goals.

In this chapter, you will learn the basic techniques of what is often called assertive communication as the key to more satisfying relationships. If you've already taken a course in "assertiveness training," "assertive communication," or "effective listening," you will likely find much familiar material here. Perhaps you are already practicing some of the techniques we describe. Use this chapter as a chance to refine your skills and to fill in the gaps in your repertoire of effective communicating techniques. What we add to conventional approaches is the use of autogenic relaxation with affirmations and visualizations, and the fact that we don't teach this Vital Life Skill in isolation but as part of a comprehensive, interactive prescription for change.

In its most essential form, self-affirming, or assertive, communication simply means asserting your *self* during communication with another person. It emphasizes the confident putting forward of your needs, opinions, claims, and rights. Assertive communication means the direct communication of your wishes while remaining sensitive to another person's feelings and position—it's a balance between speaking and listening, between sending and receiving. It means that you take responsibility for your feelings and that you let others know how you feel. The effect of this kind of communication is to affirm and reinforce the self, while reducing uncertainty—both yours and the other person's. Those actions add up to a feeling of power and self-control that produces much lower levels of stress. You can build the specific assertive-communication skills we discuss in the "Basic Training" section into your daily behavior to put you more and more frequently in the active center of your communication, not off on the sidelines.

The benefits of self-affirming communication are considerable. Since relationships are the biggest source of uncertainty in most people's lives, improving your communication dramatically reduces uncertainty and stress levels.

Self-Affirming Communication helps you clear away the obstacles and encumbrances that often make communication so difficult. It helps you reveal yourself to another person. It permits you to suspend momentarily the priority of your own reality, so that you can experience the reality of the other without losing a clear sense of your own boundaries. There's a wonderful scene in Harper Lee's *To Kill a Mockingbird* when Atticus explains to his young daughter, Scout, the essence of his philosophy of human relations. He tells her, "You never really understand a person until you consider things from his point of view . . . until you climb into his skin and walk around in it." This is the ultimate test of Self-Affirming Communication: to be able to know and assert your self while respecting and embracing the reality of the other person.

As you gain skill at communicating, you will experience fewer interpersonal problems and improved relationships at all levels, until real intimacy becomes possible. You'll become more at ease with your emotions, and you'll be more effective at work, as well as happier in more personal environments.

The example of Bill, a 48-year-old psychiatrist who entered the program with a body age of 61, shows clearly how communication and Values/Goals Clarification work together so powerfully. He had been in professional psychiatric practice for more than twenty years and was one of the most extreme Drifter-Loners we've ever seen. When he finally began to open up, he described himself as "totally cut off, trapped between the unreal and the unmotivating. I fly that [patient's] couch eight hours a day, year after year, knowing I can't relate in a fully real two-way relationship with my patients, and at the same time I find most nonpatients to be incredibly boring. I just don't make any effort with friends and colleagues. I know I should try, but it seems so artificial when I do."

Bill was a very good listener, a fact that made him a very good therapist. But like so many "service professionals," he felt phony applying his listening skills in "real relationships" in the "real world," even with his wife. It was only as he got in touch with his core values, which included the strong desire to have close friends, that he saw how he was killing himself through lack of self-expression in his nonwork life. He began to invite acquaintances he liked to his farm outside the city and consciously set about treating them as friends, using his considerable communicating skills. He explored how his hundred acres could help his new friends enjoy and express themselves. He created an environment in which friendship and openness were the norm. For the first time in years, he felt that he had real soul mates, not just intimate patients and distant acquaintances. He didn't feel phony at all. At his eight-month checkup, Bill's body age was down to 48, the same as his calendar age and an impressive gain of 13 biological years.

RATE YOURSELF

In this section, you will discover the following:

> Your current communication skills
> Your self-defeating (vitality-draining) communication styles
> Your opportunities for more self-affirming, energy-conserving communication
> Your communication affirmations and visualizations.

Effective communication requires a balance of listening skills and skills for expressing yourself. In the exercises that follow, you'll be assessing yourself in both of these fundamentals.

Your Assertiveness Checkup

Rate yourself on each of the items below, using this rating scale: 1—never; 2—rarely; 3—sometimes; 4—often; 5—always.

_____I trust my own judgment.
_____I can get in touch with my own real feelings, even in difficult situations.
_____If it's important, I let others know what I'm feeling.
_____When I disagree with someone, I express my disagreement to them.
_____If I think someone is being highly unfair, I bring it to their attention.
_____I openly object if someone interrupts me when I'm speaking.

_____When someone butts in front of my place in line, I tell them I don't like it.

_____I return substandard merchandise for repair or replacement.

_____I am not easily swayed from what I think is right.

_____I am forthright in my views.

_____I don't do something just to go along with the crowd.

_____When someone tries to manipulate me, I don't let them get away with it.

_____My actions reflect my own best judgment.

_____I don't mind rocking the boat when I disagree with someone.

_____I expect and, when necessary, insist that my landlord (repairman, mechanic, etc.) live up to his responsibilities in our relationship.

_____When someone is late in returning something they have borrowed from me, I mention it to them.

_____If I feel there is a problem building up in a relationship, I tell the other person about my feelings and ideas.

_____I feel comfortable expecting—and, when necessary, insisting— that my spouse or roommate do his or her share of household chores.

_____If I think I'm being asked to do more than I possibly can at work, I say so.

_____If the food or service in a restaurant does not meet with reasonable standards, I ask for better.

_____I'm not hesitant to ask for help when I need it.

_____I avoid outbursts of temper as a means to get my way.

_____I am not the kind of person to be sucked into doing something I don't want to do.

_____Making decisions is easy for me.

_____I like being with people I don't know in new situations.

_____If someone watches me at work, I still remain focused and comfortable.

_____I am confident and comfortable when I speak in a public discussion or debate.

_____I find eye contact easy to maintain in conversation, when speaking and when spoken to.

_____I am able to get my ideas across and make myself clearly understood.

_____I'm the kind of person others can count on for a straight-from-the-shoulder opinion.

_____Total Score

Have you been self-assertive enough to answer the questionnaire honestly? Or have you given the nonassertive "socially appropriate" responses? A perfect score on your assertiveness checkup is 150. If you scored 115 or higher, you can congratulate yourself and turn to another intervention chapter, since you already are practicing assertive communication in a significant way. In all likelihood, however, your score was well below 115. Drifters and Loners generally score well below 100, which is an average assertiveness score.

Go back over the questionnaire, paying particular attention to those items on which you scored 3 or lower. Consider how you "lose yourself" through these behaviors and attitudes. Start to imagine ways in which you could play these scenes differently, with yourself at center stage. Already you are beginning to zero in on areas for action. The next two exercises will allow you to focus these still further.

How Well Do You Listen?

Test your listening ability by answering yes or no to the following:

_____Science says you think four times faster than a person usually talks to you. Do you use this excess time to turn your thoughts elsewhere while you are keeping track of the conversation?

_____Do you listen primarily for facts, rather than ideas, when someone is talking?

_____Do certain words, phrases, or ideas so prejudice you against a speaker that you cannot listen objectively to what is being said?

_____When you are puzzled or annoyed by what someone says, do you try to get the matter straightened out immediately, either in your own mind or by interrupting the speaker?

_____If you feel that it would take too much time and effort to understand something, do you go out of your way to avoid hearing it?

_____Do you deliberately turn your thoughts to other subjects when you believe a speaker will have nothing particularly interesting to say?

_____Can you tell by a person's appearance and delivery that he won't have anything to say?

_____When somebody is talking to you, do you try to make him think you're paying attention when you're not?

_____When you're listening to someone, are you easily distracted by outside sights and sounds?

_____If you want to remember what someone is saying, do you think it is a good idea to write it down as he goes along?

If you have answered "yes" to any of these questions, then there are some ways in which you can improve your listening skills. Ponder these questions and think about the situations or people that seem to give you listening trouble. Imagine ways you could listen more effectively at these times.

Checklist of Self-Defeating Communication Styles

Unproductive stress often results from communication styles that people have developed and practiced over the years, usually in order to avoid dealing with feelings, their own and those of other people. Some of the most destructive, self-defeating communication styles are described below. Which do you practice in your relationships? Which would you like to change?

The Elusive Butterfly. The butterfly refuses to fight. When a conflict arises, he flits out of reach—by falling asleep, pretending to be busy, leaving the room, or making a joke. He is a notorious subject changer, never allowing a sensitive issue to be explored. Because this practiced avoider won't respond or fight back, it's very difficult for his partner to express feelings or to pin down just what he's feeling—about anything.

The Marshmallow. Not only does he refuse to face up to a conflict, he pretends there's nothing wrong at all: "I'm okay, really" is his response to an expression of genuine concern. This pose leads to deepened feelings of guilt and resentment from the other person. It's a bit like talking to someone who isn't there.

The Martyr (also known as the Jewish Mother). The martyr tries to get his partner to change by making him feel responsible for causing pain, rather than by coming right out with his true feelings of disapproval or nonacceptance. A typical martyr statement is: "It's okay, don't worry about me," delivered in a hopeless tone of voice and often followed by a big sigh.

The Therapist. Instead of allowing the other person to directly express his real feelings fully, the therapist launches into a detailed character analysis, explaining what's really bothering the other person and the reasons why. This makes it unlikely that either partner will get his feelings directly or fully on the table.

The Sucker Shooter. A master of misdirection, the sucker shooter sets up a "desired" behavior for his partner. Then when it's met, he attacks the very thing he requested. In response to a line such as, "Let's be totally honest and open with each other," the sucker shooter's partner gets conned into sharing his deepest feelings only to have them attacked as unacceptable.

The Sneaky Critic. This type drops all kinds of hints that he doesn't approve of something, but he never comes out and says it. If he doesn't approve of how much money his partner is spending, he says, "Gee, I didn't know we had any money left over in our budget this month" or "How much did that cost? It looks expensive." His criticism is always just below the surface, never fully expressed and never dealt with.

The Time Bomb. This person hardly ever shows the resentments he feels. Instead, he saves them up until his big and small gripes have reached critical mass. Then he explodes—usually at some insignificant provocation—and overwhelms his unsuspecting partner.

The Guerrilla Fighter. Instead of directly stating his frustrations or anger, he nibbles away at his partner in a hundred small, irritating ways. Perhaps he leaves the sink dirty, or "forgets" to pick up the laundry, or turns the stereo up too loud, or arrives late for an important date, or clips his fingernails in bed. His weapons are endless.

The Good Humor Man. He avoids conflict—or genuine contact— with another person by joking or kidding around whenever things get personal or serious. He thus manages to fend off and devalue the expression of serious feelings.

The Kidney Puncher. We all have our tender spots, areas of our personalities that just shouldn't be touched, for example, something about our past behavior, our appearance, or a previous relationship. The kidney puncher uses this knowledge to "get even" with his partner (or a co-worker or friend). Such behavior not only eliminates the possibility for adult, constructive discussion of the issue, it can also permanently damage a relationship.

The Nit-Picker. The nit-picker picks on petty details as a way of derailing discussion of the big picture or the real issue. If there is any kind of contract between two people, this type will focus on the fine print and use any small departure from this agreement as grounds for ending the argument, or the relationship. He sounds something like this: "It's your job to wash the dishes (to think this way; to feel that way). That's what we originally agreed. Otherwise our contract is totally over."

The Kitchen Sink Fighter. In an argument, this type will bring up any and every topic or perspective possible, no matter how irrelevant. This keeps his opponent off balance and the discussion unfocused.

The Withholder. "Not tonight, dear" could be the motto for this type, who indirectly attacks and punishes his partner by witholding some rewarding behavior, whether cooking, sex, approval, or laughing at a joke. This withholding is done instead of expressing anger or hurt honestly and directly.

The Saboteur. This type "gets" or gets back at his partner by placing all sorts of land mines in his path. He may encourage others to misunderstand, ridicule, attack, or discount what his partner has to say. Or he may simply fail to come to his partner's defense when needed.

Identify Your Communication Opportunities

From the styles listed above, make a list of your top five self-defeating behaviors. Under each one, list the two or three key situations in which each of these behaviors most frequently emerges. Are certain people repeatedly involved? Go back over the list to identify those behaviors and those situations that occur at least once and probably several times a week. Consider how in each of those situations you could behave in a more self-assertive way, if you had the gumption. Note which of those situations currently seem to you to be too difficult to tackle, and which appear possible to change.

Look back over the lists in "Your Assertiveness Checkup" and "How Well Do You Listen," to see if they suggest any communication opportunities you want to add.

Now identify your top five opportunities to communicate better. At the top of the list, place those situations and behaviors that occur frequently and that you feel capable of changing: Your hierarchy is thus a list of priorities based on both doability and potential benefit. As you move down the list, the items will be more challenging. If you need help in creating this hierarchy, use the following method:

Assign a frequency level to each communication opportunity based on a 1-through-5 rating system (1 = never; 5 = all the time). There will obviously be no 1s, since a "never" wouldn't have made your short list.

Assign a severity level to each item. Again use a scale of 1 through 5 (1 = a small irritant or roadblock; 5 = a very self-defeating behavior).

Assign each communication opportunity a "chances of changing" rating on a scale of 1 through 5 (1 = impossible; 3 = medium difficult; 5 = easy).

Multiply these three numbers together. The numbers that

result provide your hierarchy rankings. The higher the score, the more important yet possible it is for you to change, and the greater will be the payoff from your action. Thus your high scores are your top priorities. Tackle the important, yet doable, things first.

RANK YOUR COMMUNICATION OPPORTUNITIES
(SAMPLE SCORE SHEET)

Opportunity	Frequency		Severity		Chance of Change		Priority Level
#1	3	×	5	×	1	=	15
#2	4	×	3	×	3	=	36
#3	5	×	2	×	1	=	10
#4	3	×	3	×	5	=	45
#5	2	×	3	×	4	=	24

The chart provides a brief example of how this method was used by one of our study subjects. June, who saw her main communication problem as "not setting limits" and "being a door mat," had become upset with her inability to say no to her kids (item #4 on the sample score sheet). This happened with moderate frequency (a rating of 3), affected her quite severely (3), and was almost completely under her control (5), yielding a priority level of 45. However, when June ranked her communication opportunities, she disregarded this highest-yield opportunity, and decided instead to focus on the situation that bugged her the most (severity rating 5): her boss, "who never lets me finish a sentence—who talks over me all the time." Her scoring for this item (#1 on the sample sheet) was: frequency, 3; stress severity, 5; chance of change, 1. In other words, given her position (his subordinate) and his personality, this opportunity for communicating better was a very tough one. So June wasted a lot of stress in telling herself, "There must be something I can do about my boss," when there wasn't. Meanwhile, the golden opportunity to communicate better with her kids went untouched.

Once you've calculated the priority level for each of your top five communication opportunities, list them in order of priority.

Develop Your Self-Assertive Affirmations and Visualizations

You now should have a good sense of some specific opportunities to communicate more effectively. The skills you'll learn in the next section

will help you do this. This awareness will help you to develop the affirmations and visualizations that capture and express the major themes of
self-assertion for your four-week start-up program.

Here are some sample affirmations:

> I respect myself and others.
> My rights are important.
> My voice is calm and clear.
> I am sensitive to the needs of others.
> I listen actively and give clear feedback.
> I express my emotions easily.

Here are some sample visualizations:

> You and a significant other engaged in lively two-way
>   communication
> Hugging your wife and kids
> Setting limits on the telephone
> Receiving a handshake and smile after a boardroom pre-
>   sentation
> Responding constructively to a frequent critic
> Keeping eye contact with someone who intimidates you
> A past situation in which you and the others involved call
>   on the assertive communication resources you each
>   need

One of our study subjects was a small-town minister who loved every
aspect of his job except the Sunday sermon. He developed this affirmation:
"God's love shapes my words," and combined it with the following
visualization: "I see myself shaking hands at the back of the church after
the service, and the warmth in each hand that touches mine is appreciation
for the love and warmth I brought to my sermon."

Once you've developed your affirmations and visualizations, you are
ready to take action to improve your relationships by introducing assertive
communication into your life.

BASIC TRAINING

Understanding Self-Affirming Communication

Have you ever had a friend with whom you experienced real rapport
—a soul mate, a bosom buddy, a spiritual sister, a blood brother? Recall

what it is like to be with this person, particularly what it is like to communicate with him or her. Here are some of the things you might remember: This other person is always interested in what you have to say and makes you feel as though you are heard and understood. You feel no need to impress, to dominate the dialogue. You find it easy to listen to this other person without your mind wandering or wondering about what you'll say next. While you aren't afraid to interrupt, and you don't mind being interrupted, you don't find yourself doing either often. There's an easy conversational ebb and flow. You don't give speeches to each other. When you are with this person, you feel trust and give trust. When the conversation is over, you feel a genuine sense of completion. Underlying everything is your solid sense of self-esteem: You like yourself when you're with this person.

If you reflect on what is different or special about your interaction with this person, you may become aware that you communicate your inner thoughts and feelings, as well as mere words; that you are able to expose yourself without feeling weak; that your defenses are down because you don't need them.

This is what it is like to experience self-affirming or assertive communication. And it doesn't have to be reserved for your close friends and loved ones. There is no reason why you shouldn't be able to get more and give more in all your relationships. However, the more significant the person, the more powerful the relationship as a potential stressor—or, conversely, as a potential stress-reducing source of emotional support. It has been said that communicating is a form of caring. At its best, it is an act of love.

This talk of lowering your defenses and exposing your feelings may well have you squirming in your chair. There's a huge resistance in our culture to emotional openness: We equate it with weakness, particularly in men. But it takes a lot of energy to be always on the defensive, and a defensive posture promotes a similar posture in others. Ironically, the more you are willing to reveal your emotions and to be honest with another person, the more self-control and sense of personal power you will experience.

But don't just take our word for it. There are numerous assertive-communication skills, and we invite you to experiment with them to see what works for you.

Communicating Your Self. Do you know the real you? Does anyone else? Or are you hiding behind an elaborately constructed parapet of protective, "self-denying," self-diminishing behaviors? Behavior that denies who you are saps your confidence and contributes to high stress levels (it takes a lot of energy to keep the "real" you in check). Nowhere are these truths more evident than in the realm of relationships.

Your communication style is the key to the kind of relationship you have. And how you communicate determines the quality of your relationships. Many people "lose themselves" in interpersonal situations. They lose touch with the well-balanced, confident part of themselves. Instead they become caught up in what is going on "out there" at the expense of their own needs and values. This is particularly true for people who seek satisfaction in a constant attempt to please others. Clear and honest communication (which is, at root, what assertive communication is) can affirm your sense of self even in the most trying circumstances. If you've just missed getting a job you really wanted or just lost out on an Olympic gold medal by a fraction of a second, you could be hard on yourself ("I've failed," "If only I'd trained harder," "I'm a bad person," "I'm not as good as other people," "Others will think poorly of me") or you could turn rejection into self-affirmation ("I came close. I have achieved my personal best ever").

The solidity of your sense of self—your self-esteem—is the foundation of the way you communicate. (One gauge of this is how quickly you bounce back after hurt, rejection, disappointment, or failure.) And sound communication solidifies your sense of who you are. When you fail to assert your rights or exercise your responsibilities in interactions with other people, you start to feel powerless. When you fail to empathize with the other person's position, they feel powerless, and you feel detached and disengaged. This sense of weakness increases feelings of uncertainty on both sides, uncertainty already heightened by unclear or ambiguous messages. And, as we've pointed out before, uncertainty is the root cause of most modern stress.

When Communication Breaks Down. The sorts of questions you probably ask yourself when communication is going wrong are: Where do I stand? How will this turn out for me? What can I do to escape this situation unscathed? What does this person want from me? The posing of such questions is a fruitless, wheel-spinning mental exercise. It feeds the cycle of communication breakdown.

It takes two to tango, and it takes two to communicate. (The minute a third person comes into the room, things become even more complicated.) For starters, language is a terribly imprecise tool of communication. The 500 most frequently used words in English have a total of 14,000 dictionary definitions. For another thing, even within a fairly homogeneous culture, body language and other physical factors are open to many different interpretations. (For example, depending on who you are and how you are feeling at the moment, the person who leans toward you as you speak may appear either attentive or threatening.) In addition, the sender may be unsure of his message, unclear himself about what he wants to say or afraid to reveal his true feelings.

The receiver, or listener, must decipher the content of the words and interpret the context in which they are presented. Among the things he must "hear" are facts, feelings, intents, motivations, patterns, tone, tempo, body posture, and eye contact. To make matters worse, the receiver may also be uncertain of his position, unsure of himself in the interaction, or distracted by other thoughts, or time pressures, or aches and pains, or he may be uncomfortable expressing his own thoughts and feelings. He may have prejudices, preconceptions, or fears that interfere with his ability to concentrate—to hear what the other person is saying. In addition, you can think about four times as fast as you can speak (about 100 to 200 words a minute). This fact gives the receiver lots of time to think of something other than what the speaker has to say, and makes listening well especially difficult.

Communication breaks down in so many ways that it would be possible to fill this whole chapter with examples. When people of differing cultures encounter each other, the potential for misunderstanding is even greater. This is what happened to Lisa, a 38-year-old X-ray technician who entered the program with a body age of 44.

Lisa, a Basket Case, was a recent immigrant from Yugoslavia, a society in which physical touching is an accepted part of even the most casual conversation. Although this trait seemed to put her patients at ease in the sterile clinic setting, it made her WASP boss very uncomfortable, or so she hypothesized as a result of the Institute training sessions. He seemed to avoid her in all one-on-one situations and was becoming increasingly distant.

Lisa determined to test out her theory. She asked several co-workers about her "too much touching" hypothesis, and they confirmed they'd noticed how it affected the boss—in fact, it made them uneasy, too. Lisa had now received some enormously important feedback about the way she was undermining her communication with her co-workers. She began experimenting with a "more North American" touching style. Since touching was so automatic for her, she gave herself these guidelines: "No touching at work unless the person is a friend" and "If I do it inadvertently, I explain (not apologize) in a low-key way about my cultural background." (At her eight-month checkup, Lisa reported that her boss had just promoted her, making the following comment: "Lisa, earlier this year I really didn't think you were going to work out here. But now I'm sure I've made the right choice in making you shift supervisor."

Expressing feelings (the emotional part of your inner self) is essential to effective communication, but in our society, the expression of emotion is difficult for many people. Children who have never communicated their love to a parent who has died are often wracked with guilt. And how many of us have held back anger or tears? Or even laughter? Depression is often described as anger turned inward, a failure to express pent-up aggression. When strong feelings are left unexpressed over a long period of time, they become chronic stressors and are unquestionably a factor in physical illness. Some researchers believe that asthma attacks are connected to the earliest efforts by an infant to cry for its mother. Tension headaches are in many cases the result of difficulties in expressing pent-up anger. Eczema and other skin rashes may be related to a failure to communicate feelings of inadequacy and inferiority. Indeed, many physical symptoms may be viewed as the body's attempt to communicate when verbal communication has failed.

Self-Defeating Habits of Communication. Before you read any further, try the following "sabotage" game. It's designed to make you aware of just how skilled you can be at self-defeating communication.

> Your mission, should you choose to accept it, is to go out and sabotage a conversation. (We suggest you pick as your victim someone who will likely forgive you afterward.) During this conversation, see how often you can do some or all of the following: interrupt (inappropriately); argue (just for the sake of arguing); misinterpret (deliberately misunderstand); laugh when something isn't funny; change the subject for no reason; let your mind wander; inject distracting humor; look at the ceiling; become wrapped up in a pointless story or digression. Start a sentence with "Yes, but . . ." or "Well, you have a point, but . . ." Pick techniques you already use and exaggerate them (you should be more aware of these now that you've completed the "Rate Yourself" section). Note: Arguing and repeating yourself are the two most common self-defeating communication habits. (If this sabotage game seems too difficult, simply turn yourself into an observer of the sabotage games other people play.)
>
> During and after this act of deliberate sabotage, how do you feel? How is the other person handling it? Afterward, ask yourself what you got out of this behavior? Is any of it familiar?

If nothing else, this game shows that communicating well is difficult, given the number of pitfalls and obstacles you can put in your own way or in the way of others.

The Interpersonal Stress Cycle. Your communication style is probably mostly outside your awareness. What you notice when communication goes wrong are feelings of inadequacy, passivity, powerlessness, resentment, or anger. You may literally feel lost, confused, "hot under the collar,'' or ''sick to your stomach,'' you may think that the other person is a ''pain in the neck'' or find yourself ''getting cold feet.'' Most of us have fallen into at least some bad communication habits. Identifying these habits and the circumstances that trigger them is a first step toward replacing them with positive, self-affirming communication skills.

One of the most common subversive communication styles is to express yourself in an overinclusive, or too general, fashion. If, at the end of a hard day at the office, you exclaim, ''I hate this place,'' the people within earshot may assume you're angry with them, when you aren't. Bad communication has just taken place, potentially harming your relationships with your co-workers. If, on the other hand, you'd been more personal and specific—as in, ''I'm so frustrated. The phone hasn't stopped ringing, and I haven't managed to spend even five minutes on the report that's due tomorrow''—you might have found sympathy and received helpful feedback and even some support. This type of overinclusiveness or overgenerality is most typically found in arguments between spouses. How often have you said to your partner something like the following? ''You don't care about my feelings, just your own.'' Such an overgeneralized broadside usually disguises a specific, legitimate grievance—along with some genuinely unpleasant feelings. Perhaps what you really meant to say was something such as: ''When you made that joke last night in front of our guests, I felt hurt and embarrassed. I was thinking perhaps you were discounting what I had to say.''

The interpersonal stress cycle pictured on the next page shows how we typically fall into these self-defeating traps. It is a revolving cycle of conflict, which leads to anxiety, which leads to anger or withdrawal, which leads to loss of self-esteem, which leads to greater conflict, and so on around the cycle. It summarizes how we lose track of ourselves in interactions with other people.

This repetitive behavior pattern represents one possible way in which you respond to another person (a source of uncertainty) in your environment. It characterizes the potential for distress in all relationships. If you tend to get trapped in this cycle, relaxation techniques can help you communicate better by reducing your urge either to withdraw or to make matters worse by blowing your top.

Imagine entering into a situation in which there is potential conflict with another person. Suppose you have a meeting with one of your subordinates to go over his or her job performance. The person in question has frequently been absent from work, and his performance has been below par. Your goal is to get him to pull up his socks, become more responsible, and perform better. To do this, you know you have to communicate your perceptions of his shortcomings: You assume you have to give him a negative performance appraisal. When the fellow walks into

THE INTERPERSONAL STRESS CYCLE

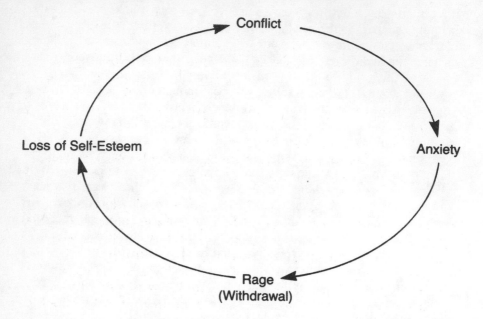

your office, you can immediately feel yourself become tense and uncomfortable (the anxiety stage). And, if you have a self-defeating communication style, this is where you go off track.

The interview passes amiably but you try so hard to be nice—this in itself raises your stress level—and to couch your criticism in pleasant tones and terms, that when the guy leaves you realize you have failed to communicate your very simple message: His work is not up to par, and he had better shape up fast. You are probably now blaming yourself, as well as feeling anger at your subordinate. You feel like a failure. As a result, more serious conflict with this employee is almost inevitable. The next time, you may dump all over him unfairly. As well, you will be walking around with a great deal of bottled-up anger that will likely be felt by people in your environment who don't deserve it.

The best time to break the cycle is the point at which you start to feel anxiety. This is when all sorts of irrational beliefs interfere with clear communication. These beliefs, which lead to rage and withdrawal, were originally identified by Albert Ellis, the creator of rational-emotive therapy. They can be boiled down to the following ten:

1. I must always be in control of every situation.
2. I must always appear strong and sure of myself.
3. I must always strive to accomplish more.

4. I must always be right.
5. I have to be liked and receive approval from everyone all of the time.
6. If I refuse a legitimate request, then I am selfish or wrong.
7. If I ask questions or make statements in a situation in which I am not sure of myself, I will appear ignorant.
8. I am not okay when I make mistakes.
9. It's not all right for me to express anger at anyone else or for them to be angry at me.
10. If I assert myself and your feelings are hurt, then I am bad and responsible for hurting you.

In the above example, the boss was clearly operating under irrational beliefs number 5 and 10. Most of you could probably go through the list and imagine a scene from your life that demonstrates each one, either in your own behavior or that of someone you know. Most people find that they use numbers 3 and 4 most often. Each of these ten basic irrational beliefs is a form of defeatist self-talk that leads to uncertainty, withdrawal, and loss of self-esteem, which in turn leads inevitably to greater conflict and still higher stress levels.

People who adhere to these irrational beliefs inevitably become adept at conversational sabotage. If you tried the sabotage experiment, you may have used some or all of the following nine self-defeating communication techniques. All are based on irrational beliefs and unreasonable generalizations; all of them diminish trust and decrease rapport. How many of them are part of your regular arsenal, especially when the communication is with someone significant about something important to you?

Giving advice (playing the parent instead of the equal adult). We all know people who prefer to tell us how to solve our problems rather than listening to what we have to say.

Changing the subject (are you really trying covertly to manipulate the situation?). For example, "You know, I think what you're talking about is even clearer in a situation that happened before you started working here."

Discouraging strong feelings (so what are you afraid of?). For example, "Let's just stay with the cold, hard facts. Okay?"

Commiserating (sympathy without empathy brings no insight). For example: "Oh, you poor thing," often said while looking off in another direction.

Suggesting without listening (''If I were you, I'd . . .''), also known as trying to problem-solve prematurely. Before you can arrive at a solution, you both need to air your views (thoughts, ideas) and feelings. Impatience with the communication process betrays your insecurity: What's your hurry? What have you got to lose? Many people are quick to offer solutions to other people's problems without really hearing the feelings involved. When this happens, the other person is likely to resent being misunderstood and to start to feel hurt or angry.

Arguing a point (what are you really gaining by arguing? are you getting any closer to mutual understanding?). Ask yourself what the likelihood is of your actually changing the other person's opinion. Aren't you really just pushing them away instead of giving them a full hearing? Are you arguing for some purpose or do you assume (were you once taught?) that disagreeing makes you seem more intelligent than agreeing? Arguing focuses attention on information and often obscures the real subject: the arguer's upset feelings.

Inappropriate joking (favored by the escape artist). Notice how this deflates emotion and distracts from the actual subject, which might be the speaker's real feelings.

Discounting or devaluing the truth, as in the phrases ''Yes, but . . .'' and ''Well, but . . .'' (this type of comment can easily hurt another person's feelings). The person who reassures you that your concern isn't really so serious discounts you, along with your problem.

One-upping (so this is a competition?). This is the art of moving the focus of attention from the speaker to yourself. Often this is done in the guise of empathy for what the speaker has to say; sometimes it is more blatantly selfish. Either way, it discounts the other person's experience completely. For example, ''Oh, that reminds me of the time I was . . .'' or ''I just had a very similar thing happen to me.'' Often it causes the listener to lose interest.

The Three Types of Aggressive Communication. Imagine yourself standing in a line in a department store waiting to be served. Just as you are about to get your turn, another customer barges in front of you. When the salesperson asks, ''Who's next?'' you immediately angrily chew out both the pushy interloper and the sales clerk. A shouting match ensues. But you've made your point and held your ground. You've been assertive—or have you?

Many people confuse assertive communication with hostile or aggressive behavior. In fact, assertive communication actually makes life easier by sharply reducing grounds for misunderstanding while increasing your sense of self-respect and control (both of yourself and the situation) and so moderating your own stress level.

In the above example, the person was actually being aggressive, not assertive. You can think of aggression as any act that deliberately invades another person's "space" or "turf." The assertive response would have been something like the following: in a firm voice to have said "I'm next," indicating to the sales clerk what you wished to buy. The non-assertive (passive, withdrawing) response would have been to boil inwardly, saying nothing.

Aggressive behavior is not assertive. There are three basic forms of aggression: direct, indirect, and passive. Unlike assertive communication, all three have in common their disregard for the other person. In fact, they are often defensive postures grounded in fear of the other person and fear of losing control of the situation. The desire to have complete control is the underlying theme of aggressive communication. Selfish or manipulative control is a very closed form of communication: It implies that only one person decides the outcome.

Direct aggression (anger, hostile behavior, physical violence). Of the three types of aggression, direct aggression is the most obvious and the most easily confused with assertiveness. Unlike assertive behavior, it completely ignores the needs and feelings of the other person. Here control and domination are achieved by means of bullying, provoking, demanding, and threatening. In our culture, direct aggression has traditionally been associated with macho male behavior. It can also be an overreaction by a weak or passive personality type, a temporary explosion before a return to a passive, nonassertive mode. In either case, it works only as long as the other person is afraid to assert his or her rights.

The stereotypic schoolyard bully is a perfect example of the direct aggressor. So is the boss who sexually harasses his secretary. In both cases, the style invites a strong response: If you stand up to the bully, he (or she) often crumbles.

Jim (age 36, body age 41), a Loner, had a recurring problem when entertaining potential clients (a frequent part of his job), since he was very anxious and introverted in social situations. He was married to Sheryl, a very attractive woman who was invariably the object of aggressive male attention at these business affairs. Whenever Jim saw someone making a pass at Sheryl (something he knew she didn't like either), he felt immobilized and did nothing, and his stress level shot up. He and his wife rarely raised the subject: They both found it "too awkward."

After starting the program, Jim decided to discuss this recurring pattern with Sheryl, to see if they couldn't do something about it—together. One evening, at a time when there hadn't been a business party for several weeks, he raised the issue in a relaxed but direct way. As it turned out, Sheryl was as anxious as her husband to get this stressor out into the open and to plan a strategy for dealing with it.

They agreed that making passes, although annoying, was usually the harmless act of an "insecure slob." But they agreed that when Sheryl was feeling uncomfortable, she would touch her right shoulder with her left hand, a signal for Jim to come to the rescue. Sheryl would then "introduce" Jim as follows: "I think you know the love of my life, Jim. Jim, this is Mr. . . . Oh, I'm sorry, I've forgotten your name—what was it again?" Mission accomplished, and aggressive behavior defused.

Indirect aggression (inappropriate criticism, sarcasm, hypocritical niceness). Indirect aggression is a technique for assuming control by making the other person feel guilty or bad. It takes the forms of deception, seduction, trickery, and manipulation. Culturally, this has traditionally been associated with the female behavior characterized as "womanly wiles." But it is by no means exclusive to the female of the species. Any time you attempt to gain control over another person by indirect means, you are guilty of this type of aggression. Your real goal is to get attention and exert control. But because you fear rejection, you resort to indirect manipulation. This approach might include withholding something you know the other person wants (sex? attention?) until you get what you want. It might include criticizing some aspect of the other's behavior other than the one you really want to change: "Don't use that tone of voice on me!" "It drives me crazy when you leave the cap off the toothpaste." "Your work station is a mess. Clean it up!" Sarcasm is a common form of indirect aggression. So is insincere niceness (as in the phrase, "kill with kindness"). Sometimes people even get sick as an indirect way of getting at someone.

Relationships between spouses are often characterized by a good deal of indirect aggression. When one half of a couple feels aggrieved or neglected, he or she often resorts to concealed or misplaced hostilities. The husband who spends too much time at work may find that his wife loses interest in sex (she wants more attention). The mother of a newborn baby may find her husband extremely critical of her housekeeping (he's really feeling jealous or neglected by her).

A nursing administrator Worry Wart named Anna (age 38, body age 49) was a master of indirect aggression. Since some of her central concepts of "good nursing" ran counter to those of the hospital's medical director (her boss), not to mention many of the other doctors, and since she did not believe that the power of her position was great enough for her to "get a fair hearing" (that is, win it all), she spent a great deal of her stress energy on indirect aggression.

For example, she formed allegiances with other department heads, misrepresenting to them, ever so slightly, the medical director's intentions. Then she would sabotage her boss by fomenting all sorts of misunderstandings at the weekly administrative meeting he chaired. She also repeatedly orchestrated the staff schedule for discord: Nurses who might agree with the director's new programs were rarely on duty when he was around. As a result, many of his initiatives "died a natural death," seemingly lacking any grassroots staff support. Finally, she punished any doctor not in her camp by jumping on his or her slightest departure from hospital procedure. Her indirectly aggressive communication style drained great amounts of her energy to no constructive purpose, but she saw it as a survival technique that gave her some sense of control over her environment.

Passive aggression (martyr behavior, playing the victim, "Poor me"). The third and possibly the most insidious form of aggression is the passive mode. This technique for gaining control usually aims to make the other person feel sorry for us or pity us. Outwardly this behavior doesn't seem like aggression at all, since the person is typically soft-spoken and low key, adopting the helpless role of the underdog. The experts at this form of aggression are the people whose lives seem to be one constant "poor me," who are always asking us to feel sorry for them and their plight. These are the people who refuse to make a clear decision, who won't ask outright for anything but simply say, "You know best" or "Whatever you think is right."

The stereotype of the Jewish Mother is a perfect example of passive aggression. Her words are "Don't worry about me, I'll be fine." Her message is "You don't pay enough attention to me." Her feeling is hurt and anger. How many of you have used the same unrewarding tactic in your relationships with others? This passive pose masks anger.

Georgina (age 36, body age 44), a Worry Wart, was a high school department head whose husband had put her into a double bind. He told her flat out, "Since you put so much energy into your work, I'm going to have affairs." In the same breath, he informed her she could keep him as her husband as long as she made enough money to pay for his favorite pastime (piloting small airplanes). Instead of punching him in the mouth and walking out, she acquiesced. Then her guerrilla campaign began.

Georgina used typical passive-aggressive tactics. She'd discovered that her husband's newest flame was a young nurse working shifts. She found out the shift rotation and then "innocently" scheduled family activities (outings with the kids, a dinner party) for the times when her husband's heartthrob had her evenings open. Then she would send him subtle messages that this wasn't a coincidence. When it came time to make payments on the small plane he had purchased, she would deliberately be late or make the check out incorrectly.

Much psychotherapy is devoted to turning passive-aggressive behavior into the direct expression of resentment. In our culture, such "negative" feelings are usually seen as being socially unacceptable. As a result, expressing legitimate anger and resentment is one of the most difficult aspects of assertive communication for most people. Often we repress these feelings until they explode as pure aggression.

Aggressive communication seldom pays off in the long run, although there are certainly times when it is appropriate to fight fire with fire. Generally, however, it muddies the message and discounts both you and the other person. But old habits die hard. Replacing open or covert hostilities with clear, self-affirming assertive communication can be very difficult. It takes considerable practice.

Self-Affirming Communication Skills

Effective communication requires skills at both sending and receiving. These skills help you to be clear about the message you are sending and sensitive to the person you are sending it to. They also help you to be sure you're receiving the message you think you are and to be sensitive to the person doing the sending. Effective communication is based on the following basic assumption: There is a grain of truth (and something I can agree with) in every comment or opinion expressed by another person. If I listen well enough, they will be able to express themselves clearly. In a sense, effective communication is the art of turning every interaction into a win-win situation: Being sure of your own ground, you are able and willing to compromise. By contrast, manipulators who always seek "total victory" invariably end up in win-lose situations, in spite of themselves. In effective communication, you keep your sense of power, but don't need to control the other person.

Assertive, or self-affirming, communication—a vital key to satisfying relationships—can be improved by focusing on guidelines and skills that can lower your stress thermostat by providing positive feedback to the self. Assertive communication is based on self-knowledge ("What do I want?") and self-affirmation ("I am an important person in this interaction; are my needs and wants being adequately met?"). The better you feel about yourself, the more able you are to. be sensitive to others, to listen well, and to respond sympathetically.

Here is the assertive communicator's bill of rights:

> I have the right to do anything I choose, as long as it does not hurt someone else.
>
> I have the right to maintain my dignity by being properly assertive—even if it hurts someone else—as long as my motive is assertive, not aggressive.
>
> I always have the right to make a request of another person, as long as I realize that the other person has the right to say no.
>
> I realize that there are certain borderline cases in interpersonal situations where rights aren't clear. But I always have the right to discuss the problem with the person involved and so clarify it.
>
> I have the right to assert my rights.

If this sounds selfish, it is, but in the best sense. You can't look after others until you've looked after yourself. A certain amount of egoism is extremely healthy—without your ego, you'd still be at an early infant stage of development. Dr. Selye called this healthy adult selfishness *altruistic egoism*, making it the basis of his personal philosophy, which he summarized as "earn your neighbor's love." This attitude is a form of enlightened self-interest in which you serve yourself through serving the interests of other people, thus "earning" their respect and love. At its core, this philosophy is based on the same principles as assertive communication. Selye argued that this principle is common to all forms of life, down to the molecular level. Therefore, to deny the natural law that "number one comes first" is to be stressfully at odds with your basic nature.

The aim of assertive communication is simple: to clarify communication in ways that affirm who you are. This clarification can be achieved in the following ways:

> Getting in touch with your own needs and taking active responsibility for meeting them. (For a complete discussion of how to develop this skill, see chapter 8, "Values/Goals Clarification.")
>
> Learning to communicate in an open, clear, direct, honest, effective, comfortable, and empathetic way
>
> Learning to listen and really hear and understand what others are communicating
>
> Managing the giving and receiving of criticism, resentment, and anger

Managing the giving and receiving of compliments; expressing
and receiving affection and caring
Changing the negative things we say to ourselves—the neg-
ative "self-talk"—into positive, self-affirming self-talk
Cutting through the manipulative games we and others play
Being able to say a clear "yes" and a clear "no."

All of us have considerable assertive communication skills—if we
didn't, we'd be living as hermits. But because we are largely unaware
of these skills, they are open to improvement. When it comes to communication, most people are like swimmers who know how to stay afloat
and can perhaps do the dog paddle, but haven't yet learned a more efficient
stroke such as the crawl. With practice, you can greatly enhance your
skill at interpersonal communication. But first you need to become aware
of just what you are already doing well, as well as your self-defeating
habits.

The following section is a summary of self-affirming communication
skills. Some apply primarily when you are speaking (or sending a message), some primarily when you are listening (or receiving a message),
and some, such as body language, apply equally to both. These are
behaviors that characterize a highly confident and self-directed person
who is not subject to unneeded stress-energy drains. Notice which are
typical of you and which are unfamiliar or alien.

Message Skills

1. Use "no" when you mean no. (If you really want to refuse a request,
then say no right at the beginning. Set your limits. Draw a line. Keep
your boundaries clear.) And use "yes" when you mean yes (as a commitment to and an endorsement of *your* choices). Sometimes it may be
necessary to say yes or no several times until you're clearly heard.

2. Be polite but firm and don't apologize for things you don't believe
require an apology.

3. Use "I" instead of "it" when talking about yourself, as in the
sentences "It would be nice if you arrived at work on time" versus "I
would like you to arrive at work on time" or the more assertive "I want
you to arrive at work on time."

4. Be direct and to the point, avoiding long explanations.

5. Respond quickly and without hesitation. This shows the other person
that you know what you want.

6. Speak fluently, using as few "ahs" and "ums" as possible. These
indicate uncertainty: They heighten your stress level and the other per-

son's. This is easier to do when you use short sentences and get into the habit of making your main point in the first sentence.

7. Give clear feedback (including about how you are feeling). If you don't let the speaker know what kind of impact he is having on you, he won't be able to tailor his message to the audience.

Two-Way Relationship Skills

1. Anticipate the feelings or needs of the other person by trying to put yourself in his or her situation. Once you have some grasp of what's going on for the other person, acknowledge his feelings. (An especially useful technique for people in sales, this is just as important in intimate relationships.)

2. Seek mutually acceptable compromises when you disagree. Many people seem determined to emerge from a disagreement with all or nothing. To them, compromise is a sign of weakness.

3. Listen actively. Keep an open posture, maintain eye contact, and reflect back to the speaker what he has said. Allow a comfortable interval before you respond.

Nonverbal Voice Skills

1. Use a volume of voice that's appropriate to the circumstances, neither too loud nor too soft.

2. Speak firmly. A firm voice indicates a firm person. Try slowing your voice down: You may feel more relaxed and in control if you do.

3. Speak in a lively tone of voice to convey your ease and your involvement with a discussion (fake boredom or reserve saps your energy and that of others). A firm, even tone (not a dull drone) is usually the most effective at communicating assertively. A soft, pleasant voice communicates warmth and affection, whereas a whining or nasal voice can easily alienate the listener.

4. Speak in a clear voice. Don't mumble. Get your message across. You can make sure you're getting through if you pause occasionally to ask your hearers if they understand what you're saying. (This is also known as soliciting feedback.)

Body Skills

1. Look directly at the person you are speaking or listening to. This doesn't mean staring; it does mean standing or sitting with your body more or less aligned to face him or her, rather than at an angle (body language that "deflects" rather receives what the other person is saying is a defensive posture that tells your interlocutor that you are expecting to be attacked). This conveys genuine interest in and attention to both what he has to say and your own point of view.

2. Face the person to whom you are speaking or to whom you are listening, and lean slightly toward him. This indicates that you are open and attentive to what he has to say and have no manipulative hidden agenda.

3. Gesture appropriately (and don't overuse gestures). Make sure your hands and facial expressions are consistent with your words. Many people smile or grin when they have something unpleasant to say. This is an essentially dishonest mode of communication and only generates mistrust. If you're sincere, don't grin, smile (or frown), or nod when you don't mean it. Being yourself and being spontaneous are as important as learning to be more direct and assertive.

4. Stay in touch with your body and try to keep your hands, arms, and legs relaxed. A high level of muscular tension not only heightens your internal stress level; it is instantly conveyed to the other person as unsureness, and possibly preparation for an attack.

5. Adopt a comfortable posture. Avoid sitting stiffly; ease of posture literally conveys a sense of ease about your position. Is your posture open and receptive, or is it closed and defensive (arms or legs, or both, crossed?).

6. Be aware of the intuitive and physical signals you are picking up from your body and from the body posture of the other person.

All of these skills are important. In the following pages, we recast them as four basic techniques that you can consciously start to phase into your daily life: nonverbal communication, self-assertive language, giving and receiving feedback, and active listening.

Nonverbal Communication. All the behaviors listed under "Nonverbal Voice Skills" and "Body Skills" are nonverbal. The importance of your body language and all other forms of nonverbal communication cannot be overemphasized. In fact, current research indicates that as much as 75 percent of what we actually communicate—what the other person understands, as opposed to what we intend—is nonverbal. Where you stand or sit (too close? standoffish?), your posture (leaning forward or back? arms folded? legs crossed?) your tone of voice and the confidence with which you speak (as opposed to the content of your words), the expression on your face, and any expression of genuine emotion (whether tears, laughter, or anger)—all these have an enormous impact on the other person. So does the way you look (do you convey a sense of self-care, of self-respect?), your handshake (is it firm? are your hands cold and clammy?), even the physical environment you create for your communication. What message is conveyed by your home, your office, your desk, your kitchen, or your car?

An extremely important, though much neglected, form of nonverbal communication is touching. It is particularly important in intimate relationships, especially within families. Touching is the child's first way of communicating, and there is no question that touching is essential to an infant's healthy maturation. The healthy development of the nervous system is stimulated through physical contact with the parents. And infant stress, especially before the child has learned to speak, is of necessity managed through touch.

Psychological illnesses have been closely linked to a lack of physical contact in the first few years of life. So have various physical complaints. Ashley Montague, in his book *Touching*, describes a considerable body of research that suggests that skin problems such as eczema, as well as various allergies, can often be traced to a lack of early physical contact. In the nineteenth and early twentieth centuries, before the importance of touching was understood, many children in orphanages died of a condition called marasmus, from the Greek word for "wasting away": They had enough food but not enough physical affection. Recent studies have shown that lonely people who own pets are less prone to depression. In sum, touch is a very powerful communication tool—for both receiving and giving (expressing yourself). A large number of our study participants reported increased touch experiences—with their spouses, in casual conversation with friends, or in having a professional massage. Gina, a Loner accountant (age 29, body age 37), reported at her four-month checkup that one evening as she was hugging her daughter at bedtime, it dawned on her why the Body Age Program emphasized "getting in touch" with your most basic values. "Hugging my children and touching my friends has literally added the third dimension I felt I was missing in my life."

Some of our study subjects made pets a part of their communication prescription—a great way to get more touching into your life. Early in the program, Sam, a Worry Wart (age 40, body age 46), started to walk dogs at the local humane society shelter. In no time, this valued leisure activity affected his overall behavior, and he became more easygoing. He shifted from being a rather prim and proper dresser to someone who proudly sported dog hairs on his blue suit. By the fourth month, he had adopted two dogs.

However, touch carries with it all sorts of social baggage and often can be misinterpreted. To use touch as a healthy form of communication, you have to be in a context in which its use is understood and accepted. Yet certainly your relationships with your closest friends and with your family can be improved and deepened through touch. If you haven't hugged your kid or your spouse today, give it a try.

Nonverbal communication is often more spontaneous than the words we use and can often present a clearer picture of what we intend to communicate than can words alone. It can also confuse the picture considerably. The person whose tone of voice and body language are out of phase with the content of his words is sending a mixed message that will cause anxiety in the hearer-observer. Certain gestures have come to have certain meanings. If you close your eyes while listening, the other person may assume you're bored, not concentrating on what he is saying. So it's important to be aware of what you are doing and of its potential impact. Ask yourself whether your expression, tone of voice, and gestures are consistent with what you are saying. Do your nonverbal signs reinforce or undercut your message? (This can be a particular problem for people delivering what they imagine to be an unpleasant message.) Avoid mannerisms that are meaningless (to you) and annoying, distracting, or open to misinterpretation.

Despite your best efforts, you likely will find that some of your nonverbal habits are hard to kick. To mitigate this, you can put the other person at ease by simply telling him what these are. If you mention that you always close your eyes when you're concentrating, he won't feel ignored. If you explain that you raise your eyebrows when you find something especially fascinating, she won't think you are disapproving.

This technique boils down to awareness. If you become more aware of the nonverbal messages you send, you'll send clearer ones. For specific things to do, look back over the behaviors listed in the sections "Body Skills" and "Nonverbal Voice Skills."

Self-Assertive Language. The way you use words and the content of those words will often be lost unless you adopt self-assertive modes of language. The rules of linguistic self-assertion are actually quite simple, but they give many people difficulty.

Use the pronoun "I" more frequently instead of impersonal constructions. The power of this simple habit cannot be overstated.

One of the common substitutes for "I" is the impersonal pronoun "it." Example: "It would be nice if you'd come to dinner." Note that this sentence leaves the speaker out entirely. Upon hearing this statement, you might well ask, "Before I decide whether or not to come to dinner, I'd like to know whether you'll be there." Other frequent substitutes for the pronoun "I" are the pronouns "we" and "you." How many times have you said, "We'll be seeing you," instead of the more assertive "I'll be seeing you"? How often do you talk about yourself in the second person, almost as if you weren't present. For example, "When that happens, you feel really awful."

Such self-defeating linguistic habits undermine efforts at assertive communication. Whenever you are the subject, put yourself in the forefront by using the pronoun "I."

Use the words "yes" and "no." These have amazing impact as a substitute for all the qualifications and circumlocutions typical of much modern communication. Here's a simple example.

> QUESTION: "Will you help me wash the car?"
> NONASSERTIVE RESPONSE: I'd love to, but I've got a lot of work to do this weekend. Besides I have a sore back from weeding the garden, so I'd better take a rain check on that unless you'd like to see how I'm feeling tomorrow.
> ASSERTIVE RESPONSE: "No, I'd rather not."

"Yes" is an equally difficult word for many people.

Don't explain or apologize without reason. In the above example, the person refusing to wash the car was making all sorts of unnecessary excuses. You can practically see the self leaking away with each subordinate phrase. The time to explain is when someone needs information you haven't provided—and asks for it. The time to apologize is only when you have acted in a way you genuinely regret. How many times have you spoken the phrase "I'm sorry to disturb you, but . . ." Presumably, if you were sorry you wouldn't be doing it. In fact, avoid all self-diminishing or equivocating language: "I guess"; "All I really meant was . . ."; "There's some truth to what you're saying."

Avoid the word "but." Example: "You're doing a good job, but I have a few questions about your work habits." In effect, the word "but" negates the clause that precedes it, proving it to have been a manipulative lie. In fact, the speaker in the example had some criticisms of the job being done and was afraid to come out with them. The assertive person would simply have said something such as, "John, I'd like to talk to you about your work habits."

Of these rules, the first is certainly the most important, and well worth experimenting with. You'll discover that every time you say "I" when you mean "I," you'll experience a difference. At first, you may feel quite awkward, even exposed. This is because you are putting your self in the center of the action—where you belong. But once you get used to it you'll feel a growing sense of personal power.

Giving and Receiving Feedback. Giving and receiving feedback is crucial to clear communication. Although it is often confused with criticism, feedback is quite different. Criticism carries with it a judgment; feedback is the exchange of information. It tells the communicator about his effectiveness in getting his message across, and it helps the listener-observer be sure that he understands the message. Because it is often difficult to separate a judgment from a factual evaluation, giving and getting clean feedback can be tricky. But it is a rewarding skill.

The best feedback you receive is the kind you solicit from others, since you are less likely to be defensive and block it out. Ask your partner (or friend, colleague, or spouse) to watch you in a situation—a meeting, a social event—and then to describe your behavior. If you're dealing one on one, let the other person know you'd like their feedback during or after the interchange. If you do, you will likely discover a number of verbal and nonverbal mannerisms that are completely outside your awareness. Many people don't notice the number of times they say ''ah'' or ''um,'' or their habit of drumming their fingers or tapping a foot. If the feedback you get is too general to be useful, get the person to be more specific. You might ask a colleague to watch you at a meeting to see if there are times when you appear bored, or whether you did anything to indicate nonverbally that you disagreed with his ideas, or to describe your tone of voice and how he felt when listening to your tone, rather than your content.

There are a number of basic rules for giving and receiving good, clear feedback. If you follow them, it is much less likely that the other person will experience what you have to say as a critical attack. Above all, remember that good feedback is self-assertive, but never aggressive.

Avoid value judgments. Describe what you see rather than your opinion of what you see. For example, ''I notice that you scratch your chin frequently when you are talking.'' Or ''Were you aware that you tapped your foot throughout the presentation?'' Or ''I noticed that you looked at the floor the entire time I was speaking to you.''

Be as specific as possible. The more general the comment, the less useful, and the more likely it will become a value judgment. For example, if you tell someone that he dominated the meeting, he will likely experience this statement as a criticism. But if you say something like, ''You know, just now when you were deciding the issue, you didn't seem to be really listening to what I and the others said,'' he may hear you and alter his behavior accordingly.

Report the impact the behavior had on you without judging the behavior. It is much easier to criticize than to express your true feelings. However, probably the most useful feedback you can give another person is to explain as simply as possible your emotional experience when the particular behavior was taking place. For example, "While you were drumming your fingers on the table I felt uneasy" will likely be heard as useful feedback, whereas "I didn't like the annoying way in which you were constantly drumming your fingers" will be received as an attack. (Note that this aspect of feedback keeps you at the center while respecting the other person.)

Useful feedback takes into account the needs of both the giver and the receiver. Feedback can easily turn into destructive criticism when it serves only your needs and fails to consider others.

Direct your feedback toward behavior that the other person can do something about. Frustration and stress are only increased when a person is reminded of some shortcoming over which he has little or no control.

The best feedback is solicited rather than imposed. But if someone could benefit from it and won't ask for it, assertive communication often requires you to give it.

Give feedback as soon as possible. In general, feedback is most useful at the earliest opportunity after the particular behavior has occurred. Don't wait two weeks or even two days.

Check with others to make sure your feedback is being clearly communicated. This means separating the value judgments and the facts.

If you are receiving feedback, it is easy to become defensive, especially if it is aggressive or judgmental. If you stay aware, you can more easily manage your stress level and can usually unmangle the message by getting down to specific facts and feelings. If, for instance, someone accuses you of dominating a meeting, ask him to be more specific about exactly what you did and when he felt excluded from the decision-making process.

Check with others on the accuracy of the feedback you are giving or receiving. The more people involved, the more accurate the feedback will be. Is it just one person's impression, or is the impression shared by others?

In sum, feedback is a way of giving help to another person as well as helping you to understand better. It functions as a corrective mechanism that helps you and the person you are communicating with learn how well behaviors match intentions and how well the message is getting across. When a person discovers that his intent and effect are out of phase, he can take steps to change what he does. The clearer the message, the lower the level of uncertainty, and the lower the level of stress.

Active Listening. Active listening is one of the most important and most easily neglected communication skills. This is because we think of listening as passive, requiring much less effort than sending a message. It isn't. If you listen actively, you hear emotions as well as words, and messages as well as facts. And you will give the speaker the greatest compliment of all—the compliment of being profoundly understood— by acknowledging his or her point of view and reality.

We all know the sure sign of passive listening: boredom. When your attention starts to wander and you have difficulty concentrating on what the other person is saying, you need active listening to rectify the situation. And sometimes interrupting is the only way of asking for and getting the communication back onto a two-way street.

Active listening is a kind of ongoing feedback while communication is in process. This approach helps you be sure you understand the meaning of what the other person is saying or doing; it confirms that what he is saying or doing means the same thing to you as it does to him. It allows you to experience the reality of the other person while keeping you very much in the center of the communication process. You can use this technique in a formal meeting or while having coffee with a friend.

There are several basic rules and tools of active listening. Here they are:

Frame the conversation. This is a good way to minimize potential distractions. It can happen at the beginning or at any stage of the encounter. Framing the conversation means defining, together with the other person, the perimeters of your dialogue: what subjects you are both willing to talk about, or how the talk should go, or what specific topics should be omitted, or how long you are willing to talk. It is especially useful if you have another commitment and time is short.

Disturbance takes precedence. How many times have you experienced that split feeling of attempting to listen to what someone is saying while your mind is somewhere else? Perhaps you've just come from an upsetting phone call and you're still going over in your head what your friend said. Perhaps you have another appointment in half an hour and you're worried about getting there on time or are rehearsing what you'll say. Perhaps you are uncomfortable with the person or with your physical position.

Whatever the disturbance or the distraction, you must attend to it before active listening is possible. If you have a plane to catch, make your time constraints clear at the outset of your meeting: "You should know I've only got fifteen minutes for this. Let's see how much we can get accomplished in that time." If you're still wrapped up in something that's just happened, say so. Keeping these disturbances to yourself out of some notion of politeness is actually the height of rudeness, since it means you will be listening with less than half an ear to what the other person has to say.

Sometimes distractions arise in the course of conversation. The most common sources are trigger words, words that are, for you, laden with strong associations. Different words trigger emotional disturbances in different people. Would any of the following cause you to lose track of what the other person is saying: abortion, peacenik, gay, terrorist, fascist, nuclear, communism? You can make your own list, which will probably change with circumstances. Something the other person is saying may trigger a memory or a thought that is simply too insistent to dismiss and that takes you far from the subject at hand.

When something triggers a disturbance that distracts you from listening, the only thing to do is to stop the conversation and admit what's going on. For example: "The sun is shining in my eyes. Let's move our chairs to a different position." Take a moment to refocus. Then return to the conversation. The simple act of bringing the disturbance out into the open will usually dispel it.

Listen to all nonverbal messages. Nonverbal messages include posture, eye contact (or lack of it), tone of voice, rhythm, and inflection. Since only a small portion of any message is contained in the words or received through the words, this aspect of active listening is crucial.

We all listen to nonverbal messages to some degree. But as part of increasing your listening skills, attempt to hone this process by bringing it more into your awareness. Begin to note each aspect of the other person's nonverbal communication and ask yourself what this communicates to you. For instance, if the person is sitting with his arms folded across his chest and is speaking in a clipped monotone, how does this make you feel? What subtext does this add to the words he is saying? By bringing these nonverbal messages more vividly into your conscious mind, you can begin to respond to the entire communication, not just some aspect of it. In fact, the nonverbal message may actually be distracting you from what the person's words seem to be saying, and you need to deal with this disturbance before you can deal with his words. The behavior itself is not bad or wrong, but if it is distracting to you, you may need to say so.

Re-create what you are hearing and play it back to the speaker. Once you have dealt with any disturbance and clearly identified the nonverbal content of the message, you are in a position to respond appropriately to what another person is saying. The technique for this, sometimes called reflecting back, has two levels: mirroring and paraphrasing. It boils down to playing back to the speaker what you are hearing—emotions and all. This approach has the additional benefit of letting the other person know you are interested in him and in what he has to say. It helps you tune in to his wavelength. If the other person really believes you understand his point of view, he is more likely to be willing to understand your viewpoint. Real communication becomes possible.

Here, in more detail, are the two levels of reflecting back:

Level 1: Mirror. Repeat back, word for word, what you have just heard the speaker say. It is useful to begin with the phrase "What I hear you say is . . ." or "What you are saying is . . ."

Level 2: Paraphrase. This is more appropriate once you are in rapport with the speaker, when a degree of trust and attunement has been attained. In this case, you first restate in your own words the content of what you think the person is saying. Then you attempt to state in your own terms the feelings that underlie what's being said, as they have been either stated or implied. The least threatening way of doing this is to use a tentative reference, such as "I imagine you were feeling very angry and frustrated when . . ."

You may be amazed at the difference better listening can make. Florence Wolff, the author of *Perspective Listening*, gives her students the following assignment: Spend twenty minutes listening to your spouse. The only requirements are to lean forward slightly, to keep eye contact, to nod occasionally, and not to fidget. One of her male students reported after trying this exercise (it meant he had to turn off the TV), "This is the first time in six years that my wife and I have really communicated."

Celeste, a Worry Wart professional artist (age 39, body age 46), found that active listening transformed her relationship with her son: "As I listened to my teenage son—actively—I was so shocked by the contrast to what I'd heard before (almost nothing). My mind could not escape the awareness that previously I had 'heard' his experiences as if they were grainy black-and-white photos. What I was hearing now was a series of fully realized paintings rich in colors and tones (and feelings). My Action Diary Planning Page now focuses on appreciating these 'unveilings' as they are offered to me."

Assertive or self-affirming communication is a function of your degree of emotional and intellectual openness. As you reveal your self, you affirm your self. The more you are willing to speak not only facts and opinions but also inner thoughts and feelings, and the more you are willing to listen with both your mind and your heart, the more successful you are at communicating. As you raise the emotional stakes, you discover that relationships you previously found difficult or impossible become rewarding and nurturing. As you improve your assertive-communication skills—both speaking and listening—you build relationships founded on openness and trust. The amount of uncertainty in your life is thereby greatly reduced. And so is your stress level.

YOUR FOUR-WEEK START-UP PROGRAM

Week 1: Get Ready. Deepen your awareness of your communication strengths and weaknesses by keeping an interaction diary. Use this information to refine your "top five opportunities for better communication" from the "Rate Yourself" section. Plan for concrete action.

Week 2: Take Your First Step. Work on one specific, recurring situation or behavior you want to change. Handle it differently this week.

Week 3: Build on Your Success. Continue working on your week 2 priority by improving your communication in this situation.

Week 4: Consolidate Your Gains. If you are starting to feel more comfortable with the new behavior or situation, try your new skills elsewhere. Continue to deepen your practice of self-affirming communication.

In the "Rate Yourself" section, you identified your top five opportunities to communicate better. This priority list forms the basis of your start-up program. In the first week, you will work on deepening your awareness and refining your list. In the subsequent three weeks, you will concentrate on one situation or behavior that occurs frequently or seems most open to change. Later, as you gain in self-confidence, you will tackle those self-defeating habits that are more deeply rooted and more difficult to dislodge.

Regardless of where you begin, you'll likely find that putting assertive communication into practice provokes considerable anxiety. Let's face it, most of us have been doing a lot of hiding for a long time. So even peeking out occasionally from behind the protective wall you've built will be difficult. That's why it's important to start small and to concentrate initially on what seems most doable. You'll quickly discover the very different and more satisfying quality of the experience each time you assert yourself. Over time, your old, bad habits will simply wither away.

Your primary focus during this four-week start-up program is to build on your existing communication strengths and to start to develop new skills.

Week 1: Get Ready

During this week, you will deepen your awareness of the ways in which your communication style undermines your sense of self, and you will become clearer about opportunities for introducing new behaviors. This awareness will help you plan the small, specific, concrete change you will make in week 2.

Fill out your Action Diary Planning Page. Agree that in the coming week you will introduce the following new behaviors into your life:

1. *Autogenic relaxation plus affirmations and visualizations.* At the beginning of this week, find some quiet time in which to listen to the autogenic tape and then introduce the affirmations you've chosen as your themes for more self-affirming communication. While you are still in a relaxed state, visualize yourself successfully putting assertive communication into practice in some situation or situations in which you habitually sit on the sidelines or feel like the least important member of the team. Enjoy the feelings of confidence and power that go with this success. Practice autogenic relaxation at least three more times this week.

Choose to use your affirmations at least once each day, ideally two or three times daily.

2. *Keep an interaction diary.* Many of you will be eager to try out some assertive communication techniques right away. Don't. Use this week to deepen your awareness of the ways in which you defeat yourself when you communicate with others. The best way is to keep a daily interaction diary. In it, record each interpersonal situation in which you "lose yourself," in which you feel dissatisfied, diminished or incomplete in terms of the communication that's going on. Attempt to identify exactly what was happening for you in the situation, including your feelings during and after the encounter. And note what the other person was doing to contribute to the communication breakdown. Is he, too, an accomplished saboteur?

For instance, after an unsatisfactory meeting with your boss, you might write the following entry: "Wanted feedback from boss about current project. Talked instead about various problems in the organization. Then discussed last night's Blue Jays game. Began to feel hot under the collar. Realized I always allow my boss to 'run' our encounters. Result: We seldom if ever get to my agenda. Boss is an avoider type. And I'm not looking after my own needs.

"Possible solution: Try framing the interview beforehand by telling my boss the specific subject I want to talk about and setting up a formal appointment instead of just dropping in on him unscheduled."

Your entries don't need to be this long or detailed. And you can use point form instead of prose. The main thing is to get down the key things about the event so that you can recall them later.

At week's end, go over your interaction diary. Look for the recurring patterns and themes that stand out. Now refer back to your top five opportunities for communicating better in the "Rate Yourself" section. Use the additional awareness you've gained from your diary to refine these priorities for action. Pick one and plan what you will specifically do next week to communicate more effectively.

3. *Check in with your partner.* Let him or her know how your week of self-discovery is going. Share what you've learned about your communication style and the way you get trapped or sidetracked. Get all the support you need as you get ready to make some real self-affirming changes.

4. *Record your progress in your Action Diary and plan for action.* At the end of each day, summarize what you've learned about yourself: the way you communicate and your opportunities for change. Congratulate yourself for each new awareness.

Week 2: Take Your First Step

The size of this step is up to you, but we strongly recommend that you keep it small. Whatever you choose, remember that this is your first move. It may feel awkward, and it may not seem very successful. It is a concrete step nonetheless.

Fill out your Action Diary Planning Page. Agree to do the following during the coming week:

1. *Continue using autogenic relaxation with affirmations and visualizations.* Use the relaxation tape at least four times this week. Modify your affirmations and visualizations as you wish. Your deepening awareness in week 1 may have suggested more powerful self-themes for positive thinking. Repeat your affirmations daily, ideally two or three times each day.

2. *Act on your plan.* At the end of last week, you picked a behavior or situation that you feel confident you can change (you planned for success, not failure) and resolved to handle it differently. Here are a few possibilities that will suggest the wide range available to you.

Plan a get-together with a friend whom you love dearly but who always leaves you feeling as though you haven't had a chance to talk about what's important to you. Experiment with one of the techniques of active listening, perhaps paraphrasing.

Schedule a meeting with your boss, and tell him ahead of time the subject you want to discuss.

The next time your boss asks you to do something that isn't part of your job—and that you object to doing—tell him or her. And explain why. Then propose a doable win-win solution.

Experiment with using the pronoun "I" more frequently (and banishing the impersonal "it," we," and "you").

Reduce your use of self-diminishing or equivocating language, such as "I guess I feel . . ." or "All I really meant was . . ." or "There's some truth to that . . ."

Experiment with saying no when you mean no, and yes when you mean yes.

Plan how (specifically) to cut short the next phone call from a boring acquaintance you really don't want to talk to.

Hug your wife and kids at least once a day.

Compliment your subordinates on work well done.

Ask for feedback from a co-worker.

Go back to that restaurant where you always feel you don't get as good service as the other patrons, and experiment with getting your needs met (plan in advance).

Decide to renew your marriage vows (this can be a tangible expression of what you want to continue doing day by day in your relationship).

Experiment with body language and eye contact during a one-on-one interview.

Sarah (age 44, body age 51) was regional sales manager for a major pharmaceutical firm. She liked her job and got along well with her boss. The only trouble was that, as she put it, his management style was "slightly to the right of Genghis Khan." Her particular gripe was their weekly review meeting, invariably scheduled for 10:30 A.M. each Friday. Her boss never told her what was on the meeting agenda until she got there, usually kept her waiting fifteen minutes in his outer office, and then during the meeting would go off on so many tangents that she always ended up being late for the noon lunch meeting she held with her sales force.

In week 2, Sarah decided to arrange to do this meeting differently. On Wednesday, she asked her boss for an agenda before Friday so that they could be finished in time for her staff meeting to begin as scheduled. She explained that this would enable the sales force to have a full afternoon for getting all its end-of-week phoning done, which could only help sales volume.

Sure enough, she got a handwritten agenda from Genghis in time. Then, halfway through the Friday meeting, she reminded him of the noon target. They met it. As a result, Sarah was less frazzled and didn't have to apologize to her own staff for being late. This was a successful behavior change she could build on in week 3.

3. *Check in with your partner.* You'll probably have lots to talk about. How successful were you? How did it feel to be a bit more self-assertive in your communication?

4. *Record your progress in your Action Diary.* Noting your missed opportunities for self-assertion is almost as important as actually adopting new self-affirming communication behaviors. You are still learning about the ways in which you discount your self when you communicate with others. Each time you become aware of how you downplay your hand in an interaction, you take an important step toward giving yourself a more central role in your own life story—as long as this awareness is accompanied by a clear picture of the positive alternative (doing it better and how much better you'll feel when you do). Just noticing how you avoid assertive communication can be an act of self-affirmation. Every time you note a missed opportunity to ''do it differently,'' you are making it more likely that the next time you'll try something new.

Here is a sample Action Diary Planning Page for week 2 of Self-Affirming Communication. Your planning page will reflect the assertive-communication technique(s) you want to emphasize and when. Find ways to incorporate each new behavior into your life without major dislocations. Don't overdo. Remember: Change is stressful, so take it one step at a time. Above all, remember to give each behavior you undertake on this self-care contract the SMART test. Ask yourself whether it is Specific, Measurable, Acceptable, Realistic, and Truthful.

FOR WEEK OF Sept 23 TO Sept 29

Planning Page

Affirmations (My self-themes for this week in key words and phrases)

I _am sure of myself when I communicate with others_

I _feel good about myself when I say what I mean_

(Other) _I listen well and respond clearly_

Opportunity Visualizations (I clearly see myself . . .)

I clearly see myself going into my boss's office and asking for a raise (which I deserve and which is long overdue) My voice is calm and firm and even, and my breathing is regular. He listens respectfully to what I have to say. I feel heard.

I choose to deepen this Vital Life Skill as follows (My specific behavioral objectives this week)

I choose to _do a fifteen minute autogenic relaxation, followed by affirmation and visualization, at least 4X's during the coming week_

Under the following circumstances: _Monday, Wednesday and Friday before dinner in the den with the door closed. Saturday morning before breakfast_

I choose to *repeat my communication affirmations at least once each day this week*

Under the following circumstances: *On first waking up in the morning, before getting out of bed.*

I choose to *use the paraphrasing or reflecting-back technique of active listening with my friend Jane*

Under the following circumstances: *I will invite Jane to dinner on Saturday evening (I'll feel more confident on my own turf)*

I choose to _____

_____

Under the following circumstances: _____

_____

I choose to _____

_____

Under the following circumstances: _____

_____

My other opportunity situations for skill practice are:

1. *Dealing better with my secretary.*
2. *Finding out what is really going on in my kids lives*
3. *Finally asking my mother whether or not I was adopted.*

_____

I have arranged to check in with my partner . . .

When?	About . . .
Sunday around noon	*How the dinner with Jane went*

Week 3: Build on Your Success

Fill out your Action Diary Planning Page. In the next three weeks, choose to do the following:

1. *Continue to practice autogenic relaxation plus affirmation and visualization.* Modify your affirmations or introduce new ones to suit your deepening sense of self. Continue to practice autogenic relaxation at least four times a week. Use your affirmations daily—ideally two or three times each day.

2. *Build on your week 2 behavior change.* Whatever you did in week 2, keep doing it, and look for additional opportunities and ways to deepen your practice of this assertive skill. Perhaps you've noticed that you have particular difficulty with assertive language. In this case, you might plan for specific opportunities to get the pronoun "I" into your daily speech. Or maybe there's a weekly meeting at work in which you have always felt helpless and weak. Look for new ways to be more assertive at the meeting this week. Plan ahead.

In week 3, Sarah took the next step. She stressed to her boss just how helpful last week's agenda had been, and again he had an agenda to her in advance, this time by Wednesday. When she gave it back to him Thursday morning, she had added two items to it that were important to her. Realizing what a difference this improved communication was making with her boss, she invited her subordinates to do the same with her: to propose items for the agenda of their Friday noon meeting.

Until this point, Sarah had always felt so overwhelmed by her boss's style, and so caught up in simply reacting to the developing situation, that she had felt incapable (no time) of being open to new ideas from her sales force (they would only mean more work for her and even more stress, and would likely be blocked by her boss, in any event). Now, after only two weeks, she was feeling a little more control in her job and confident enough to begin to really listen to her staff—and to take her changing relationship with her boss a step further in week 4.

3. *Check in with your partner.*

4. *Record your progress in your Action Diary.* As you congratulate yourself for your successes and for noting missed opportunities, you will see more clearly where you need to concentrate your attention.

Week 4: Consolidate Your Gains

Fill out your Action Diary Planning Page. During the week, agree to do the following:

1. *Continue to practice autogenic relaxation plus affirmation and visualization.* Your self-themes for assertive communication are gaining potency as you take action to express your real self. This positive self-talk is becoming a larger part of your inner dialogue.

Use your relaxation tape four times this week. Repeat your affirmations daily, ideally two or three times each day.

2. *Consolidate your new self-affirming behavior(s).* If your are becoming more comfortable with ''I'' language, then get into it even more. Perhaps start to use it in a situation in which you are usually quite unsure of yourself. Have you tried active listening with your boss, but not with your spouse? Now may be the time to tackle this more challenging relationship. Whatever you choose to do this week, consciously build on the successes you've had in the previous two weeks so that your new skills really take root.

In week 4, Sarah's new openness with her staff paid off. One of their ideas was to move the Friday sales meeting to Monday (when they wouldn't be wasting valuable follow-up time): They too were becoming more assertive. When she considered this suggestion, Sarah realized that her Friday meeting with the boss would also make more sense on Monday, since sales figures for the previous week would have been tabulated.

But there was a problem: Friday review meetings had been part of ''company culture'' since the dawn of time. And since her boss was an arch-traditionalist who'd been with the company forever, the idea looked like a real recipe for conflict. Sarah felt her stress thermometer rise. Then she made a plan.

First, she checked to see if anyone had ever proposed a Monday meeting before (no one had). Over the weekend, she drafted a memo to her boss carefully outlining the rationale for the change. This was on his desk on Monday, they had a follow-up discussion on Tuesday (boss resistant, no resolution), then Sarah added it as an item of discussion on the Friday agenda. It took two Friday discussions before the boss came around. The tactic that finally melted his resistance was Sarah's framing the issue in a ''win-win'' way, suggesting a six-month pilot project to see how the new system worked.

3. *Check in with your partner.* Are you still encountering obstacles? Are you letting others sabotage the communication process? Discuss these obstacles with your partner and brainstorm solutions.

4. *Record your progress in your Action Diary.* Look back at how far you've come since week 1, and pat yourself on the back for the progress you've made. You aren't such a Milquetoast after all. Continue to give yourself credit for each new behavior you've introduced and each opportunity you've noticed. Savor your success.

Continuing Your Prescription

Now that you've completed your four-week start-up program for Self-Affirming Communication, it's up to you what you do next. Are you feeling better about yourself? Do you still feel that you have a long way to go? You have now laid the cornerstone of lasting change.

As you continue this intervention, you can use the start-up structure as a model or prototype for successful behavior change. It takes about three weeks for a new behavior to take root, to move from being an awkward novelty to a grounded part of yourself. So plan to introduce one new behavior every three weeks and gradually reinforce it, as Sarah did. You will soon be on your way to living in a more self-affirming way.

When you feel ready (the sooner the better), begin phasing in the next intervention on your Prescription Pad. (We recommend, however, that you don't start to do this before week 8 of your program.) The sooner you do, the sooner your total prescription can interact to accelerate your body age reduction and increase your vitality.

At the heart of successful stress regulation is a sense of increased "life control." As Sarah reported at the eight-month checkup (her body age having gone down 9 years to 42, below her calendar age by 2 years), "I had always felt a little embarrassed or inadequate by my title of manager, because as a typical 'driven dog,' I was anything but managing. Now I am *a manager* ['I manage my work' was one of her affirmations]. Now that I use the power of my position in a forceful, caring way, I'm no longer intimidated by its responsibilities. Once I began standing up for my rights, they began standing up for me. The way I feel this most days now is that when I give people—at work and in my personal life—the opportunity to respect me, they do . . . with surprising regularity."

CHAPTER 11
Essential Exercise

SECONDARY INTERVENTION: Basket Case
ALSO IMPORTANT FOR: Cliff Walker

Core Message

A sound exercise program has a balance of exercises for suppleness, strength, and stamina. It includes a minimum of three twenty- to thirty-minute aerobic workouts a week.

Your exercise program should start small, be geared to your fitness needs and lifestyle, and, above all, be simple and fun.

Root your changes in exercise behavior through the use of affirmations and visualizations. These techniques will also help you focus, conserve, and self-pace your expenditure of energy.

Exercise contributed most to the body age reduction of the Basket Case stressotype, where it was the second most effective intervention, and of the Cliff Walker stressotype, where it ranked third. In general, it proved most effective when used in conjunction with at least one other Vital Life Skill. For both of these stressotypes, exercise was more potent when undertaken in combination with High-Performance Nutrition. True physical fitness results from a balance of good nutrition and adequate exercise.

Regardless of your stressotype, there are many benefits of regular, balanced exercise. Here is a short list of the payoffs you can expect from a sound exercise program:

1. *Exercise is a natural stimulant that promotes the optimum efficiency of certain crucial bodily systems.* Regular exercise of the kind recommended here improves the operating efficiency of your muscles, lungs, circulatory system, and heart. It aids digestion and cuts down on the bone-mineral loss associated with aging. It can actually restore lost efficiency to these systems, thus directly contributing to body age reduction and reducing your risk of degenerative diseases of the heart and circulatory system.

2. *Aerobic fitness means more efficient use of stress energy.* The higher your level of aerobic fitness, the more efficiently your body uses oxygen. (We'll be talking about what aerobic fitness is in the "Basic Training" section.) This means you need to rely less often on your stress hormones and that you will recover more quickly from physical exertion or high-stress situations. A person who is out of shape will use a lot more stress energy getting through a normal day than a person who is fit. And he or she will have little stress energy in reserve when a big demand comes along.

Any exercise that raises your heart rate to "training range" (discussed below) for more than one minute and that is immediately followed by relaxation breathing will improve your stress recovery, the time it takes you to return to a lower stress level following a high-stress event.

3. *Exercise helps lower your stress level.* In chapter 2, we explained how stress is a primitive bodily mechanism preparing you to fight or flee, readying you for intense physical action. If you've spent the entire day in this high-stress state of red alert, a strenuous workout (which can be anything from a brisk walk to a several-mile run, depending on your level of fitness) sends a signal to your body that it's okay to lower the stress thermostat. In short, exercise provides the action your hyped-up body craves. Thus a very good time to exercise is during or after a high-stress day.

4. *Exercise purges your body of stress-induced fatigue acids.* Fatigue acids, notably lactic acid, build up in your body because of stress. Your muscles become tired and heavy, your energy level drops, and you feel you've "taken a beating." An intense aerobic exercise session lowers the level of these fatigue acids in your body, which is why many people experience a second wind after a good workout.

5. *Exercise relaxes your body and your mind.* In a stress reaction, your muscles tighten, ready to ward off an attacker. Unfortunately for many people, this stress-induced muscle tension becomes chronic. And when tight muscles become very uncomfortable, they begin to affect your performance.

Stretching exercises are particularly good at relaxing tense muscles, whether the tension results from stress or from unbalanced exercise. In fact, any intense physical workout followed by an appropriate cool-down should leave your muscles more relaxed than before you started.

Exercise also relaxes your mind by allowing you to focus on something other than your problems and worries, helping you release pent-up emotions as well as physical tension. In short, exercise can be one of the most effective relaxation techniques.

6. *Exercise helps you avoid injuries and recover from injuries.* Because any physical injury is very stressful, anything you can do to prevent bodily mishaps will reduce your stress demands. For most people who lead a sedentary lifestyle, a regular and balanced exercise program is a good way of avoiding injuries. It can also help you avoid or cure chronic back problems.

7. *Exercise makes you feel and look younger.* Appropriate exercise is fun and leaves you with a pleasant sense of physical well-being. People who exercise regularly tend to sleep better, and use less sugar, caffeine, alcohol, nicotine, and other drugs. Regular exercise tones your muscles, improving your appearance.

Above all, exercise makes you feel good about yourself, especially if you do it in a self-affirming way. For most people, exercise is one of the most obvious self-respecting behaviors; it reinforces the positive self-behavior cycle. Nothing can beat the pleasure of seeing your performance improve. And the more solid your sense of self, the less often you will perceive a threat that isn't there, or overreact to uncertainty or something new. That means you'll spend less unnecessary stress energy and have more stress energy when you really need it.

Essential Exercise works for you because it is an active expression of your increasingly positive sense of self. We aren't interested in muscle building, we're interested in self building. Each time you jog, visit the gym, or play a game of squash, you are building your positive self-image—a physical, mental, emotional, and spiritual foundation for your growing self-esteem.

Many people in the Body Age Study found that exercise almost immediately made them feel better about themselves. Sharon (Basket Case, age 32, body age 38) noted that by the end of her third evening of swimming, ''although most work days left me feeling totally beat, I took the leap of faith into the pool and found I literally had more energy and felt less tired after a vigorous half-hour swim.'' In her first week, Sharon experienced one of the beneficial effects of exercise—the purging of fatigue acids. Other fitness payoffs, such as increased energy reserves, would come a bit later.

The first step in learning this Vital Life Skill is to find out how fit you now are.

RATE YOURSELF

In this section, you will learn the following:

> If you are ready to begin exercise right now
> Your level of fitness in each of the three key
>   exercise areas: suppleness, strength, and
>   stamina
> Your exercise goals
> Your exercise affirmations and visualizations

Are You Ready for Exercise?

This simple questionnaire, closely based on the widely used Physical Activity Readiness Questionnaire (or Par Q), helps you decide how to go about beginning a regular exercise program. For most people, increased physical activity poses no health problems, especially when it is phased in slowly. This questionnaire will help you find out if you are one of the small number of adults for whom physical activity might be inappropriate or who should get medical advice before starting an exercise program. Answer the following questions carefully with either yes or no for each one.

Has your doctor ever said you have heart trouble? _____
Do you frequently have pains in your heart and chest? _____
Do you often feel faint or have spells of severe dizziness? _____
Has a doctor ever said your blood pressure was too high? _____
Has your doctor ever told you that you have have a bone or joint
    problem, such as arthritis, that has been aggravated by exercise
    or might be made worse with exercise? _____

Is there a good physical reason not mentioned here why you should
   not follow an activity program, even if you wanted to? _____
Are you over age 65 and not accustomed to vigorous exercise? ___

If you answered yes to one or more questions, you should consult your
physician before increasing your activity or taking a fitness test. Your
physician can advise you on an appropriate exercise program or refer to
you to a fitness professional who will do so.

If you answered no to all questions, you are probably ready for either
a graduated exercise program or fitness appraisal.

The key to physical fitness is a balance of suppleness, strength, and
stamina. The following exercise tests allow you to gauge your current
level of fitness in each of these three crucial areas. If you want an even
more precise measure of how fit you are, we recommend that you take
a clinical fitness test conducted by a physician. Ask your doctor to refer
you to a clinic that can perform such a test.

Test Your Suppleness

Suppleness is perhaps the most easily neglected exercise area, yet one
of the most important. Suppleness, or flexibility, is the range of motion
of a joint; it underlies your ability to perform all physical activities with
ease, whether reaching for the telephone or bending to pick up a pencil
off the floor. Suppleness exercises prevent joint problems associated with
aging and help other body systems, such as digestion and circulation, to
work better. With regular exercise and regular use of relaxation techniques, you can be as supple as a 3-year-old.

The following tests measure your flexibility in eight key muscle groups.
You'll need a partner to get an accurate score for some of them.

Shoulder Stretch Test. Bring one hand around and place it on the back of your neck. Bring the other hand around to small of your back. Now try to touch the fingertips of your two hands. Have a friend measure the distance between your fingertips. Your fingers should be able to touch or overlap.

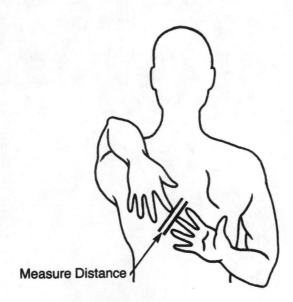

Measure Distance

Side Stretch Test. Stand upright with your arms dangling at your sides. Slide one hand down the side of your body toward the knee, without shifting your hip bones. Measure the distance between your fingertips and the side of your knee (a partner will make this easier). Is there a difference on one side or the other? If so, you are more muscle-bound on one side than on the other. You should be able to reach to or below your knee.

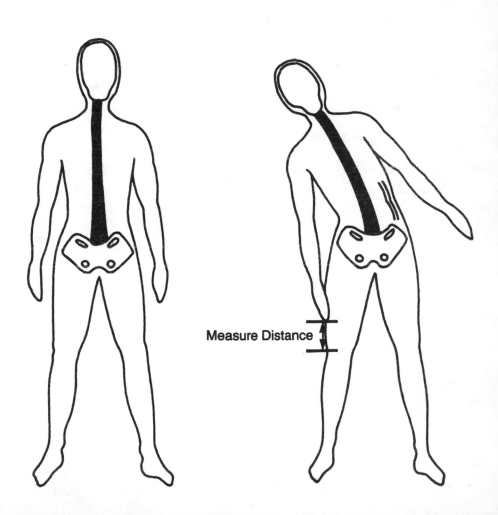

Measure Distance

Back Flexibility Test. Lie on the floor with your feet flat on the ground (knees will be at about a 45-degree angle). Your feet should not be held down in any way. Now put your hands beside your head. Try to sit up slowly, without raising your feet off the floor. If you can't sit up without your feet rising off the floor, try the test with your arms folded over your chest. If your feet still lift off, try the test with your arms stretched out in front of you.

The illustrations below indicate how fit your back is in descending order from grade 1 (very flexible) to grade 4 (very stiff). Note that this test also measures the strength of your stomach muscles.

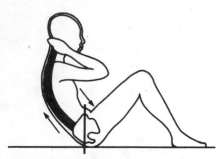

Grade 1: Able to sit straight with knees bent and hands behind neck.

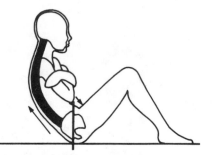

Grade 2: Able to sit up with knees bent and arms folded across chest.

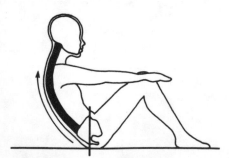

Grade 3: Able to sit up with knees bent and arms held out straight.

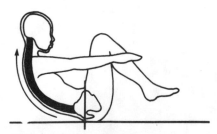

Grade 4: Unable to sit up with knees bent.

Hip Flexibility Test. Lie on your back on the floor with your legs stretched out and with your knees bent comfortably. Bend your right knee to your chest and hold it there firmly. Now straighten your left leg out along the floor as far as it can comfortably go, but without moving your right leg away from its position against your chest. Repeat this exercise on the other side. Your grade on this test is determined by the position of the straightened leg in relation to the floor. (Grade 1 is most flexible; grade 4, least flexible.)

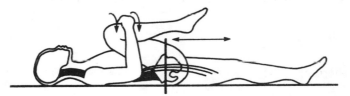

Grade 1: Able to hold one leg firmly against chest with other leg flat against floor.

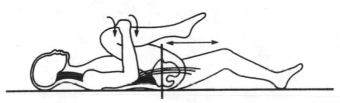

Grade 2: With effort able to hold one knee against chest while straightening other leg flat to floor.

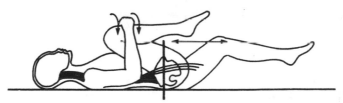

Grade 3: With one knee fixed firmly against chest, the other leg will not reach floor.

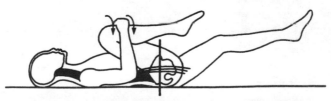

Grade 4: Unable to get one leg firmly against chest without causing pain or discomfort and/or other leg raises off floor significantly.

Hamstring Flexibility Test. Sit on the floor with one leg bent so that the foot is near the knee of the straight leg (it can be touching). The knee of the straight leg is on or close to the floor. Gently curl your upper body toward the knee of the straight leg. Hold your maximum comfortable stretch. Now have a partner measure the distance between your head and your knee. Women should be able to touch their knees. Men should be able to get within about 2 inches of the knee.

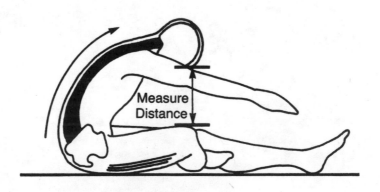

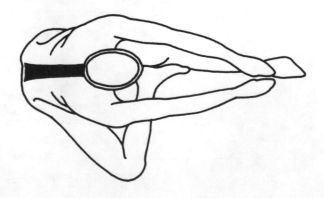

Groin Flexibility Test. Sit on the floor with your knees bent and the bottoms of your feet together. With your hands gently clasping your ankles and your forearms resting on your calves, push both knees down and out as far as possible (without pain). Have your partner measure the distance between your knee and the floor. Men should be able to get their knees as close as 4 inches; women, 8 inches.

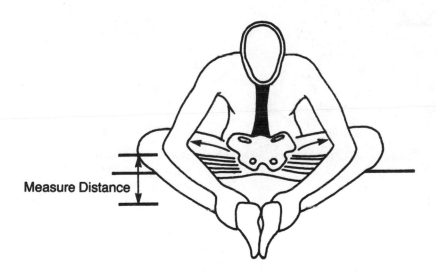

Measure Distance

Thigh Flexibility Test. Lie face down on the floor. Bend your right leg and grasp the ankle with your right hand. Bring your heel as close as possible to your buttock without pain. Have your partner measure the distance from heel to buttock. Repeat with the left leg. Most people can touch the heel to the buttock.

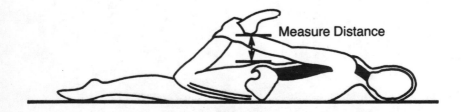

Measure Distance

Calf Flexibility Test. Sit on the floor with your back straight and your feet flat against a wall. Bring your toes and the ball of your foot away from the wall. Have your partner measure the distance from the ball of your foot to the wall. Repeat with the other foot. You should be able to move the ball of your foot at least 2 inches from the wall.

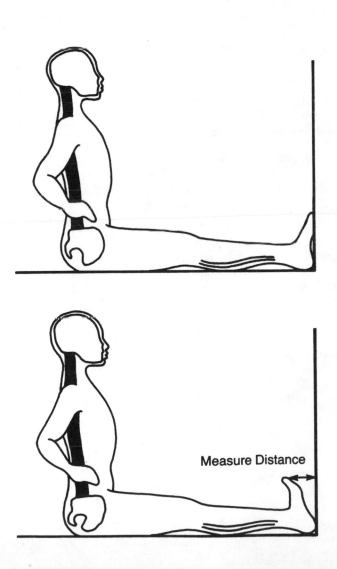

Measure Distance

Test Your Strength

Strength consists of two elements: the maximum force or tension that a muscle can exert, and muscle endurance, the length of time a muscle can continue to exert force. Strength underlies the ability of a muscle to perform the same action repeatedly (chopping wood, hitting a squash ball, climbing the stairs). It is a function of the length of the muscle, not just its size or bulk. (For more on the relationship between length and strength, see the section "Balancing Your Exercise Budget.")

The following three tests will give you an idea of the strength of your most important muscle groups: the strength foundation you need for daily life and for all exercise. Most back problems stem from weak trunk muscles.

As soon as something starts to hurt or you become uncomfortable, stop the test. The point is to see how strong you are, not to injure yourself trying to exceed your limit.

Stomach Strength Test. Your stomach muscles are particularly important, since weak stomach muscles often contribute to poor posture and lower-back problems.

Lie on the floor with your legs bent to 45 degrees and your feet on the floor. Put one hand between your lower back and the floor. Tighten your stomach muscles, and flatten the arch in your lower back so that it presses your hand to the floor. Now straighten your legs and raise your feet until they are about 6 inches above the floor. Hold this position for ten counts, if you can. Keep your back flat, pressing firmly on your hand, throughout the test. If your lower back begins to curve away from the floor, don't continue to hold your legs up—back strain may result.

Compare your performance with the illustration. Grade 1 means your stomach muscles are in excellent shape. Grade 2, average, means you need more stomach-muscle strength. Grade 3 (fair) and grade 4 (poor) mean that the stomach-strengthening exercises such as the Sit-Down, described in the "Basic Training" section, are very important for you.

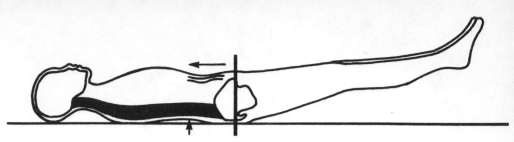

Grade 1: Able to keep back flat against floor while raising legs 6 inches for a count of 10.

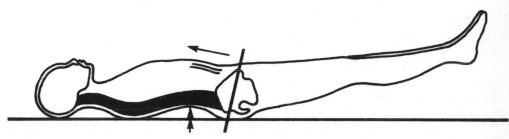

Grade 2: Able to raise legs for several counts, but back curves partway through the test.

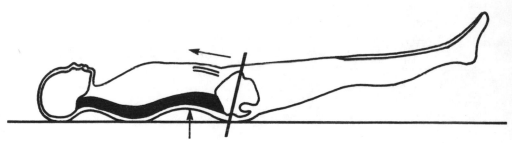

Grade 3: Able to lift legs, but back curves immediately when legs are raised.

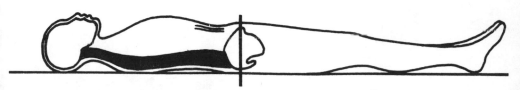

Grade 4: Unable to lift both legs for 10 counts and/or lifting legs causes discomfort.

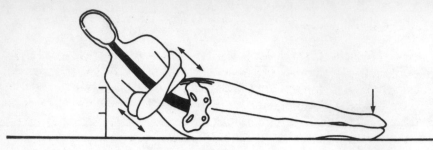

Grade 1: Able to raise shoulder 12 inches off floor without difficulty, and hold for 10 counts.

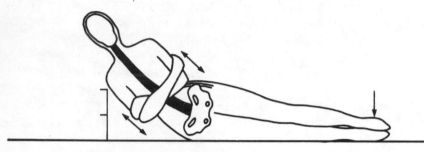

Grade 2: Able to raise shoulder 12 inches off floor only with difficulty; cannot hold for 10 counts.

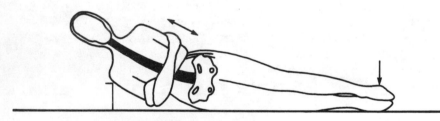

Grade 3: Able to raise shoulder only slightly off the floor and with difficulty.

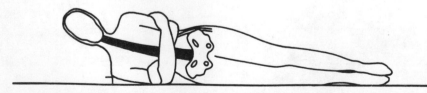

Grade 4: Unable to raise shoulder off the floor.

Lateral Muscle Strength Test. This test of the strength of your lateral trunk muscles (along the sides of your torso) also will tell you if there is any imbalance between your right and left lateral muscles.

Lie on your side, with your legs and body in a straight line and your arms crossed in front of your chest. Have your partner grasp your feet at the ankles and hold them firmly to the floor. Now raise your shoulders and trunk slowly from the floor without twisting your body backward or forward. Hold this position for ten counts or as long as you can without pain. Repeat the test on the opposite side.

Add together your grades for the right and left side, and divide the total by two for your overall grade. Grade 1 is excellent; grade 2, average; grade 3, fair; and grade 4, poor. The lateral leg lifts described in the "Strengthening Exercises" section of "Basic Training" will help you strengthen these important muscles, which also help with back fitness.

Arm and Shoulder Strength Test. This test is nothing more than the common push-up. But since push-ups are often done incorrectly, be sure to follow these instructions to the letter.

Men: Lie on your stomach with your legs together. Position your hands beneath your shoulders, palms down and pointing forward. Push up from the floor or mat by fully straightening your elbows, keeping your body straight (without straining), and using your toes as a pivot point. Keep your body in a straight line throughout the exercise, finishing each push-up with your chin touching the floor (neither your chest, stomach, nor thighs should touch). Keep breathing in and out as you do the push-ups and do as many as you can until you begin to strain or are unable to continue the proper push-up technique. (Your partner can monitor this for you.)

Men

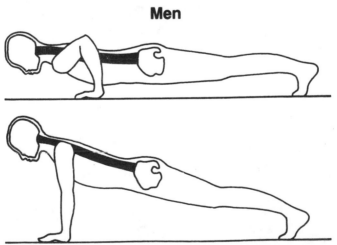

Women

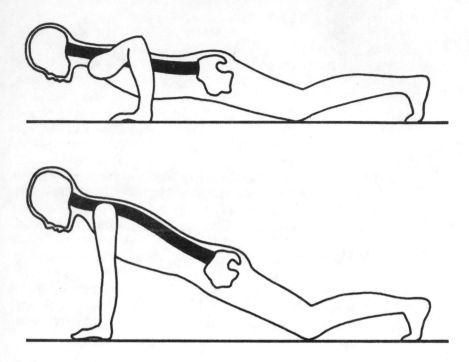

Women: Lie on your stomach with your legs together. Position your hands under your shoulders, palms down and pointing forward. Now push up from the mat by fully straightening your elbows, keeping your back straight, and using your knees as the pivot point. Keep your upper body in a straight line as you complete the push-up. At this point, your chin should be touching the floor, but your stomach should not. Continue your push-ups until you are straining forcibly or can no longer keep your upper body straight. (Your partner can monitor you.)

The chart below shows the number of push-ups the average person can do, depending on age and sex.

	Age 15–19	Age 20–29	Age 30–39	Age 40–49	Age 50–59	Age 60–69
Men	23–28	22–28	17–21	13–16	10–12	8–10
Women	18–24	15–20	13–19	11–14	7–10	5–11

Test Your Stamina

In simplest terms, stamina is a measure of the efficiency with which your heart and lungs transport oxygen to your muscles and organs. Thus stamina is often referred to as cardiorespiratory fitness. Aerobic exercises promote stamina (*aerobic* simply means requiring air or oxygen). You are probably aware of your stamina in two ways: how long you can keep up an extended period of exercise (a game of tennis, a hike in the woods, climbing a flight of stairs), and your reserves of energy during a normal day.

The goal of testing your stamina is to find how much activity it takes to raise your heartbeat to your training heart rate, which is the number of heartbeats per minute that is equivalent to between 70 and 85 percent of the maximum heart rate for your age. This training range is the level of activity at which you begin to condition your heart and lungs to deliver oxygen to your muscles and organs more efficiently (that is, with less effort). Note that there is no benefit to exceeding this range, and there could be some risk.

Use the chart below to see the training heart rate range for your age.

CALCULATE YOUR TARGET HEART RATE FOR THE TRAINING EFFECT

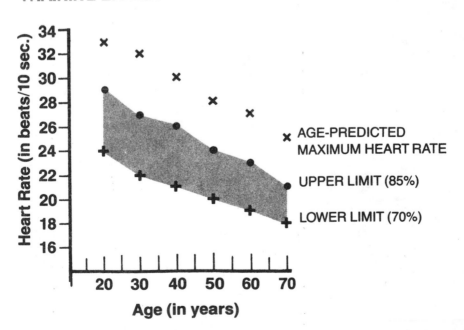

To check your heart rate, do the following:

Find a spot where you can feel your pulse. The two most common spots are at the wrist and at the neck. For the wrist pulse, place your first two fingers just below the base of your thumb and just above the tendons running up the arm. Move your fingers around until you find a steady pulse. You should need to press only lightly. For the neck pulse, place your first two fingers in the groove between your Adam's apple and the muscle running vertically down the side of your neck.

Count the number of pulses in a ten-second period. Multiply the number by 6 (this gives you your beats per minute).

Is this number within the training range for your age group?

Now that you know your training heart rate and how to check your pulse, you are ready to test your stamina. The simplest test is to go for a walk, stopping periodically to test your pulse. Keep increasing your walking speed until your training heart rate is reached. (Note that you should do this test when you are well rested and at least an hour after your last meal.) If walking won't get you up to your training heart rate, then try jogging or some other activity you enjoy. If you are already regularly doing some exercise that you assume increases your stamina, test yourself during the exercise to see if you're really enjoying the training effect. Most people find that they tend to exceed the recommended rate when exercising and so must deliberately slow their pace.

This test will give you a good idea of what level of activity you should aim for as you start your exercise program. If you are aerobically fit, you should be able to easily maintain your training heart rate (without going over it) for twenty to thirty minutes of continuous exercise, whether this is cycling, swimming, jogging, dancing, or some other activity.

What Are Your Motivations for Exercise?

As preparation for developing the affirmations and visualizations you will use as you get your exercise program under way, identify your underlying motives for undertaking Essential Exercise. You probably decided to read this chapter because your prescription showed exercise to be an important intervention for you. But you likely have some other motives and images of your more fit self. These will help drive your behavior change. The following list has been drawn from the Body Age Study participants who worked on exercise. It is by no means comprehensive, and we've left space at the end for you to write in additional reasons for exercising.

At the left of each item, assign it a value on a scale of one (low) to ten (high).

_____I want to look better: slimmer, more shapely, "bright-eyed," bright-faced, more vital.

_____Sports are a way I enjoy being with friends and family.

_____Exercise is a great way to meet new or casual acquaintances.

_____I want to have more stamina: stronger heart and lungs.

_____I want to strengthen my heart muscle to avoid a heart attack.

_____Exercise feels good, during and after.

_____Exercise relaxes me through release of muscle tension, by taking my mind off distracting and worrying thoughts, and by damping down my stress hormones.

_____I want to get in shape for a particular sport.

_____Exercise helps me control my appetite.

_____Regular exercise gives me self-confidence. It shows I can look after myself.

_____I want to have more "pep and endurance" throughout the day.

_____I want to overcome fatigue at the end of the day.

_____Exercise gives me a sense of time mastery; it is "my time for me."

_____Exercise allows me to measure my progress, to see I'm getting a return on my investment.

_____Exercise is a "third space," a place that is neither work nor intimate personal life.

_____When I exercise, I get respect from others, and I feel more respect for myself.

_____Exercise is a good topic of conversation: new exercises, accessories, progress in a particular sport.

_____When I maintain a constant weight, I spend less money on clothes.

_____I like to be a role model for my kids.

_____I want fun and excitement.

_____I want to challenge my abilities and stretch my limits.

_____I want to learn new things.

_____

_____

_____

There are many good reasons to exercise. So how come you're not doing it? For most people, the biggest roadblock (excuse) is time: "My schedule is too busy—maybe when my workload eases off." If you really want to exercise, you will find the time. (For help in this endeavor, see, in chapter 8, "Pinpoint Your Time Wasters" and "Investing Your Time Capital.")

Your Exercise Affirmations and Visualizations

You are now ready to develop affirmations and visualizations that capture the essence of what you want to achieve through your new exercise behavior. Draw on what you've learned about your fitness gaps and your exercise goals to come up with one or two affirmations—words or phrases—that express meaningful self-themes for your exercise program. Develop visualizations that portray your exercise success—either in the act of exercising or in the way you will look and feel after exercising. Or you may wish to use a more general vitality affirmation.

Here are some possible affirmations with which to begin week 1 of your start-up program:

> I can count on myself three times a week.
> I am lean energy.
> I am as supple as a cat.
> Ready and able.
> I am a lean machine.
> I've got what it takes.
> Energy on tap.
> Feeling stronger, lasting longer.
> Curves where I want them.

Here are some sample visualizations:

> I see my heart pumping blood through the veins to my muscles.
> I see myself going to the club and taking an aerobics class.
> At the end of my exercise session, I see myself glowing with good health and energy.
> I see energy (oxygen) releasing or exploding in my body.
> I see myself sweating heavily; as each drop falls to the ground (or evaporates), I see the cares and worries being flushed from my whole being.
> I feel my muscles "smiling at me" as I go through my workout.
> As I jog, I see high-octane fuel being pumped into my reserve tank, for use when I need it.
> As I work out on the weights, I see myself as a sculptor slowly shaping each muscle group to make the ideal me.

BASIC TRAINING

In the "Rate Yourself" section, you learned how fit you are and the areas you want to improve. In this section, we'll explain some underlying principles and teach you the basic skills of Essential Exercise. As with all five Vital Life Skills, it is important to keep exercise simple, doable, and fun.

Fit for What?

Fitness tests are useful, but perhaps the best measure of your fitness is a much more subjective one: Can your body do what you want it to do and still have something left in reserve? Do you have the capacity to meet the demands of your daily life, including the occasional crisis or peak demand, without undue strain on your muscles or your ability to manufacture stress energy when you need it? Is there still gas in your tank even after a peak demand has been met? Remember: Fitness is your capacity to perform when you want to.

The first step in figuring out exactly what kind of fitness investment you want to make is to answer the question "Fit for what?" Most of you probably have no ambition to run the Boston Marathon or to climb Mount Everest. If you're like the vast majority of our study subjects, your main interest is in becoming more fit for everyday life. Just what is the life you want to become fit for?

Among the participants in the Body Age Study were a number of people who exercised regularly but were not really up to the basic demands of ordinary living. One of them was a 41-year-old Drifter high school teacher (body age 46) who worked out five times a week power-lifting. He could bench-press 345 pounds, but if asked to run down the block, he would have been out of breath. Another was a Loner stockbroker (age 32, body age 39) who regularly ran 3 miles after work. But he complained of lower-back pain and chronic stiffness in his neck and shoulders. At the end of a tough day, he was a wreck, exhausted mentally and physically. Being truly fit for everyday life requires a more balanced exercise program than most people realize.

If you work a ten- to twelve-hour day, you probably need exercises that increase your stamina. If you work at a sedentary job, you need exercise that keeps up the strength and flexibility of muscles you don't use a lot and that maintains an efficient level of blood circulation. In particular, you need exercise to strengthen weak abdominal muscles. If your job is one that demands an occasional burst of high-energy activity during an otherwise uneventful day, you need to have a high level of aerobic capacity.

Many people become quite obsessive about exercise without stopping to consider whether the program they've chosen really prepares them for the activities they want to do. A twenty-minute jog in the morning is better preparation for a stressful day than a 6-mile run (and it will keep you in good shape for the game of tennis you want to play at the top of your form). What sort of return are you getting on your exercise investment? Here's how to get more back for the energy you spend.

Balancing Your Exercise Budget (Suppleness, Strength, and Stamina)

Depending on your lifestyle, you may benefit from giving special emphasis to one of the three Ss of Essential Exercise: suppleness, strength, and stamina. But no exercise program is complete without a *balance* of these exercises, just as no total fitness regimen is complete without a balance of good nutrition and regular exercise.

Suppleness (the range of motion of your joints) is in many ways the foundation of Essential Exercise, yet many fitness fans neglect it. How often do you go for a jog or play a game of tennis without a warm-up that includes a complete set of stretches? And does your morning ritual include five to ten minutes of stretching before breakfast? If not, you are neglecting this basic exercise skill.

One of the main benefits of suppleness exercises is to lengthen muscles that are short and therefore weak. There are four basic ways that muscles become too short: from chronic muscle tension due to stress; from too much unbalanced exercise (for example, weight training without stretching); from disuse and aging; and from injury or spasm. Short muscles can be restored through specific stretching routines that lengthen the weakened muscles. Stretching exercises also help lubricate your joints and promote blood flow to essential organs.

Exercises for strength (the ability to apply force) complement suppleness exercises by working to shorten muscles that are too long (and therefore weak). If you've been pregnant, you know what long, weak stomach muscles feel (and look) like. If you have lower-back problems, it's probably because your stomach and other trunk muscles are long and weak.

Muscles usually become too long because of injury or disuse. Long muscles can also result from unbalanced exercise, usually because stretching is neglected. They can also result from too much stretching (for example, if you practice Yoga and nothing else).

Strength and suppleness are two sides of the same coin. When muscles are too short (muscle-bound), they need to be stretched through suppleness exercises. When they are too long (flabby), they need to be shortened through strengthening exercises. The object of the strengthening and suppleness exercises we'll teach is to balance your muscles at their optimum length, neither too short nor too long. Balanced muscles are powerful muscles.

Once you have toned your muscles so that they are in optimum balance, the only way you can increase your muscle power is by building their bulk, which requires increasing the load when you do strengthening exercises; this is the principle underlying all weight training. Muscle power is a combination of muscle balance and muscle bulk.

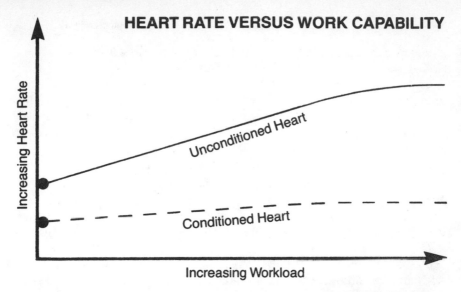

HEART RATE VERSUS WORK CAPABILITY

Increasing Heart Rate

Unconditioned Heart

Conditioned Heart

Increasing Workload

An unconditioned heart works harder at rest than does a conditioned heart, and as workload increases, an "out of shape" heart's rate rises much more quickly. In short, the unconditioned heart works harder to do the same amount of work as a conditioned heart.

The third S, stamina (aerobic or cardiorespiratory endurance), balances the first two Ss. To increase your stamina, you need to choose an activity that raises your heart rate into your training range and keeps it there for between twenty and thirty minutes.

As you condition your heart muscle, it is able to pump more blood with less effort. This means that it actually beats more slowly when at rest and doesn't have to pump as hard when called on to increase blood flow. Conditioning your heart makes its job easier, helping it last longer. An important side effect of a stronger, more efficient heart is better circulation of the blood, which is pumped more forcefully to your muscles and other tissues; that is, more blood flows with each squeeze of the heart muscle. More blood pumping more forcefully through the arteries and veins helps keep them clean and unblocked, which in turn makes the heart's job easier.

If you have suppleness, strength, and stamina, you're physically fit in the specific ways that exercise can promote. But the potential return on your exercise investment is considerably greater than any narrow measurement of your fitness level.

The more you make exercise a part of your life—the way you work and the way you spend your leisure (including your stress patterns)—the more your exercise success will spill over into other parts of your existence. The pleasure of seeing your performance improve with practice encourages improved performance elsewhere, especially if you exercise as a positive expression of your self-image, using the reinforcement of autogenically rooted affirmations and visualizations. Each success is proof that you are becoming the person you really want to be.

This section provides you with the basics of a sound, balanced exercise program—one you can follow without joining an expensive health club or purchasing fancy equipment. The program has four building blocks: warm-up and cool-down; suppleness exercises; strengthening exercises; and stamina exercises.

But first consider the Stretch-Relaxation Formula. Use it whenever you are doing a stretching exercise, whether as part of a warm-up or cool-down, or by itself.

The Stretch-Relaxation Formula

You should begin every stretching exercise by adopting gentle, slow relaxation breathing, which is explored in detail in chapter 9, "Effective Relaxation." Here is a simple summary of the basic breathing technique.

If you perform this breathing exercise by itself, you can sit in a comfortable chair and let your head and arms dangle. Since here you are doing relaxation breathing in the context of stretching exercises, simply remember to let all the parts of your body that aren't involved in the stretch stay relaxed. Important spots to monitor include the jaw (is it relaxed or clenched?), the knees (are they locked or slightly bent?), and the shoulders (are they relaxed or tight?). The essentials of relaxation breathing are as follows:

1. Breathe in deeply, first expanding your belly and then your chest. Your shoulders will naturally rise a bit at this point.
2. Breathe out *slowly*, consciously letting go of muscle tightness, first releasing the air from your chest, then letting your belly fall.
3. When your breath has fully expired, your muscles are more relaxed. The muscle you are stretching will elongate on its own.
4. Continue breathing in this way throughout the stretching exercise.

Here is how to combine relaxation breathing with stretching to produce the Stretch-Relaxation Formula.

1. Begin to breathe in a slow, relaxed manner. Stretch the muscle to the point just before pain. If it starts to hurt, stop the stretch. Pain means you are overstretching. Hold this position for the duration of at least one slow out-breath. On a long, slow out-breath, consciously let go

of the tightness in the muscle you are stretching. Don't bounce.

2. Take up the slack in the muscle by stretching it a little further, to a point just before pain.

3. Repeat the movement while continuing relaxation breathing.

4. You can work on increasing your maximum stretch still further by holding the stretch and breathing in and out several times, allowing the stretch to lengthen on each long, slow out-breath.

With the Stretch-Relaxation Formula firmly in mind, you are now ready for the four building blocks of Essential Exercise.

Warm-Up and Cool-Down

This important and often-neglected aspect of exercise deserves to be highlighted. Do a five-minute warm-up before every aerobic exercise session and before every session that works primarily on building strength. Always cool down for five minutes after any intense exercise.

A warm-up consists of limbering movements and stretching exercises to get the blood flowing to all the muscles, and to stretch and loosen tight muscles while lubricating the joints. As the name implies, a warm-up literally warms you up, by increasing your blood flow to your tissues and muscles. It raises muscle temperature to allow for more efficient muscular contraction while gradually increasing your heart and lung activity. At the end of a proper warm-up, you should feel warmer and ready for more intense activity. Many minor aches and pains are created when a cold or stiff muscle is forced to exercise. Thus a proper warm-up definitely reduces the risk of injury.

Five minutes is the minimum time needed for an adequate warm-up. Ten minutes is ideal. If you are just beginning to get back into shape, allow ten minutes for your warm-up before more strenuous exercise. As your flexibility and muscle strength increase, you can warm up in as little as five minutes. A warm-up routine is also a great way to start the day.

The Shakeout (see p. 207) is a wonderful limbering-up exercise that you can use as part of your warm-up. Dancing, jogging lightly in place, or riding a bicycle at a gradually increasing pace are all suitable limbering exercises as part of your warm-up.

For your warm-up stretches, use the eight basic suppleness exercises in the next section.

A good cool-down consists of about five minutes of easy movement that allows your heart rate to slow down gradually. You might begin by walking, then do some simple strength exercises, and then end with a few favorite stretches.

Suppleness Exercises

Exercises that improve and maintain body flexibility are often the most neglected aspect of an exercise program, because many people equate exercise with working up a sweat or building muscle size. Yet for people over 30—and especially those over 50—flexibility exercises are just as important as exercises for the heart and lungs. They will also give you the quickest return on your exercise investment (as you regain flexibility, you'll feel younger). The stretching exercises that follow should be a part of every warm-up and can be part of any cool-down.

Stretching exercises to increase your body's suppleness should be performed at least once every day for between five and ten minutes, ideally the first thing in the morning. They are also a good preparation for a relaxation session (see chapter 8, ''Effective Relaxation'').

The basic rule for suppleness exercises is the opposite of the old jock adage ''No pain, no gain.'' If it hurts, stop doing it, or do it more gently. Pain is your body's way of telling you to stop before you cause injury.

The following eight flexibility exercises require no equipment and can be done almost anywhere. They belong in your basic kit of fitness skills. Any good aerobics class or other professionally led exercise session should include flexibility exercises that cover all the key body areas. If you like, add your own exercises before and after the session. Ideally the exercises that follow should be done wearing loose or stretchable clothing, but many can be done in office clothes, especially if they aren't too tight.

We've highlighted those exercises that improve back flexibility and help alleviate or prevent back problems.

Shoulder Stretch-Relaxation. Let your arms dangle at your side. As you breathe in deeply, slowly raise your arms over your head, crossing them in front of you as you do. As you slowly breathe out, rotate the arms out while pressing backward as you make a broad arc to return to the starting position. (You will feel the loosening in your shoulders.) Repeat the sequence three to five times, gradually enlarging the arc each time.

Side Stretch-Relaxation (good for backs). Clasp both hands on top of your head. Bend your body to one side and a little forward until you feel a stretch on the opposite side. Don't shift your hip bones. Hold this position as you breathe out slowly and feel the stretched muscles relax. Increase the stretch. Do this three to five times on both sides.

SHOULDER STRETCH-RELAXATION

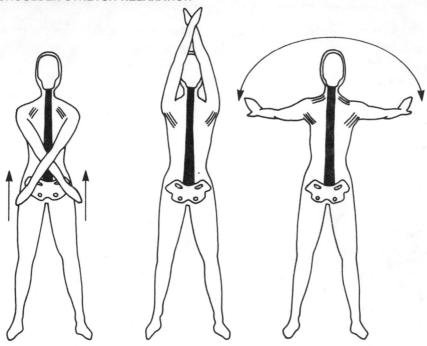

SIDE STRETCH-RELAXATION

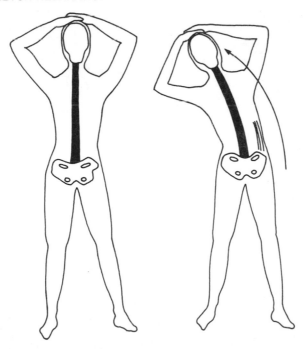

Back Stretch-Relaxation (good for backs). This exercise is sometimes known as the Mad Cat or Cat Back. Get down on all fours, with your back level. As you breathe in, arch your back upward, touching your chin to your chest. Hold this position and breathe out deeply. Increase the stretch. Now return to the level-back position, breathe in, and bend your back toward the floor. Hold this position and breathe out deeply. Increase the stretch. Return to the level position. Repeat three to five times.

Dome Position

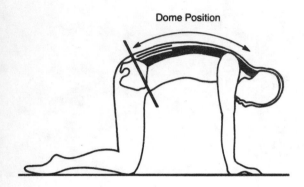

Level Position

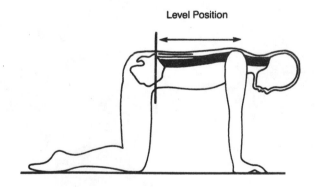

Suspension Bridge

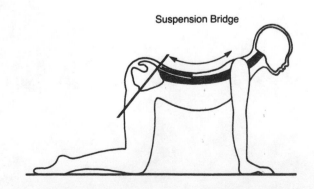

Sling Stretch-Relaxation (lengthens hip flexors). Lie on your back with legs straight out. Bring your right leg toward your chest by grasping the knee with both hands. Stop as you feel tightness but before the point of pain (do not jerk or force the muscle). Hold this position and slowly breathe out for a count of 10. You should feel the muscle loosen. Lengthen the stretch. Hold this new position and repeat, breathing out slowly. Repeat this exercise three to five times on each side.

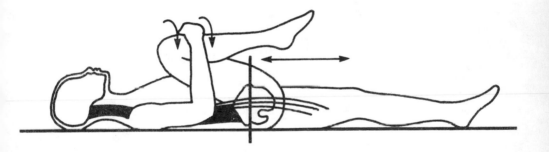

Hamstring Stretch-Relaxation. Sit with one leg bent and with the foot near the knee of the straight leg (it can be touching). The knee of the straight leg remains on or near the floor. Gently curl your upper body toward the knee of the straight leg and reach forward with the hands so that your arms are outstretched. Hold this position and breathe out slowly. Feel the hamstring muscle relax. Extend the stretch. Repeat three to five times. Then switch sides and do the exercise again.

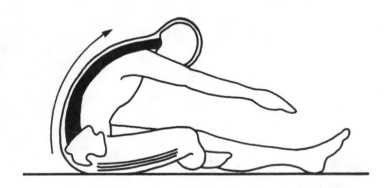

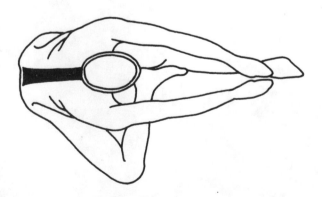

Groin Stretch-Relaxation. Sit on the floor with knees bent and bottoms of feet together. With your hands gently clasping your ankles and your forearms resting on your calves, push your knees down and out as far as they will comfortably go. Now bend your head toward your feet, stopping when you feel resistance. (Don't use your hands to pull yourself forward.) Breathe out deeply and feel the groin muscles relax, bending further forward and dropping your knees as you do so. Repeat three to five times.

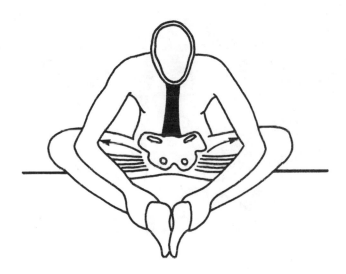

Thigh Stretch-Relaxation. Stand in a well-balanced position (you can use a desk or railing for support). Bend your right knee, grasp the foot at the ankle, and pull gently toward your buttock. Hold and breathe out slowly, increasing the stretch as you feel the muscles loosen. Be conscious of keeping your stomach pulled in and your pelvis level (this position is known as the pelvic tilt). Repeat three to five times on each leg.

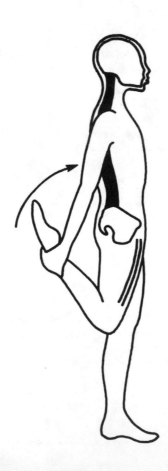

Calf Stretch-Relaxation. Place one foot ahead of the other, with the front leg slightly bent and the rear leg straight (but not locked). Bend your front leg further while keeping your rear leg straight and your rear foot flat on the floor—you'll feel the stretch in your calf. Hold the maximum stretch, and breathe out slowly. As you feel the muscle relax, bend your front knee a bit more to increase the stretch. Repeat three to five times. Then change legs and do it again.

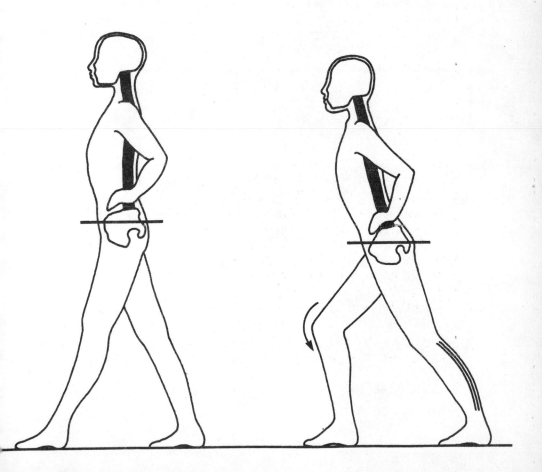

These eight exercises are by no means the only good techniques for increasing the length and flexibility of your key muscle groups. If you prefer another type of stretch, that's fine. Just remember that you need a stretch for each area of your body and that whatever technique you choose, it should be practiced using a formula that combines relaxation breathing with a slow, careful lengthening of the muscles.

Exercises for Strength

The suppleness exercises just described increase flexibility and work to lengthen short, tight muscles. The strengthening exercises in this section work to shorten muscles that are too long. Exercises that promote strength generally involve either pushing (for example, push-ups) or pulling (all lifting exercises). If you want to increase the bulk of your muscles, you must also gradually increase the load.

In this section, we have included exercises for all the main muscles groups, exercises that complement the eight basic stretches. If you combine the stretching exercises with the strengthening exercises, you will have a balanced muscle workout that you can do almost anywhere. You can use the stretches as part of your warm-up for a strength workout. Or you can do the strengthening exercises immediately after an aerobic workout that has included stretching. In addition, many physical activities, from jogging to playing tennis, have a strengthening component. (For advice on how to balance your exercise activities, see "What, When, and How to Exercise," below.)

If you want to build your muscle bulk rather than make the most of the muscles you now have, you should consult a fitness professional who can design a suitable weight-training program for you. Any weight-training program consists of the following basic elements: application of a load, or weight, to the particular muscles you wish to strengthen; multiple repetitions of the exercise; multiple sets of repetitions; and appropriate rest intervals between sets. In our strengthening exercises, your body is used as the weight.

Make strengthening exercises part of every complete workout. (Most fitness classes include a series of strengthening exercises as part of the cool-down following the aerobic section.) You may want to combine some strengthening exercises with your morning set of stretches as a perfect way to start the day. Regardless of when you do exercises for strength, aim for three to five times weekly.

As with suppleness, we've highlighted those strengthening exercises that benefit your back.

Shoulder Dips (shoulder strength). Place two sturdy chairs far enough apart that you can kneel between them with a little space to spare. Grasp the corners of the chair seats firmly with your hands. Slowly lift yourself up and hold for two counts. Remember to keep breathing throughout the exercise. Slowly lower yourself back down to the floor. Repeat this exercise five to ten times. If you are just starting, stop as soon as you have trouble lifting yourself off the floor.

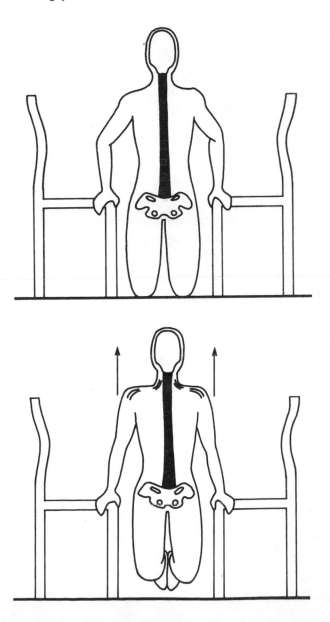

Wall Sits (upper thigh strength). Stand with your back flat against a wall, your knees slightly bent, your feet flat on the floor, and your heels about 6 inches from the wall. Slowly slide down the wall until you have reached a "sitting" position. Hold this position as long as comfortable (your upper thigh muscles will start to burn). Don't forget to keep breathing and to keep your upper body, including your neck and shoulders, relaxed. When the burning sensation begins or your thigh muscles tire, stand up again. Repeat five to ten times.

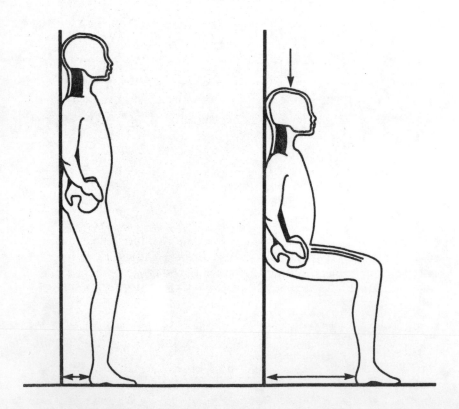

Calf Raise. Stand up straight with your hands on your hips and your feet parallel and slightly apart. Make sure your head, neck, shoulders, and back are straight, and that you feel well balanced. (If you have trouble keeping your balance when you first attempt this exercise, steady yourself by putting one hand lightly on a table or chair.) Now rise slowly up onto the balls of your feet as high as you can go. Keep breathing fully as you hold this position for a count of 2. Then slowly lower your heels back to the floor. Repeat five to ten times.

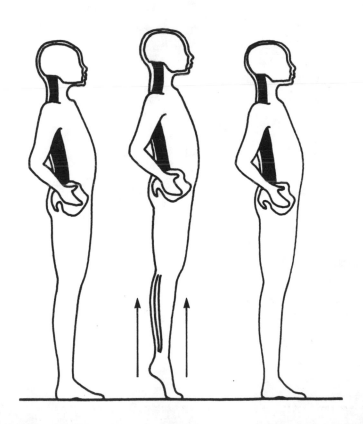

Hamstring Push-Pull. Lie on your stomach, turning your head to one side and resting it on the floor or on your hands. Keep your thighs resting on the floor as you bend your legs at the knees and raise both feet so that your legs below the knees are roughly at a right angle to the rest of your body. Cross your ankles, and push with one foot as you pull with the other. You should feel this in your hamstring muscle of the pulling leg. Hold the push-pull as long as you are comfortable. Then switch legs so that the former pulling leg is the pusher and the pushing leg is the puller. Hold as long as comfortable. Repeat five to ten times for each leg.

Throughout this exercise, keep breathing and relax the parts of your body that are not involved.

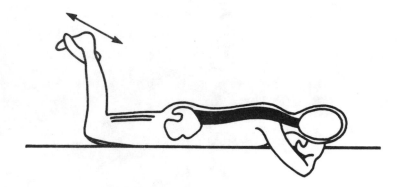

The Sling Push-Pull (hip strength; **good for backs**). Lie on your back and flatten it against the floor. Bring one leg up so that the knee is roughly at a right angle and the lower leg is parallel with the floor. Place both hands on your knee (contract your stomach muscles to keep your back flat on the floor). Now push forward with your hands as you pull your knee forward. Increase the pressure in both directions so that the knee stays in the same place. You will feel this exercise in the area of your hip socket. Hold this push-pull as long as is comfortable. Repeat five to ten times, then change legs and repeat.

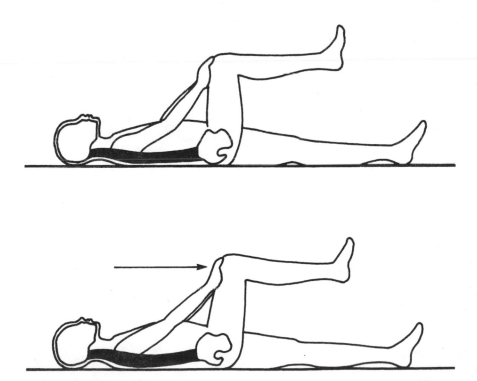

Sit-Down (stomach muscles, **lower back**). Sit on the floor with your hands out in front of your body. Curl back slowly as you count to 7. Do not hold your feet down or tuck your feet under any object; if they rise up off the floor, let this happen as you roll back gently. Sit up again; if you need help to roll back up, use your elbows to push back to the starting position. Repeat five to ten times. Throughout the exercise, don't forget to practice relaxation breathing.

You can make the exercise harder (increase the load) by crossing your arms in front of your chest or by placing your hands beside your head.

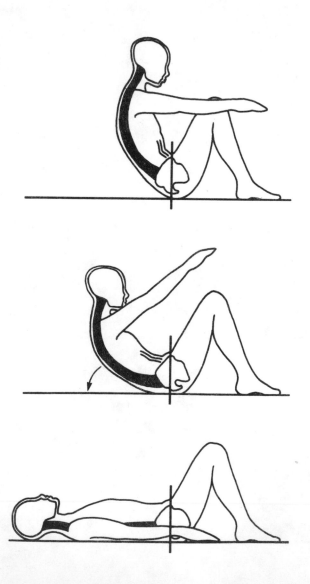

Lateral Leg Lift (sides, buttocks, **lower back**). Lie on your side with one hand behind your head like a pillow and the other hand in front of your body like a tripod for support (see drawing). Keeping your feet together, raise both legs off the floor a distance of about 2 inches.

Keeping your body straight (no twisting) and your head resting in a relaxed way on your arm and hand, slowly raise your upper leg 12 inches, while holding the bottom leg stationary. Lower the upper leg slowly, again holding the bottom leg stationary. Repeat ten times.

Turn over and do the exercise on the other side.

You can make the exercise more difficult by raising the bottom leg higher than 2 inches off the floor. You can make it easier by moving the bottom leg closer to the floor.

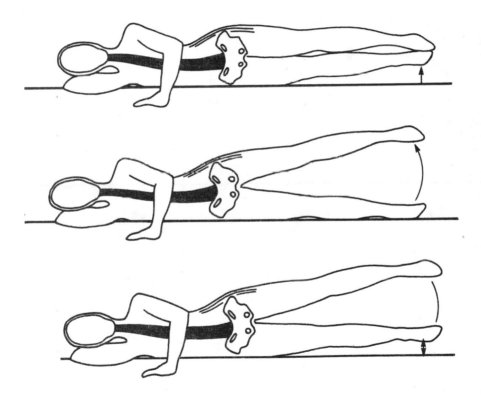

Push-Ups (chest, triceps). For instructions for this exercise, see the Arm and Shoulder Strength Test (Push-ups) on p. 283–284. Note that both men and women who are out of shape can start with the easier push-ups (pivoting from the knees), then graduate to the more difficult type (pivoting from the feet) when able.

Stamina Exercises

Every exercise program should contain a regular aerobic workout that raises your heartbeat to its training range, simultaneously increasing your body's requirement for oxygen taken in through the lungs. You don't fully benefit from the "training effect" unless you continuously maintain your target range for at least twenty minutes. To find out your target training range and for instructions on how to take your pulse, see pp. 285–286.

When exercising, you'll need a watch or a clock with a second hand to check if you've achieved your. training heart rate. If you check your pulse in the middle of intense exercise, remember to keep moving while you're counting; this prevents the pooling of blood in one part of the body, and thus eliminates the risk of fainting.

If you forget your watch or if you're in the middle of a sequential activity and don't want to stop, there's a simple rule for ensuring that you don't exceed your training heart rate. This is the Talk Test, which says that you should be able to carry on a normal conversation while continuing your exercise. If you can't, slow down. And, if you start to feel uncomfortable for any reason, slow down or take a breather. The most important rule of all is: Listen to your body. When it says to stop or slow down, heed its advice.

Regular aerobic exercise is the simple route to increased cardiorespiratory stamina. On at least three nonconsecutive days each week, plan an exercise session that includes an extended aerobic section (at least twenty, optimally thirty, minutes at training heart rate). Exercise programs tend to be most successful for people who set aside a period each day to work out, ideally at the same time and in the same place.

Aerobic exercises are all rhythmic activities that increase your heart rate to its training range and keep it there. They include walking (an underrated form of exercise), jogging, running, dancing, swimming, rowing, cycling, and rebounding. (Racquet sports, because they have many stops and starts, often don't give you a continuous aerobic workout.)

If you join an exercise class, remember that even the beginner level may be far too intense for you at the start. Monitor yourself and go at your own pace. Don't worry about competing with your classmates.

What, When, and How to Exercise

Here is a thumbnail guide to the exercise program that's right for you.

What. The exercise program you design depends on you and your lifestyle. It should be simple and fun. It should make you feel good— before, during, and after. It should be flexible enough to be adaptable to unplanned changes in your schedule, whether you're a high school teacher, a house husband, a traveling salesman, or a desk-bound executive. So, as much as possible, pick a regime of activities that you enjoy and that you know you can do. If you find that variety works for you, mix different activities in a single week. If consistency is your strong suit, then pick your favorite physical activity and stick to it.

Above all, make sure your exercise program provides you with the right balance of suppleness, strength, and stamina. The chart on the next page lists a number of sports and other physical activities broken down according to their fitness benefits. Use it to help you design the program that's right for you.

When. Many people find that it helps to schedule regular times for their workouts. Exercising with a friend will help you keep to your schedule. But if you miss a scheduled workout, have a backup in place. You should be able to exercise in several different settings and at different times of day.

Suppleness exercises do you the most good at the beginning of the day (and as a part of your warm-up). In fact a complete warm-up is an ideal way to start the day, since it gets your blood going and lubricates stiff joints. An aerobic workout is especially effective during or at the end of a high-stress day, since it not only purges fatigue acids but helps you lower your stress thermostat. Strengthening exercises are ideally done in combination with suppleness exercises or as part of a complete, balanced workout that includes aerobic exercise as well.

Finally, exercise does you the most good if you have had a solid night's sleep. Don't exercise when you are physically exhausted.

How. It is very important to phase in your exercise program slowly, especially if you are out of shape. You'll find specific suggestions in the four-week start-up program below.

As a general guide, use the FITT formula to design the program that's right for you. FITT stands for Frequency, Intensity, Time (duration), and Type. In other words, you should be exercising often enough to do some good, at a level of intensity that will have the training effect, during individual sessions of adequate duration, and using a program that balances the three Ss.

Frequency. Plan for a minimum of three balanced exercise sessions a week, sessions that involve all three Ss. Schedule your full workouts for nonconsecutive days so that your muscles have time to recover. If you want to get fit faster, increase the number of complete, balanced workouts you do. But even if you are exercising every day, give yourself one day off each week.

BALANCE YOUR EXERCISE

Activity	Suppleness	Strength	Stamina
Walking (golf, hunting)	Tightens leg muscles (calf, hamstring, hip flexor)	Leg muscles	At target heart rate
Jogging/running	Tightens leg muscles (calf, hamstring, hip flexor)	Leg muscles	At target heart rate
Dancing	Good for whole body	Leg muscles	At target heart rate
Cross-country skiing	Arms	Leg muscles	At target heart rate
Racquet sports	Medium	Arms/lower body	At target heart rate
Swimming	Arms and legs	Whole body	At target heart rate
Bicycling	Hamstrings, thighs	Leg muscles	At target heart rate
Weight-training	Low (needs warm-up)	High (whole body)	If target rate maintained
Aerobics class (with strength section)	High	Moderate	At target heart rate

NOTE: The key when balancing exercise activities is to emphasize flexibility in the muscles that you use most (for example, leg stretches are needed to warm-up for jogging or running).

Intensity. The intensity of your exercise is related closely to how you feel while doing it. If it hurts or you feel real discomfort, you should stop, slow down, or reduce the level of resistance or the range of motion. With stamina exercises, the range of intensity can be determined by monitoring your training heart rate and making sure you stay within the safe range for your age. A less precise gauge is the Talk Test (if you can talk normally, you aren't working too hard). When you exercise, you should aim for the maximum *comfortable* level of intensity.

Time (duration). The cardiorespiratory part of your routine should last at least twenty minutes and ideally thirty minutes. For suppleness exercises, at least five minutes is needed to do a complete set. Don't rush your stretches. Enjoy them.

Type. Any exercise session that works on strength or stamina (or both) should be preceded by a warm-up and followed by a cool-down. This is always a good idea, but it becomes increasingly important as you grow older. Finally, the type of exercise you do—whether walking, jogging, or playing tennis or other sports—must suit your tastes and your lifestyle.

A PICTURE OF A COMPLETE AEROBIC WORKOUT

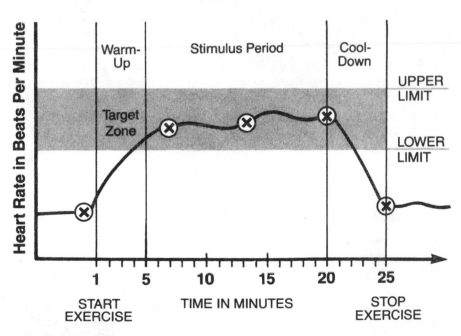

⊗ **Possible Recording of Pulse**

The illustration of a complete aerobic workout shows you the perfect pattern for an exercise session that trains your heart as well as your muscles. The warm-up should include your eight basic stretches, followed by more vigorous movement (for example, an easy jog gradually increasing in intensity). During the stimulus period you must be exercising strenuously enough to maintain your heart rate within the target zone. The cool-down consists of gradually slowing exercise (always keep moving) and ends with some easy stretches.

Focus and Conserve Your Exercise Energy

Once you've decided on your basic program, and have FITT it to your life, the final step is to make the most of every exercise session.

The following three exercise principles are derived from the philosophy of stress-energy efficiency that underlies the Body Age Program. In essence, the more efficiently you exercise, the greater the return on your exercise investment. These principles apply whether you are training to be a competitive power lifter or an effective telephone receptionist.

Conserve energy. Many people confuse exercise with exhaustion. They think that the only good workout is one that leaves them with nothing to spare. That's wrong. And for anyone who is starting on an exercise program after a long layoff, it could be downright dangerous.

In particular, conserve your stress energy for worthy exercise applications. Don't chase the bus if you've got time to spare. Don't (as some fitness experts recommend) use the stairs at the office instead of the elevator. Save your valuable energy for your 2-mile jog, your twenty-minute swim, or your after-dinner walk—when the expenditure will actually do you the most good. The principle of warming up before strenuous exercise and cooling down afterward dovetails with the principle of energy conservation.

Focus your energy on the activity, and use affirmations and visualizations while you exercise. If the task is worthy, then do it fully. If you have chosen to do this workout, do it with complete concentration and total involvement. That way you'll get the most return for your energy expenditure.

Affirmations and visualizations are especially useful to enhance your exercise. You don't have to be a competitive power lifter or an Olympic swimmer to visualize the perfect workout—for you. Affirmation and visualization are techniques for helping you make each exercise session a meaningful expression of your positive self-image. Use these techniques before, during, and after you exercise.

Pace yourself. If you're going to run 3 miles, don't start off at a sprint. If you feel you're overdoing it, slow down or take a breather. That way your tank won't be empty for the final dash to the shower. But be sure you do reach your target heart rate zone. If you have any doubts, check your pulse.

If you're going to exercise, do it right. Get the maximum return on your investment. You deserve it.

YOUR FOUR-WEEK START-UP PROGRAM

Week 1: Get Ready. Plan your first step toward Essential Exercise. This can be nothing more than taking a walk around the block three times next week.

Week 2: Take Your First Step. Act on your plan. The simpler and more doable it is, the more likely you will be successful.

Week 3: Build on Your Success. Increase the quality, duration, or intensity of what you did last week. For instance, your one-block walk might become two blocks.

Week 4: Consolidate Your Gains. You've now been exercising for two weeks. Keep at it and find ways to do what you're doing better. For instance, your walk around the block may become a half-mile stroll three times this week.

This four-week start-up program for Essential Exercise is only an outline. It suggests ways that you can phase in balanced exercise, taking into account the wide range of fitness levels among our potential readers. Many of you (especially those who have scored highly in the Cliff Walker and Basket Case stressotypes) are now doing little or no regular exercise, and we've tilted the start-up program in your direction. But we've also included suggestions for people at other exercise levels.

If you are phasing in exercise after a long (lifelong?) layoff, you will probably find the start-up program very difficult. Your body will feel sluggish and your exercise sessions, especially those involving an aerobic workout, will seem like a real struggle. The first few times you exercise, you may actually feel worse. Your body has a tendency to resist what it experiences as a revolution. And you may feel a lot of anxiety as you actually start to *do something*. Don't despair. As long as you gradually phase in your new behavior and gradually increase the intensity, it won't be long before exercise becomes a pleasure in itself, which is, after all, why most people do it and continue to do it.

The theme of the start-up program is to make a series of small, specific, concrete changes. Add exercise to your lifestyle in small, doable increments. Make just one change each week, and you'll be on the road to success. If you are starting from scratch, we recommend that you begin with suppleness exercises, then add stamina or strengthening exercises as you aim toward a balanced program. Above all, don't go too quickly.

Week 1: Get Ready

Fill out your Action Diary Planning Page. Make a contract with yourself to do the following during the coming week:

1. *Practice autogenic relaxation with affirmations and visualizations.* Before you do anything else this week, find some quiet time to listen to your autogenic tape and introduce your exercise affirmations. Follow this by visualizing images and feelings of a fitter you. (Plan for three more autogenic sessions this week.) Use your affirmations and visualizations while you exercise. For example, if you're a swimmer, as you take each stroke, picture your heart pumping oxygen-filled blood to your muscles. Or repeat to yourself a simple affirmation such as "power," "strength," or "speed." Repeat your affirmations two or three times each day.

2. *Plan for your first change.* The only new exercise you're introducing this week is to push a pencil on a piece of paper as you plan your first exercise steps for next week. Analyze what you are doing now in the way of exercise (don't forget that gardening and walking are excellent exercises), and pick just one concrete way in which you can do something new. Then plan to do it. For example, if you choose to go for a swim this week, get out your datebook and schedule your swim.

One of our program participants was a Drifter named Marty (age 41, body age 45) who was already swimming regularly and had good stamina. But as he got more in touch with his exercise goals, he realized that he wanted to look more powerful. So he decided to take up weight lifting three times a week. To do this, he scheduled three workouts in his diary, based on the times several of his friends would be in the weight room. Then he told them he'd see them there. He also subscribed to a popular weight-training magazine to provide him with new ideas and motivating images. Finally, he traced out in his mind the two ways he was most likely to sabotage his commitment, and planned in advance how he'd respond if these happened. He was determined to get to the gym.

3. *Check in with your partner.* Set a time to call your partner or to have your partner call you. Discuss your plan. If you're having trouble deciding where to begin, get your partner's feedback.

4. *Record your progress in your Action Diary*. Has your use of autogenic training helped you get clearer and feel more confident about your proposed exercise program? Have you noted opportunities for increasing the amount of exercise in your life? Have you identified the roadblocks (for example, not enough time) that you use as excuses for not getting down to exercise? Congratulate yourself on whatever progress you have made this week in awareness and planning for change.

Week 2: Take Your First Step

Fill out your Action Diary Planning Page. Agree with yourself to do the following during the coming week:

1. *Continue to practice autogenic relaxation with affirmations and visualizations*. Take time for four autogenic sessions again this week. You may want to try out some new affirmations and visualizations, but if you feel good about the ones you're using, stay with them. And don't forget to use affirmation and visualization while you exercise. They will help enhance the pleasure and satisfaction you gain from taking care of your body. Repeat your affirmations preferably two or three times each day.

2. *Act on your plan*. Where you begin will depend on what you are already doing, especially if you now do little or no regular exercise.

If you are completely out of shape and haven't exercised at all for quite a while, begin very slowly and very simply. Make a contract with yourself to introduce some daily suppleness exercises during this week. If you're feeling more ambitious, introduce some stamina exercises as well—perhaps a ten-minute walk three times this week. If all eight stretching exercises seem too much, then pick four (ideally the four on which you scored most poorly in the suppleness self-tests) or even two. Stretch five mornings this week—or three, or one.

If even this level of exercise appears too daunting, design a more modest beginning. If you take public transit to work, choose to get off one stop before your usual one and walk the rest of the way. Do this three days this week—or two, or one. In later weeks, you can build up gradually by doing it more often or getting off at an earlier stop. Soon you'll be ready for a more strenuous aerobic workout.

If you are already exercising fairly regularly, look for ways to balance your weekly exercise better. Your new behavior might be to start each exercise session with a warm-up that includes all eight relaxation stretches. Or perhaps you already do lots of stretching before and after your daily jog but have been neglecting some basic exercises for strength, especially in the upper body, where jogging provides little strength benefit. Or, if you are now exercising properly, but sporadically, choose to exercise three times over the coming week.

If you are out of shape and want to increase your stamina, start with low-demand aerobic activities such as walking, gardening, or easy bicycling. Over the next three weeks, gradually increase the amount of time and the degree of intensity. At the beginning, don't worry about attaining your training heart rate. The main thing is to get moving. Only after the activity begins to come more naturally should you begin to experiment with a level of intensity that gets you into training range. Gradually increase the amount of time you can sustain your training heart rate until twenty minutes is no problem.

Many of our program participants were doing little or no exercise when they entered the study. One of these was Mary (a Cliff Walker, age 37, body age 45), who had not done any exercise on a regular basis since graduating from high school. Like so many nonexercisers, she was trapped into the all-or-nothing view of fitness: Either I run 6 miles a day, at least six times a week, or I'm a slob. Therefore she did nothing.

At the end of week 2, Mary reported that she had just broken the world's record in the "Tour de Block" (her residential block) "gentle saunter competition." Once she discovered that brisk walking and building toward twenty minutes of aerobic exercise is a viable middle ground—and discovered how good this self-caring activity made her feel—she was a hooked block tourer.

3. *Check in with your partner*. This and every week throughout your exercise Start-Up Program, get some support from your partner. Maybe you can plan to exercise together. At the very least, plan a phone call to discuss problems and report successes.

4. *Record your progress in your Action Diary*. Whatever your progress, take pleasure in the first concrete step(s) you've taken. If you were already exercising regularly, notice the small ways in which you are exercising better or improving your exercise balance. Look for opportunities to make exercise more fun for you—and more effective. If you started from zero, pat yourself on the back for breaking out of your rut, however small the change. Enjoy your successes and congratulate yourself for noticing missed opportunities to make Essential Exercise part of your life.

Here is a sample Action Diary Planning Page for week 2 of Essential Exercise. Your own planning page should suit your lifestyle and schedule. Find ways to incorporate each behavior without major dislocations. Don't overdo, especially if exercise is new for you. Remember: Change is stressful, so take it one step at a time. Above all, remember to give each behavior you undertake on this self-care contract the SMART test. Ask yourself whether it is Specific, Measurable, Acceptable, Realistic, and Truthful.

ACTION DIARY FOR WEEK OF _Oct 2nd_ TO _Oct 8th_

Planning Page

Affirmations (My self-themes for this week in key words and phrases)
I _am growing stronger everyday_
I _feel my blood bring Oxygen to my muscle_
(Other) _I am lean energy_

Opportunity Visualizations (I clearly see myself . . .)
I see the leaner, fitter me - no paunch, no sags I am aware of the compliments and admiring glances I get as I walk down the street. I feel strong and self - confident I am proud of my body

I choose to deepen this Vital Life Skill as follows (My specific behavior objectives this week)
I choose to _do a 15-minute autogenic relaxation followed by affirmation and Visualization, at least 4x's during the coming Week_
Under the following circumstances: _Monday, Wednesday + Friday before dinner in the den with the door closed. Saturday morning before breakfast_

I choose to _repeat my exercise affirmations twice each day this week_

Under the following circumstances: _in the morning as soon as I wake up; in the car as I'm driving to work_

I choose to _go for a ten-minute walk 3x's this week. I won't worry about trying to get up to training heart rate. While I'm walking I'll repeat my affirmations._

Under the following circumstances: _Sunday evening after dinner, Wednesday evening after dinner, Friday evening after dinner_

I choose to _____

Under the following circumstances: _____

My other opportunity situations for skill practice are:

1. Weekdays after work
2. I could walk part of the way to work instead of taking the bus all the way
3. I could join the health club near the office (I have a good friend who's a member)

I have arranged to check in with my partner . . .

When?	About
Monday, Wednesday and Friday	How my walks are going

Week 3: Build on Your Success

Fill out your Action Diary Planning Page. Agree to do the following during the coming week:

1. *Continue to use autogenic relaxation with affirmations and visualizations.* Give yourself at least four fifteen-minute autogenic sessions each week, modifying your affirmations and visualizations as you see fit. And don't forget to use affirmations and visualizations while you exercise, to help you focus on the activity and increase your sense of pleasure and satisfaction. Repeat your affirmations daily, preferably two or three times each day.

2. *Build on your first step.* Keep doing what you've been doing, but look for ways to modify and expand your new behaviors so that you do them better. This may simply mean increasing the duration or the intensity of what you've been doing. Perhaps last week you went for three ten-minute walks. See if you can now last for fifteen or twenty minutes. Or try increasing your pace. Perhaps last week you swam three times but were well below your training heart rate. You can experiment with getting closer to the training level, or even sustaining it for a few minutes. Look for ways to improve or deepen what you are already doing right. If you are already exercising regularly, continue to improve your balance of suppleness, strengthening, and stamina exercises.

If you were playing three games of squash but neglecting to stretch before and after, phase in some stretching exercises. If you stretched and took three walks last week but did no strengthening exercises, add some of these. If you've been stretching each morning but avoiding working on your stamina, get started now. Perhaps you scheduled three exercise sessions and then found an excuse to miss your date with yourself. Are you trying to move too quickly? Would it help to plan to go to a scheduled fitness class? Maybe you should make a date to go with a friend (or your partner). Simply getting going can be the most important behavior change of all.

Finally, this and every week of your start-up program, ask yourself if you are having fun. If exercise still seems like drudgery, ask yourself what you could do to make it more enjoyable. Can you turn it into a recreational or social activity by involving friends or family? Perhaps your daily walk will be more pleasant if you invite your spouse or your kids to come along. What about choosing a new route you've never tried? Maybe you can plan an easy hike in the woods this weekend. Have you thought of combining your daily jog with some relaxation techniques? Remember to use your affirmations and visualizations while you're exercising to increase your pleasure and sense of satisfaction.

In week 3, Mary established a "masters" category in her Tour de Block event, and invited her husband Jack to join her. By the end of this week, she had mapped out five alternative "gentle saunter/brisk walk" routes to provide variety. Then she talked Jack into taking pictures of her at the most distant points in her tours, locations that each week were farther from home.

3. *Check in with your partner.* Don't neglect this important source of support and feedback.

4. *Record your progress in your Action Diary.* You may already be feeling better, but don't be discouraged if you're still experiencing the teething pangs of your new physical activity. Even if you haven't yet felt the physical payoff in increased energy and flexibility, you can feel better about yourself. Just the act of getting more exercise shows that you can make a meaningful change. Congratulate yourself for the progress you've made. And keep up the good work!

Week 4: Consolidate Your Gains

Fill out your Action Diary Planning Page. Agree with yourself to do the following during the coming week:

1. *Continue using autogenic relaxation with affirmations and visualizations.*

2. *Consolidate your gains.* You've now been exercising for two weeks. Even if you started from scratch, you are getting more exercise. As you consolidate your gains, work on refining what you are already doing. Maybe this means lengthening your walk from twenty minutes to a half hour, or finally getting around to those morning stretches. Maybe you've reached the stage at which you want to lengthen your cardiorespiratory workout from twenty to twenty-five minutes. Perhaps you are finally getting around to doing those strengthening exercises you've been avoiding. Or perhaps your goal this week is simply exercising in a more focused and self-paced way.

Are you enjoying yourself? If not, what creative solutions can you bring to the challenge?

Mary kept at her gradually increasing exercise program in week 4. And kept it up in the coming weeks until her Tour de Block became a 2-mile jog four mornings a week. At eight months, her body age was down from 45 to 36.

3. *Check in with your partner.* Your partner is your bottom-line support system. Don't neglect her or him.

4. *Record your progress in your Action Diary.* Continue to keep track of your progress and to congratulate yourself for every success.

Continuing Your Prescription

You now know that you can do it. Are you prepared to continue on the road to making balanced exercise a part of your life? As the weeks pass, regular exercise will cease to be a novelty and will become a self-affirming habit. More and more, the act of exercising will be pleasurable in itself. Many members of our study group reported dramatic changes in their lifestyles, largely as a result of adding balanced exercise.

Now that you've completed your start-up program, you may feel ready to phase in your next intervention. But we recommend you don't do this until week 8 at the earliest, to give yourself time to make Essential Exercise a self-affirming habit.

As one of our study subjects found, Essential Exercise can lead you to reconsider considerably more than your waistline. When Sheila entered the program, she was an accountant Cliff Walker, age 32, but with a body age of 42. She was thirty-five pounds overweight, felt lousy much of the time, and had borderline high blood pressure. We didn't have to tell her that exercise was part of the answer for her. The problem was that she devoutly believed that "being attractive was a real liability" for a woman in the business world. She felt that the less her clients thought of her as a woman, the more she could "concentrate on business." It was a matter of honor with her "not to get ahead by womanly wiles and acting sexy." But she had translated this creed into a justification for neglecting her body almost totally, even dressing in clothes that made the most conservative male partner in her accounting firm "look like a peacock."

Not surprisingly, Sheila's first breakthrough was mental, not physical. During the training sessions, she was greatly relieved to discover that two of the most important themes of Essential Exercise are: Whatever you choose to do for yourself must fit with who you are and be motivating to you personally; and, There are many different ways of being fit (you don't have to aim to look like Jane Fonda).

This perceptual shift led her to design her personal fitness program around the following goals: to gain a "competitive edge"; to look energetic and capable, rather than "mindlessly curvaceous"; and to increase her capacity (energy) to achieve at a high professional level. With these goals firmly fixed, her affirmations and visualizations followed naturally.

Her affirmations were "My energy means business" and "Top quality in the gym and on the job."

Her visualizations were "I see myself at the end of the tax season leaving on vacation with plenty of energy to enjoy it" and "I see myself striding along to a meeting step-for-step with the office jock."

At Sheila's eight-month checkup, she was regularly doing four aerobic/weight-training workouts a week, combined with nutritional changes she'd phased in once exercise had begun to make her feel better. She had brought her weight down twenty-four pounds. Her body age was 10 years lower at 32, the same as her calendar age. She looked wonderful (her appearance age was down 12 years from 45 to 33). And her blood pressure reading was down by 18 points.

Sheila's comments about her progress in the program should inspire anyone who's out of shape and contemplating Essential Exercise: "We accountants tend to see things as black or white (or red!). Now, having gotten in shape *on my terms*, doing it my way, I've begun to see (and believe in) a lot of other options too. For example, I can accept compliments on my appearance without feeling I'm being conned or that I'm incompetent. And I no longer believe that just because high blood pressure runs in my family I'm bound to get it."

CHAPTER 12
High-Performance Nutrition

PRIMARY INTERVENTION FOR: Cliff Walker and Basket Case

Core Message

Sound nutrition is basically very simple. You can achieve it by following these guidelines:

Eat a variety
of unprocessed (and little-processed) foods
with high nutrient density
in moderate amounts
during at least three regular meals a day, including breakfast,
combined with smart snacking patterns (including beverages)
while drinking at least six glasses of fluid daily, two of them water,
and taking a broad-based vitamin-mineral supplement.

Our emphasis is on nutrition for vital health and high performance, not merely on nutrition for disease avoidance (the conventional approach).

Small diet changes rooted autogenically lead to major changes in the way you eat.

High-performance nutrition turned out to be the most effective intervention for the Cliff Walker and the Basket Case stressotypes. These types are prime candidates for more sensible eating habits since both are at an advanced stage of lifestyle abuse: poor eating habits, overuse of alcohol and other drugs, and inadequate exercise. As a result, their bodies cope with stress poorly, and they have insufficient energy to meet the normal challenges of everyday life.

The Cliff Walker and Basket Case demonstrate in a very dramatic way the perils of poor nutrition, not only in terms of their high susceptibility to disease, but in terms of their stress efficiency. Poor nutritional habits (for example, skipping breakfast) cause your body to burn more stress energy to compensate. Adrenalin instead of calories must pull you through the nutritionally bankrupt periods of your day. And when poor nutrition is combined with foods that are actually stress-producing (for example, caffeine, chocolate, sugar), your body becomes accustomed to operating at an even higher stress level.

With all the dietary advice that's available today, you may sometimes feel bewildered by the sheer mass of nutritional information. We've boiled it all down to the basic guidelines listed above.

However, what we say here is different from standard nutritional advice in the following crucial respects:

We emphasize nutrition for vital good health rather than nutrition for disease avoidance or weight loss. Conventional nutritional standards (for instance, the U.S. Recommended Daily Allowances of vitamins and minerals) are based on the minimum intake required for the average person to avoid disease. In the Body Age Program, we were interested in achieving the highest level of energy and performance (the maximum health possible). Thus any desirable weight loss (or gain) is not a goal of good nutrition but an inevitable by-product. Our nutritional program is aimed at promoting your optimum bodily efficiency.

Our focus in helping you choose the right foods is on nutrient density, not calorie counting. Old-fashioned calorie counting is daunting, and it neglects the nutrient value of foods. We prefer to look at each food from the point of view of the quality of nutrition it provides per calorie. More than 50 percent of an average North American's calorie intake comes in the form of "empty calories," food that delivers little or no nutritional value. Foods that are high in refined sugar, animal fat, or salt and that are low in fiber generally deliver less nutrition per calorie.

Small, concrete dietary changes make a big difference. Something as small as substituting an apple for a candy bar or drinking a cup of decaffeinated coffee is major progress.

You root your dietary changes in your unconscious mind. As with each of the five interventions, nutrition works best when you combine it with autogenic relaxation plus affirmations and visualizations, in order to root the changes you are making in your mind and feelings. Many of our study subjects had previously tried and failed to lose weight permanently by "going on a diet." In the Body Age Program, they found to their delight that the pounds disappeared while they affirmed and made a series of small, specific changes geared toward healthier eating.

In addition to the obvious health advantages of good nutrition—including the fact that you'll be conserving your stress energy for when you really need it—this chapter offers the following benefits:

> You'll experience more energy, less fatigue. If you eat right, you'll be able to draw on food energy when you need it. You won't need three cups of coffee to get started in the morning, and you'll be less likely to experience an energy letdown in the middle of the day.

> Since your stress levels come down when you eat right, you'll find it easier to relax.

> Physical activity will be more fun. Nutrition accounts for one-half of physical fitness. Without it, exercise is less effective, just as without exercise, nutrition is less effective. With good nutrition, you'll enjoy all physical activity more, and your exercise will do you more good.

> Each new nutritious behavior "beefs up" your self-esteem. Every time you choose to eat better, you are sending yourself a self-affirming message. As these positive eating behaviors accumulate, they build your self-esteem, just as the good food you are eating improves your physical health and promotes your bodily well-being.

High-Performance Nutrition had a major impact on many of our study subjects. Doris, a computer systems analyst, is one good example.

Doris was a Basket Case for whom the battle of the bulge had become a war without end. When she entered the program at age 36 (body age 46, appearance age 44), she was almost forty-five pounds over her ideal weight. Despite having tried almost every fad diet, since her teenage years her weight had steadily risen. Each time she dieted, she would take off fifteen to twenty pounds, then gain it back within the next six months. At her entry interview, she told us that, when dieting, she "always felt like a soldier carrying my little bag of C rations, and running the risk of court-martial if I cheated once."

Our approach to nutrition made Doris very uneasy. It was common sense, demanded no radical change (unlike her diets), and, perhaps most threatening of all, it respected her "mature adult" right to select where she would begin and how she would continue. As she developed her affirmations and visualizations, she focused on the image of a sports car running on a "lean fuel mixture for best performance," with more frequent, smaller fill-ups. She decided to begin her program by starting to eat breakfast every day and resolving to enjoy her hunger pangs as signs of progress.

These two simple changes complemented each other beautifully. Previously she'd been skipping breakfast as a calorie-saving strategy. Now her small, high-protein meal at the beginning of the day sharply reduced her craving for sugary snacks and dampened her morning dependency on elevated adrenalin (a major Basket Case vitality drain). After four months, she had lost seventeen pounds "without dieting," and she was more energetic than she had been since her teens. At eight months, she was down a total of twenty-eight pounds and was having no difficulty keeping the weight off. "That autogenic tape plus my affirmations really got my lean machine flying on auto pilot," she commented. "I began to make the best choices naturally, including a regular aerobics class. The slim me just somehow gradually took over." At graduation, Doris's body age was down 9 years to 37.

RATE YOURSELF

This section is divided into four parts: You will find out how your current weight compares to your ideal body weight; you will rate how well you now eat in terms of the eight basic nutritional guidelines used by our study subjects; you'll identify the main habits, attitudes, and roadblocks that determine how you eat now, and prioritize your opportunities for eating better; you'll develop nutrition affirmations and visualizations that are right for you.

Your Ideal Body Weight

One indication of how well you are eating is your current body weight as compared to your ideal body weight. If you are overweight, usually you are eating extra calories. If you are underweight, your body probably could use additional nourishment. There is no perfect way of calculating your ideal weight, but you can come up with a good estimate using the Metropolitan Life Height and Weight Tables. Note that ideal weight varies with your sex and the size of your body frame. Use the Frame Size Measurement Chart before you look for your ideal weight.

FRAME SIZE MEASUREMENT CHART

To make a simple approximation of your frame size:

Extend your arm and bend the forearm up at a 90-degree angle. Keep the fingers straight and turn the inside of your wrist away from the body. Place the thumb and index finger of your other hand on the two prominent bones on *either side* of your elbow. Measure the space between your fingers against a ruler or a tape measure. Compare the measurements on the following tables.

These tables list the elbow measurements for medium-framed men and women of various heights. Measurements lower than those listed indicate you have a small frame, and higher measurements indicate a larger frame.

Men

Height in 1" heels	Elbow Breadth
5'2"–5'3"	2 1/2"–2 7/8"
5'4"–5'7"	2 5/8"–2 7/8"
5'8"–5'11"	2 3/4"–3"
6'0"–6'3"	2 3/4"–3 1/8"
6'4"	2 7/8"–3 1/4"

Women

Height in 1" heels	Elbow Breadth
4'10"–4'11"	2 1/4"–2 1/2"
5'0"–5'3"	2 1/4"–2 1/2"
5'4"–5'7"	2 3/8"–2 5/8"
5'8"–5'11"	2 3/8"–2 5/8"
6'0"	2 1/2"–2 3/4"

METROPOLITAN HEIGHT AND WEIGHT TABLES

All weights are in pounds for ages 25–59. Men's weights include clothing weighing five pounds and shoes with 1" heels. Women's weights include clothing weighing three pounds and shoes with 1" heels.

Men

Height Ft.	Inch.	Small Frame	Medium Frame	Large Frame
5	2	128–134	131–141	138–150
5	3	130–136	133–143	140–153
5	4	132–138	135–145	142–156
5	5	134–140	137–148	144–160
5	6	136–142	139–151	146–164
5	7	138–145	142–154	149–168
5	8	140–148	145–157	152–172
5	9	142–151	148–160	155–176
5	10	144–154	151–163	158–180
5	11	146–157	154–166	161–184
6	0	149–160	157–170	164–188
6	1	152–164	160–174	168–192
6	2	155–168	164–178	172–197
6	3	158–172	167–182	176–202
6	4	162–176	171–187	181–207

Women

Height Ft.	Inch.	Small Frame	Medium Frame	Large Frame
4	10	102–111	109–121	118–131
4	11	103–113	111–123	120–134
5	0	104–115	113–126	122–137
5	1	106–118	115–129	125–140
5	2	108–121	118–132	128–143
5	3	111–124	121–135	131–147
5	4	114–127	124–138	134–151
5	5	117–130	127–141	137–155
5	6	120–133	130–144	140–159
5	7	123–136	133–147	143–163
5	8	126–139	136–150	146–167
5	9	129–142	139–153	149–170
5	10	132–145	142–156	152–173
5	11	135–148	145–159	155–176
6	0	138–151	148–162	158–179

You don't really need to look at a chart to know whether you weigh too much or too little. In fact, a self-test that may motivate you even more effectively is what we call the Naked Mirror Test.

Take off all your clothes and stand in front of a full-length mirror. Are there rolls around your waistline? Is there any waistline at all? What happens when you jiggle your body? How do you feel about that stomach, those thighs? Give yourself an honest appraisal (but don't be too harsh). Do you like what you see? Few of us were born with the bodies of athletes or fashion models, so if you are comfortable with what you see, you are probably eating about the right amount for you. If you don't like what your mirror shows you, then start eating differently.

How Well Are You Eating?

The simple nutrition program we taught our study subjects consists of eight simple eating guidelines. In this section, you will rate yourself in each of these areas. The guidelines are:

Eat a variety
of unprocessed (and little-processed) foods
with high nutrient density
in moderate amounts
during at least three regular meals a day, including breakfast,
combined with smart snacking patterns (including beverages)
while drinking six glasses of fluid a day, at least two of them water,
and taking a broad-based vitamin-mineral supplement.

Before you do these self-tests, you may find it helpful to keep a food record for a day or two—ideally one weekday and one weekend day (people tend to eat differently on weekends). On these two days, carry a notebook and record in it *every* item of food you eat, including drinks (even a glass of water or a cup of clear tea). This food record will give you a much more accurate picture of how you are eating and will enable you to do the self-tests that follow much more accurately. (In the first week of your start-up program, you'll refine your nutritional self-awareness even further when you keep a one-week diet diary.)

How Varied Is Your Diet? Variety makes eating pleasurable and gives you the best chance of getting all the nutrients you need in the right amounts. You can ensure variety by eating a balance of servings from the four food groups and varying what you eat within each food group. The four groups are: the milk group, the meat group, the vegetable and fruit group, and the bread and cereal group.

Examples for each are given in the table.

THE FOUR FOOD GROUPS

Milk Group (protein, fat, calcium): 2 servings daily

Milk, buttermilk, yogurt, cheese, cottage cheese, powdered milk

Meat Group (protein, fat): 2 servings daily

Red meats, white meats, all fish, dairy products, eggs, legumes (including peanut butter), nuts and seeds

Fruit and Vegetable Group (high in carbohydrates and fiber, vitamins and minerals, some protein): 4–5 servings daily

All fruits and vegetables, cooked or uncooked (including legumes)

Bread and Cereal Group (high in carbohydrates and fiber, protein, vitamins and minerals): 3–5 servings daily

Bread, dry cereal, cooked cereal, pasta, rice, millet, buckwheat, bulgur wheat, oats, and bran

YOUR DAILY FOOD BALANCE
(THE FOUR FOOD GROUPS)

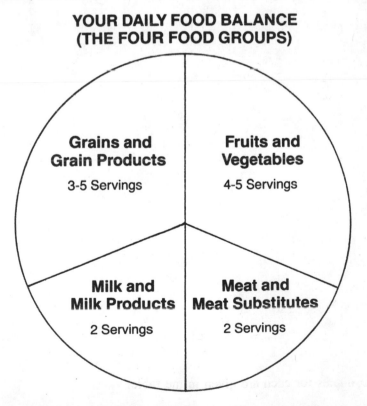

Grains and Grain Products — 3-5 Servings

Fruits and Vegetables — 4-5 Servings

Milk and Milk Products — 2 Servings

Meat and Meat Substitutes — 2 Servings

Take a look at the pie chart, a visual portrayal of the ideal balance between the four groups. Each segment represents the overall proportion of your diet (including snacks) that should come from that group. A quick glance will tell you whether you're anywhere close. The number of daily servings recommended from each group is based on the calorie requirement for a normally active person of average height and weight. (These requirements vary with individual weight, age, and level of physical activity.) Most North American diets are heavy in the meat and dairy groups (and thus high in fat and protein), and too light in bread and cereals and in fruits and vegetables (and therefore low in complex carbohydrates).

Variety is especially important when it comes to fruits and vegetables, the sources of many important vitamins and minerals. They are best consumed raw as well as cooked (raw vegetables retain more nutrients). And your diet should include dark green vegetables (for example, broccoli and spinach) and deep yellow or deep orange vegetables (for example, carrots, winter squash, and turnips) several times a week.

How varied is your diet? Consult your two-day eating diary, then circle the rating letter on the scale below that best describes your diet right now (A is good, B is medium, and C is bad). If you are eating the ideal balance between the four food groups, or close to it, give yourself an A. If you're out of balance, but not drastically so, score yourself B. And if your diet is badly off kilter (concentrated in one or two of the four groups), give yourself a C.

A B C

How Processed Is Your Food? Many of the good foods you eat are processed to some degree: whole-wheat bread, pasta, water-packed tuna, frozen (unsalted) vegetables. But, as a general rule, the more processed a food, the less nutritious it is. Food processing usually involves the addition of salt, sugar, or fat (often all three), as well as the "refining" away of many vitamins and minerals and much of the fiber found in fresh food.

How processed is the food that makes up your diet? Estimate the proportion of your diet that is fresh (meat, vegetables, grains, fruit) or little processed (whole-grain breads and cereals, brown rice, unsweetened juices, unsalted frozen vegetables, tuna packed in water).

If 50 percent or more of your diet is in the form of fresh or little-processed food, give yourself an A. If your diet is well below 50 percent in this area, though less-processed food is still a sizable proportion, score yourself B. And if fresh and little-processed food is a small portion of your diet give yourself a C.

A B C

How Nutrient Dense Is Your Food? Nutrient-dense food delivers the maximum nutritional punch per calorie. The more fat, salt, and sugar in your food, the less nutrient-dense it is. The more processed a food is, the emptier its calories are likely to be.

Use the Nutrient Density Chart on the next two pages to analyze the food you eat. It is divided into six sections, representing the four food groups, plus condiments and liquids. The chart is structured as three columns that group individual foods by their nutrient density. Column A contains foods that provide substantial nutrition for every calorie (lots of vitamins, fiber, and complex carbohydrates). Column B lists foods that are reasonably nutritious per calorie. Column C consists of foods that have empty calories, that deliver many calories but very little nutrient value per calorie.

How nutrient-dense is your diet? Refer to your two-day diet diary, then look over the chart and estimate where your food mostly falls. (Don't worry about being too precise: You'll have an opportunity to keep a detailed diet diary in week 1 of your start-up program.) If most of the foods you eat are in the A column, give yourself an A on the rating scale below. If you occupy the middle ground (many people do) and most of your food shows up in the B column, circle B. If most of your food is listed under C (be honest!), then rate yourself C.

A   B   C

How Much Do You Eat? Most people eat more food than they need or is good for them. An 8-ounce sirloin steak is actually more than twice the suitable serving for a person of average size and weight. A tall glass of orange juice is actually two servings of fruit (a single juice serving is a half-cup). A heaping plate of pasta is probably more than double the grain serving you require.

If you are overweight or always putting on weight (and then "going on a diet"), you probably tend to eat more than you need. Do you feel you have to stuff yourself to have a good time? While you probably have a pretty good sense of whether or not you eat too much, the chart on pages 336–337 can help you be more precise. It lists some common foods and the serving size appropriate for an adult of average height and weight.

How much do you eat? You needn't rigorously count your total servings in each food group to get a very good idea. If you generally eat moderate amounts and don't usually pig out on seconds or dessert (and if you are close to your ideal weight and have no trouble staying there), then you can probably score yourself A. If you know you eat more or less than you need (or tend to gain weight in spite of yourself, or are perenially underweight), then you should probably score B. If you generally eat

NUTRIENT DENSITY CHART

A. Nutrient Dense (Eat anytime)	B. On the Fence (Eat in moderation)	C. Empty Calories (Eat now and then)

* = high in fiber   Na = high in salt   F = high fat   S = high in refined sugar

Fruit and Vegetable Group (4–5 servings daily)

Fresh fruit*	Dried fruit	Jams, jellies (S)
Unsweetened fruit juice	Coconut (F)	Fruit in syrup (S)
Frozen or fresh vegetables*	Sweetened fruit juice (S)	
Unsalted vegetable juice	Avocado (F)	
	Salted vegetable juice (Na)	
	Pickles, (Na, S)	

Bread and Cereal Group (3–5 servings daily)

Whole grain (bread, pasta, cereal, matzoh)*	Refined grains (white bread, unsugared cereal, white pasta)	Very refined grains, (donut, croissant, crackers, sweetened cereals) (F, S)
Brown rice*	White rice	

Milk Group (2 servings daily)

Skim milk	2% milk (F)	Cream
Skim milk products (cottage cheese, yogurt)	2% milk products (yogurt, cottage cheese, low-fat cheese) (F)	Cream products (sour cream, cream cheese) (F)
	Whole milk and whole milk products (4% fat) (cheese) (F)	Sweetened milk products (ice cream, egg nog, chocolate milk) (F, S)

Meat Group (2 servings daily)

Egg whites	Whole egg (F)	Fish packed in oil
Lean fish	Oily fish, shellfish (F)	Red meat, untrimmed (F)
Poultry (without skin)	Poultry with skin (F)	Processed meat (sausage, salami, hot dog, pâté, ham, bacon) (F, Na, S)
Legumes (dried beans, peas)	Red meat (fat-trimmed) (F)	

A. Nutrient Dense (Eat anytime)	B. On the Fence (Eat in moderation)	C. Empty Calories (Eat now and then)
* = high in fiber	Na = high in salt	F = high fat	S = high in refined sugar

A. Nutrient Dense (Eat anytime)	B. On the Fence (Eat in moderation)	C. Empty Calories (Eat now and then)
Tofu (soy beans)	Nuts and seeds Unprocessed peanut butter (F)	Hydrogenated peanut butter (F, S)

Condiments and Sauces

A. Nutrient Dense	B. On the Fence	C. Empty Calories
Herbs and spices (except salt)	Salty condiments (salt, soy sauce, mustard)	Creamy salad dressing (F)
Lemon juice or vinegar dressing	Dressing with vegetable oil (F)	Butter, margarine (F)
Water-based sauces and vegetable purée-based sauces	Unsaturated vegetable oil (F)	Fat-based sauces (hollandaise, unskimmed gravy, mayonnaise) (F)
Unsweetened condiments (tomato sauce, apple sauce, skim milk yogurt)	Milk-thickened sauces (F)	High-fat condiments (whipped cream, chocolate sauce, cream, butter, margarine, prepared salad dressings) (F, S, Na)
		High-sugar condiments (ketchup, sweet relish, jam, jelly)

Other Drinks and Liquids

A. Nutrient Dense	B. On the Fence	C. Empty Calories
Fat-skimmed soup	Clear soup (broth) (Na)	Cream soup, most canned soups (F, Na)
Water	Sugar-free soft drinks	Sugared soft drinks (S)
Decaffeinated coffee or tea	Caffeine drinks (coffee, tea, cola)	Alcoholic beverages
Herbal tea		

SAMPLE SERVING SIZES

(NOTE: A serving can be eaten by itself or used as an ingredient in other foods.)

Milk Group (2 servings daily)

Milk	1 cup
Yogurt (plain)	1 cup
Hard cheese	1-1/4 oz. (about 1-1/2" square by 1" thick)
Cottage cheese	2 cups

Measure out a cup of liquid and pour it into a glass of the size you usually use. This will give you a visual sense of one serving of liquid. Weigh a portion of hard cheese to get a visual sense of what a serving looks like.

Meat Group (2 servings daily)

Red meat (lean)	2–3 oz. (cooked)*
Poultry (lean)	2–3 oz. (cooked)*
Fish (lean)	2–3 oz. (cooked)*
Liver (lean)	2–3 oz. (cooked)*
Eggs	2 or 3
Hard cheese	2–3 oz. (3 oz. = about a 2" square, 1" thick)
Cottage cheese	1/2 cup
Dried peas, beans, or lentils	1-1/2 cups cooked*
Nuts and seeds	1/2–3/4 cup
Peanut butter	4 tbs.

*Meat shrinks in cooking; legumes increase in volume.

A single serving of meat is much smaller than the typical restaurant portion. A medium-sized hamburger patty or small chicken breast is about 3 ounces of meat. Four tablespoons of peanut butter is more than enough to spread on a slice of bread.

Fruit and Vegetable Group (4–5 servings daily)

Vegetables (small or cut-up)	1/2 cup
Fruit (small or cut-up)	1/2 cup
Potato	1 medium-sized
Carrot	1 medium-sized
Fruit (whole)	1 medium-sized (tomato, apple, peach, orange, banana)

Fruit or vegetable juice	1/2 cup
Salad	1 bowl (1 cup, but depends on contents)
Lettuce	1 wedge (1 cup)

A single piece of fruit or a single medium-sized vegetable is one serving. For juices and cut-up or small vegetables and fruit, measure out a half cup and see what it looks like on the plate. Do the same for a half cup of fruit juice.

Grain Group (4–5 servings daily)

Bread	1 slice
Rolls, muffins	1
Cereal (cooked)	1/2–3/4 cup
Cereal (dry)	1 oz.
Pasta (cooked)	1/2–3/4 cup
Rice (cooked)	1/2–3/4 cup

A single slice of bread or a single roll or muffin is one serving from the grain group. A bowl of cooked or dry cereal is one serving. For rice or pasta, measure out three-quarters of a cup onto a plate to get a visual sense of the size of a serving.

---

big portions or always have seconds and dessert (or are very over- or underweight), give yourself a C.

A   B   C

How Regularly Do You Eat? Your brain needs a constant supply of energy to work properly, and your greatest requirement for calories is during the day, when you are physically active. If you miss breakfast, you're asking for fatigue and trouble concentrating during the day. (Not eating at the beginning of the day means that by lunchtime you will have gone roughly sixteen hours without nourishment.) If you skip lunch or just eat a salad, as many dieters do, you'll need stress energy to get you through the afternoon, to compensate for the calories you didn't eat. In sum, the old adage, "Breakfast like a king, lunch like a prince, and dine like a pauper" still applies.

However, not everyone prefers the traditional three meals a day. No matter. Five or six smaller meals may even be healthier than three large ones. (This eating pattern is sometimes called grazing.) The key, along with food variety, is regularity.

How regular are your meals? If you always eat a hearty breakfast, a good lunch, and a modest dinner (or eat a balanced diet spread over a number of smaller meals), give yourself an A. If you eat three meals every day, including breakfast, but eat lighter early and heavier late, score yourself a B. If you regularly skip any meal, give yourself a C.

A   B   C

How Smart Is Your Snack Pattern? Most people eat three meals a day plus a number of smaller "snacks," which include all the beverages they consume. The simplest way to rate your snacking pattern is to analyze it for nutrient density. To do this, look back at the Nutrient Density Chart.

How smart is your snack pattern? If you always choose nutrient-dense snacks in moderate amounts, you are an A. If most of your snacks come from column B, score yourself B. And if most of your snacks come from the high-fat, high-sugar, and high-salt column C, rate yourself C.

Lower your self-rating a notch for each of the following that is true for you:

> You drink more than two glasses of alcohol per day.
> You consume more than three cups of a caffeinated beverage (cola, coffee, tea) each day.

A   B   C

How Much Fluid Do You Drink? Water is a nutrient necessary to maintain life, and although it is found in many solid foods, including fruits (watermelon is 95 percent water), vegetables, and even cheese (40 percent water), roughly 50 percent of your daily water intake should be in the form of fluids. For the average person, this translates into six cups of fluid each day, at least two of which should be drinking water (including any kind of salt-free bottled water).

How much fluid do you drink? (Don't count any alcoholic or caffeinated beverages.) If you drink six glasses a day, at least two of them water, give yourself an A. If you drink fewer than six glasses, you score a B. If you drink little liquid (and no water), give yourself a C.

A   B   C

Do You Take a Broad-based Vitamin-Mineral Supplement? Based on the results of the Body Age Study, a vitamin-mineral supplement that includes the following ten vitamins can play a significant role in slowing the aging process: vitamin C, vitamin A, vitamin B_1, vitamin B_2, vitamin B_3, vitamin B_6, vitamin B_{12}, vitamin E, folic acid, and biotin. (See chapter 3.)

If you take a supplement, does it include every one of these ten essential vitamins? And do you follow its dosage recommendations? If so, score yourself A. If you take a vitamin-mineral supplement that lacks any of the essential ten, give yourself a B. If you take no supplement, you score a C.

A   · B   C

You can use your self-ratings as a departure point for designing your four-week start-up program, as follows: Each area in which you rated yourself C is a high-priority area for action. B items are lower priority, though still important. And any item for which you rated an A is a nutritional strength you can build on.

Deepening Your Nutritional Awareness

The three tests that follow help you identify the habits that may make it difficult for you to change the way you eat, and they enable you to spot more clearly the specific opportunities you have to eat better.

How, When, and Why I Eat. Increasing your awareness of how, when, and why you eat is a necessary first step in the change process. This simple checklist will help you identify your main eating behaviors and feelings. We've left space at the bottom for you to add additional items you're aware of. In the space to the left of each statement, rate its importance on a scale of 1 to 10, with 1 as "never" and 10 as "very true." Not all the items listed below are negatives; some are attitudes and behaviors on which you can build.

FEELINGS (Beliefs, Attitudes)
_____I eat when I'm anxious or worried.
_____I eat when I'm under stress.
_____I eat when I'm depressed.
_____I eat when I'm bored.
_____I eat when I'm angry or upset.
_____I eat when I need a reward.
_____I eat when I'm hungry.
_____I crave sweet snacks.
_____I crave salty snacks.
_____I crave fatty snacks.

_____I need a drink to help me unwind at the end of the day.
_____I'm almost always hungry or thinking about food.
_____I love fried foods and can't get enough of them.
_____I eat when I need a lift.
_____I'm not hungry first thing in the morning.
_____When I see or smell food, I get hungry and usually eat.

_____

_____

BEHAVIORS

_____I eat only when I'm at the table.
_____I eat whenever I'm within reach of food.
_____I eat food quickly or swallow food before it is completely chewed.
_____I eat nutritious snacks, low in fat and sugar.
_____I eat three meals a day, including a hearty breakfast.
_____Caffeine helps me make it through the day.
_____I eat until I'm stuffed.
_____I usually eat lean meat or fish and trim away fat or skin.
_____I eat while doing other things (working, reading, watching TV).
_____I often need a snack to get me through the morning or afternoon.
_____When I start eating sweets, I can't stop.
_____I seldom use butter or margarine.
_____I always clean my plate, no matter how much food is on it.
_____Food doesn't usually taste good unless I add salt to it.
_____I eat second helpings when available.
_____A meal isn't complete without dessert.
_____I read labels and try to avoid unhealthy additives.
_____I am constantly on a diet or watching my weight.
_____I am conscious of nutritious ways of cooking and strive to practice
       them.
_____I eat when there is nothing else to do.

_____

_____

Look most closely at those items on which you scored 7 or higher.
Are they positive or negative feelings and behaviors? What small concrete
steps could you take to modify your negative feelings and behaviors in
the direction of high-performance nutrition?

Now focus on your nutritional strengths. What are the strong points
in your diet? Congratulate yourself on the things you're doing right (and
remember to keep doing them while you're making modifications in other
areas). It's a good idea to make a list of your sound nutritional practices.
This helps underline the ways in which you are affirming your self through
the way you eat, and it may give you some ideas for nutrition affirmations.

My Roadblocks. The exercise you've just completed was a first step toward identifying the negative beliefs that stand in the way of lasting change. In order to identify your belief barriers, start asking yourself how you feel about certain positive nutritional behaviors. For example, how do you feel about giving up coffee? Would your answer be, "I'd never get through the day?" Once you've discovered your negative beliefs, you can change them to positive beliefs. For example: "Caffeine is a stimulant and contributes to my feelings of anxiety while artificially elevating my stress level. I choose to discover how I feel with less."

But remember: The positive beliefs you substitute for your tired, old negative beliefs must be true. They must be ones you believe in, not merely ones you pay lip service to. Here are a number of samples, which may or may not be appropriate for you. We've left room at the bottom for you to add any other important roadblocks you've discovered and their positive antidotes.

Negative Beliefs	Positive Beliefs
1. High-performance nutrition means giving up all the foods I enjoy.	**1.** Because tastes in food are learned, new tastes can be acquired. Many of my favorite foods are nutrient dense. And I can learn to enjoy new flavors.
2. There are so many additives in food and so much pollution in the air that it doesn't make much difference what I eat.	**2.** By eating better, I can greatly reduce the harmful additives I eat. There's lots of evidence that sound nutrition can make a difference.
3. Changing my eating habits just seems too difficult.	**3.** Change is possible. And the small, concrete steps recommended in this book mean I can change gradually and at my own pace.
4. My friends don't eat this way.	**4.** I can't control what others do. I can look after myself. Who knows? Others may follow my good example.
5. My family and I are healthy enough. We have no major diseases or chronic health problems.	**5.** Our diet is high in salt, sugar, and saturated fat. We could be developing health problems that are not yet obvious.

6. Eating out is my favorite pastime. And it's impossible to eat well while enjoying myself.

6. Restaurant food can be nutritious if I choose wisely. I don't have to overeat to have a good time. And I don't have to drink wine with every restaurant meal.

7. In the long run, we all die anyway, so why bother?

7. I'm not worried about dying. I am concerned about the quality of my life.

8. When eating out, I just can't find anything that isn't cooked in fat or dripping in grease.

8. Most restaurants will put the dressing on the side and leave the butter in the kitchen, if you ask them.

9. _____

9. _____

10. _____

10. _____

My Opportunities for Eating Better. You now have a much clearer idea of some of the gaps and imbalances in your current diet. Do you skip breakfast? Skimp on lunch? Eat a huge dinner (and a rich snack just before bed)? Do you drink too much or use too much caffeine to keep you going? Is your diet high in fat and sugar but low in fresh fruits and veggies?

What eating behaviors would you like to change? Which of the eight basic guidelines did you score lowest on? Are you prepared to do something to change your eating for the better?

Make a list of your five most promising opportunities to eat better. (If you have difficulty, look back over this self-rating section for ideas.) These will form the basis of your start-up program, once you've refined them further in week 1 by keeping a diet diary.

Identify Your Nutrition Affirmations and Visualizations

You now know a lot more about what you eat, when you eat, and why you eat. Whatever your eating habits, undoubtedly some of them have begun to stand out even more starkly as examples of poor nutrition. You should now be able to identify more specifically your short-term nutritional goals: the eating behaviors you want to change and your specific opportunities each week for changing them.

These goals and opportunities lead you directly to your nutritional affirmations, which will capture and summarize the behavior changes you make during your nutrition action program. To give you some ideas, following is a list of possible nutrition affirmations and visualizations. But remember: The most effective affirmation or visualization is one you've chosen for yourself.

Sample affirmations:

> My food fuels me.
> I eat for me.
> I fuel myself.
> Energy in, energy out.
> I feel my food energy.
> I power up at meals.
> I get out of my day what I put into it.
> I bubble with energy.
> I eat nutritious food.
> Nutrition-dense for energy-intense.
> Health is my ''just desserts.''
> My body knows what to eat.

Sample visualizations:

> I see my body as a highly efficient warehouse that I stock well, making sure all the (nutrient) shelves are filled by my meals. Throughout the day, I feel my body taking over as warehouse manager, making sure all (my) orders (for energy) are filled right on time, and nothing unneeded is left on the shelf.

> I see my body as a laboratory beaker filled with just the right ingredients to keep the energy reactions happening, bubbling along at just the right level throughout the day.

> After or while I'm eating a meal, I feel and see an intense ball of bright glowing light in my stomach, radiating energy beams to every cell in my body.

> I see myself about to order from a menu. I'm floating lightly above it, enjoying finding foods that are light as I feel, with no desire to be pulled down by the heavy, rich foods.

> I see myself fitting into my wedding suit [dress].

Find or create the affirmations that fit you. Use them as part of taking action to achieve high-performance nutrition.

BASIC TRAINING

The basic training in this section is of two kinds: nutritional background information that will hone your understanding of the eight key guidelines and why they are so important; and tips on how to put each of the guidelines into daily practice. For more detail on the fascinating and complex field of nutritional science, explore the list of recommended books in ''Further Reading'' at the back of this book.

The Building Blocks of Sound Nutrition

There are three essential building blocks of sound nutrition: carbohydrates, fat, and protein. (Fiber, which many nutritionists talk about separately, is not a nutrient.) If you achieve a healthy balance between the three essential nutritional elements, you will eat well and be getting more than enough fiber.

The typical North American of today eats a much less healthy balance of the three building blocks than did North Americans at the turn of the century. In fact, our eating habits have changed so significantly that the overwhelming evidence suggests that our diet is largely responsible for the increase in many diseases, from diabetes and hypoglycemia to high blood pressure, heart problems, and certain types of cancer. Just how bad is our diet? The chart below begins to provide an answer. The first two lines show the proportions of protein, fat, and carbohydrate in the North American diet as it was in 1910 and as it is today. The third line shows the proportions now eaten in less-developed countries, where degenerative diseases, such as heart disease, are rare. The fourth line is the diet currently recommended by the American Heart Association, a diet we consider conservative.

NUTRITIONAL GROUPS AS PERCENT OF TOTAL CALORIES CONSUMED

	Protein	Fat	Complex Carbohydrate	Simple Carbohydrate (Sugar)
1910	15–20	20–30	40	10
1980	**20**	**40**	**10**	**30**
Developing countries	10–15	10–15	70–80	[negligible]
AHA	20	30	40	10

The effect of the eight guidelines we gave our study subjects was to move them back toward the diet their parents and grandparents ate.

Carbohydrates: The Cornerstone of a Healthy Diet. One of the most enduring myths about carbohydrates is that they are fattening. But it is actually the butter on your bread, the rich cream or meat sauce on your spaghetti, or the sour cream on your baked potato that spike up the calorie count of starchy foods. In fact, a gram of carbohydrate delivers the same number of calories as a gram of protein (4 calories), while a gram of fat delivers more than twice the calories (1 gm. of fat = 9 calories).

The foods that are high in natural carbohydrates—whole grains, legumes, fruits, and vegetables—form the most important nutritional building block, your most useful source of nutritional energy. These foods come loaded with vitamins and minerals; in the case of grains and legumes, they are also high in protein. Most are low in fat content. In addition, carbohydrate foods are the *only* source of dietary fiber.

Glucose, the primary form of carbohydrate your body uses, is derived from both simple and complex carbohydrates. Glucose is vital for all organs and tissues of the body, particularly the brain, which under normal circumstances relies exclusively on glucose as fuel.

There are two types of carbohydrates. Complex carbohydrates, or starches, come exclusively from plants. A particularly attractive feature of the complex carbohydrates is that your body digests them slowly so that the glucose is released gradually into your system. (A slower rise in blood glucose levels after a meal also puts less stress on your body.) The energy in complex carbohydrates is thus available to your body over a longer period than the quick energy fix you get from simple sugars.

HIGH-CARBOHYDRATE FOODS THAT ARE GOOD FOR YOU

Complex Carbohydrates

Fresh (or frozen) vegetables
Legumes (for example, lentils, dried
  peas, peanuts)
Whole grain (for example, brown rice)
Whole grain products (for example, whole-wheat bread, whole grain cereals)

Simple Carbohydrates

Fresh fruits
Fresh (or frozen) vegetables
Skim milk (also high protein)

Note: 1 gm. of carbo = 4 calories

Benefits: Best source of energy (release is gradual); only source of dietary fiber; nutrient dense. (In their unrefined state, carbohydrate foods are high in fiber and low in fat, and have no salt.)

Simple carbohydrates, also known as simple sugars, are found in fruits, vegetables, and milk (lactose is a simple carbohydrate). Simple carbohydrates that occur naturally in food also come with a healthy dose of dietary fiber and useful nutrients. All refined sugars are also simple carbohydrates. Sugar comes in many guises, but all deliver empty calories. Refined sugar includes the following: sucrose (table sugar), brown sugar, honey, molasses, corn syrup, and maple syrup. On package labels, in addition to the names just listed and others, sugar is called dextrose, fructose, and lactose.

The most recent studies have concluded that sugar is not actually bad for you, suggesting that sucrose and its siblings have an undeservedly poor reputation. Nonetheless, the more calories you eat as refined sugar, the less room there is in your diet for nutrient-dense foods.

The best way to look at carbohydrates is to emphasize the positive. A diet high in natural carbohydrates is delicious and loaded with fiber. If you eat more fresh fruit, vegetables, legumes, and whole grains, you'll find you have fewer cravings for refined sugars. The American Heart Association recommends that we aim to make carbohydrates at least 50 percent of the food we eat, and that no more than 10 percent be in the form of simple carbohydrates, with refined sugar a very small proportion.

Fat, the Main Offender. Fat is an important part of your diet, but you need only a tiny amount of fat in food to ensure good health. (Don't confuse dietary fat with body fat. Body fat—the way your body stores excess calories—results from eating more calories than you burn, regardless of their source.) Since most North Americans have far too much fat in their diets, if you set out to reduce your overall fat consumption by eliminating or cutting way down on obvious fats (such as butter, lard, margarine, and mayonnaise) and to shift away from animal fat to vegetable fat, you'll be taking a big step in the direction of sound nutrition. We don't expect you to give up all fat; it is one of the things that makes food taste good. But a little fat goes a long way. You will get more than enough of the essential polyunsaturated fatty acids by eating a variety of less-processed food from the four food groups.

Dietary fats do serve some important functions. They help the body manufacture necessary body fat for insulation and as protection for your vital organs. Dietary fats are also a source of the essential vitamins A, D, E, and K.

Naturally occurring dietary fats consist of two basic types of fatty acids: saturated and unsaturated. The basic dietary guideline is: Unsaturated fats are okay in moderation, but avoid saturated fats as much as you can.

Since saturated fats have a higher melting point than unsaturated fats, you can usually guess what kind of fat predominates by how solid it is at room temperature: the more solid, the higher its content of saturated

HIGH-FAT FOODS

Saturated Fats (Usually solid)	Unsaturated Fats (Usually liquid)	
	Polyunsaturated	**Monounsaturated**
Red meat (liver*, pork* worst)	Corn oil	Olive oil
Poultry	Safflower oil	Peanut oil
Shellfish (shrimp* worst)	Soybean oil	
All processed meat*	Sesame oil	
Coconut (coconut oil)	Margarine	
Butter	Avocado	
Egg yolk*	Nuts	
Dairy products (except skim)	Seeds (for example, sunflower seeds)	
Mayonnaise	Fatty fish	
Creamy salad dressing	(sardines*	
Margarine	worst)	
Lard		
Palm oil, coconut oil, palm kernel oil		

Note: 1 gm of fat = 9 calories

* = very high in cholesterol

fats. Any solid fat, such as butter, lard, or margarine, is high in saturated fats.

Saturated fats are not essential to good nutrition, yet they constitute a very high proportion of the modern North American diet, because saturated fats dominate the fat in food from animal sources, and because the properties of saturated fats add the tasty texture to many processed foods (from potato chips to creamy salad dressings). In addition, the three vegetable oils most often used in food processing—palm oil, coconut oil, and palm kernel oil—are very high in saturated fats.

Unsaturated fatty acids are found in both animal and plant foods.

Monounsaturated fatty acids are present in many foods, including eel, halibut, avocados, rapeseed oil, peanut oil, olive oil, and soybean-based margarines. Current research suggests that the monounsaturates have neutral effects on your blood lipids: the form in which fat is carried in your blood. They are neither good nor bad for you.

Polyunsaturated fatty acids dominate the fats found in vegetables, fish, and shellfish. Most vegetable oils, as long as they haven't been hydrogenated (check the label), are high in polyunsaturates. (Hydrogenation is a process that converts unsaturated fat into saturated fat.) These include safflower oil, corn oil, sesame oil, soybean oil, and sunflower oil. Polyunsaturates in moderation are good for you. They form an essential part of every diet.

Among the polyunsaturates is one fatty acid family that has recently received a great deal of attention. The omega 3 fatty acids—found in fatty fish such as salmon, tuna, trout, mackerel, herring, and lake whitefish—are believed to lower blood triglycerides (fat levels) and to make your blood clot less easily (possibly lowering your risk of a heart attack). Some research even suggests that inflammation from arthritis is reduced by these fish oils.

The final chapter of the fat story involves cholesterol, a controversial chemical that is found in *all* animal tissues (including fish and shellfish)

HIDDEN FATS

Food	Specific Examples/Fat Percentages
Nuts	Cashews 70%; pistachios 90%
Peanuts	76% (including peanut butter)
Seeds	Sunflower seeds 68%
Avocado	85%
Coleslaw	74%
Olives	Green olives 98%
Coconut (fresh)	86%
Fatty fish	Tinned salmon 61%
Shellfish (some)	Fried clams 68%; broiled lobster 36%
Beef	Broiled sirloin steak 75%; hamburger 64%
Chicken	Broiled chicken breast 56%
Pork	Broiled pork chop 52%
Ham	Baked ham 69%
Liver	Liver paste 87%
Processed meats	Hot dog 80%; salami 68%; bologna 76%
Sauces	Gravy 72%; white sauce 72%; tartar sauce 96%
Eggs	Boiled egg 68%
Chocolate	Baking chocolate 93%
Whole milk products	Ice cream 54%; cheddar cheese 72%; cream cheese 91%
Chips, crackers	Potato chips 63%; cheese crackers 53%
Nondairy creamer	59%
Salad croutons	51%
Pastry	Piecrust 60%; brownie 61%; pound cake 57%

Derived from *"Neuropsychology of Weight Control,"* SyberVision Systems, Inc. Newark, California: 1985.

and which is most easily absorbed by your body in the presence of saturated fats (the majority of animal fat). Since your liver manufactures all the cholesterol your body needs, there's no minimum requirement for cholesterol in a healthy diet. However, cholesterol is found in many nourishing foods, such as eggs, liver, kidney, and shellfish. For most people, the key is to cut down on unnecessary cholesterol (for example, a well-marbled steak) rather than to attempt to eliminate it from your diet, and to eat the leanest meat and the lowest-fat dairy products.

If you set out to reduce your overall fat consumption and to shift away from animal fat to vegetable fat, you will have taken a big step in the direction of sound nutrition.

Protein, the Ubiquitous Nutrient. You need protein every day (its amino acids are the basic building blocks of your body, essential to everything from cell membranes to the creation of antibodies), but unless you are a strict vegetarian, who also eats neither egg nor dairy products, there is little danger you'll lack protein. All meat and dairy products contain what is known as complete protein, protein that has all the essential amino acids your body can't make itself. Your body needs protein every day, but most North Americans eat twice as much as they require, and far too much of it is consumed in foods that are also very high in saturated fats: meats, eggs, and dairy products. However, as you increase your consumption of complex carbohydrates and decrease your consumption of foods high in saturated fats, you will almost automatically eat more protein in healthier ways: from lean red meats and poultry (no skin) and less-processed vegetable sources. According to the American Heart Association, protein should account for no more than 20 percent of your daily calorie intake. You can thrive on considerably less.

As you decrease the amount of fatty meat in your diet and increase the foods rich in complex carbohydrates, you will need to become more conscious of the foods that contain complementary proteins, foods that

---

HIGH-PROTEIN FOODS

Animal (Usually complete)
Red meat
Poultry
Fish (sometimes incomplete)
Shellfish
Eggs
All dairy products

Vegetable (Usually incomplete)
Legumes (dried beans, peas,
   peanuts)
Nuts, seeds
Whole grains
Soy beans/tofu (complete protein)

when eaten together provide you with a serving of complete protein. Vegetable foods contain incomplete protein, protein lacking one or more of the essential amino acids. But by combining vegetable foods whose incomplete proteins complement each other you can ensure yourself a serving of complete dietary protein from non-meat sources. Keeping track of this is really quite simple. One basic rule is to combine legumes (dried beans or peas, soybeans, peanuts, black-eyed peas, kidney beans, chickpeas, navy beans, pinto beans, lentils, split peas, and lima beans) with whole grains (corn, wheat, rice, barley, or oats). The Latin American staple dish of black beans and brown rice is a perfect example of nutritious protein complementarity, as is a slice of whole-wheat bread with peanut butter. Another tip is to combine a serving of incomplete plant protein with a small amount of complete animal protein. That's what you're doing when you pour (low-fat) milk over your (unsweetened) whole-grain breakfast cereal, or mix a little (lean) hamburger into the (sugarless) tomato sauce for your spaghetti, or bake with (skim) milk powder.

If you remember to eat complete protein when you're eating protein from primarily vegetable sources, you'll get more than enough complete protein in your daily diet.

One footnote to this brief discussion of protein is its sensitivity to stress. In periods of prolonged high stress, your body loses protein much faster than normal. In such periods, while doing everything in your power to reduce unnecessarily heightened stress levels (see chapter 9, ''Effective Relaxation''), it may be appropriate for you to consume a slightly higher proportion of protein as a temporary measure.

The Micronutrients. There are 13 vitamins and 21 minerals that are essential to health. The table below lists these key micronutrients and some of the good foods they're found in. (Only 17 minerals are listed. The other four are required in such tiny trace amounts that you will invariably eat enough of them if you have a balanced diet.)

A brief word about salt: Technically salt (sodium) is a mineral, vital to good health. Your body needs salt: In effect, your tissues swim in a sea of salt water. But the average North American eats three times the salt he needs. Too much salt contributes to high blood pressure, can cause migraine headaches, and can increase the risk of heart disease. It causes your body to retain fluids and so is implicated in weight problems. Even if you studiously avoided salt in all its forms, you'd probably unwittingly eat more than enough.

The most obvious form of salt is sodium chloride, or table salt, but a disconcerting array of ''flavor enhancers'' containing sodium are used in food processing. One of the prime culprits is MSG (mono *sodium* glutamate). Any ingredient with the word *sodium* in its name is a form of salt.

GOOD SOURCES OF VITAMINS

Vitamin	Source
A	Liver, kidney, egg yolk, yellow and green vegetables, fruits
D	Fortified milk, fish liver oils, sunlight on skin
E	Vegetable oils, most meats, fish, leafy vegetables
K	Green leafy vegetables, cheese
B_1 (thiamine)	Lean pork, beef, whole or enriched grain products, legumes
B_2 (riboflavin)	Milk, organ meats, whole or enriched grain products, vegetables
B_3 (niacin)	Meats, peanuts, beans and peas, enriched grain products
B_6 (pyridoxine)	Grains, seeds, organ meats
Pantothenic acid	Organ meats, eggs, milk
Biotin	Corn and soy meals, egg yolk, organ meats, tomatoes
B_{12} (cobalamin)	Organ meats, lean meats, milk, egg, cheese
C (ascorbic acid)	Citrus fruits, tomatoes, cabbage, potatoes
Folic acid	Liver and kidney, asparagus, bean sprouts, beets, broccoli, spinach

GOOD SOURCES OF MINERALS

Mineral	Source
Calcium	Milk, cheese, green leafy vegetables
Phosphorous	Milk, cheese, meat, whole grains
Magnesium	Milk, cheese, meat, seafood, whole grains
Sodium	Table salt, sodium compounds
Potassium	Fruits, vegetables, legumes, nuts
Chlorine	Table salt
Sulfur	Meat, egg, milk, cheese, legumes
Iron	Liver, meat, egg, whole grains, dark green leafy vegetables
Iodine	Iodized salt, seafood
Zinc	In many foods (meat, seafood, whole grains, legumes)
Copper	In many foods (meat, seafood, whole grains, legumes)
Manganese	Cereals, whole grains, legumes, leafy vegetables
Chromium	Cereals, whole grains, animal proteins
Cobalt	In vitamin B_{12}
Selenium	Varies with soil (whole grains, legumes, low-fat meats, milk products, vegetables)
Molybdenum	Legumes, whole grains, milk, leafy vegetables
Fluorine	Fish, tea, fluoridated water

HIGH-SALT FOODS (PROCESSED FOODS)

Most condiments (for example, mustards and relishes)
Most processed meat and fish (ham, hot dogs, bacon, sausage, luncheon
   meat)
Most snack food (potato chips, pretzels, taco chips, crackers)
Most canned foods
Most frozen foods

Like sugar, the easiest place to cut down on salt is at the table. If you're in the habit of salting your food, gradually use less until you need to add little or no salt (and *never* salt food before tasting it). If you do the cooking, gradually reduce the amount of salt you use in recipes and eliminate it entirely in cooking vegetables and meats. Cut down on condiments such as Worcestershire sauce, soy sauce, and mustard, which are high in salt. And start singling out the saltier processed foods, such as sausages, hot dogs, ham, luncheon meat, and bacon.

Some Tips on Making the Eight Guidelines Work for You

In this section, we provide some simple advice on how to put the eight essential nutritional guidelines into practice in your daily life.

Eat a Variety. Once you've learned to balance the four food groups, you've taken the first big step toward eating a variety of food. The second step is to eat as wide a variety as possible within each group. If you are like most people, you have probably gotten into a number of eating ruts. Perhaps you always eat a certain kind of bread, you eat rice but never pasta (or vice versa), or you eat some vegetables but not others, or you always have the same kind of fruit with your morning cereal. Many people claim they ''just don't like fish,'' for example, or that they ''can't'' eat bread without butter. In many cases, the problem is in what they think of as bread (tasteless white) or as fish (frozen fish sticks) or vegetables (canned). The fresh or less-refined alternatives often taste better, especially when properly cooked. If you try, you can almost certainly find many foods you like in every group.

Not everyone finds it easy to eat enough from the milk group. There are millions of people who can't tolerate the lactose in milk and who must find milk alternatives, including lactose-free milk and other milk substitutes, as well as other food sources of calcium. Alternative high-protein drinks include the various soybean milks. If you are a vegetarian or partial vegetarian, these can function as milk substitutes.

Many study participants found that by only slightly modifying their favorite dishes, these could become part of a fully balanced meal. For example, this recipe for nachos can be transformed easily from a C to an A dish: white flour nacho chips; salty tomato sauce (with sugar added); guacamole (pure avocado paste); regular cheese; regular ground beef. The alternative looks like this: whole-wheat nacho chips; tomato pieces with slivers of green pepper, plus kidney (or other) beans as the base ingredient in the topping sauce; a·small serving of lean ground round or diced cooked chicken breast; low-fat melted cheese on top. Most people in the study found that at least three of their favorite dishes could easily be tinkered into a balanced meal. For food ideas, they looked through cookbooks.

One study participant, a Basket Case whose early affirmation was "Balanced meals for a balanced me," made a self-care commitment in week 2 to eat a balanced breakfast. In week 3, he added at least five balanced dinners. In week 4, he explored restaurants near his office, checking out menus for the most balanced lunch options.

Eat Unprocessed or Little-Processed Foods. Know and use the nine whole grains: brown rice, millet, oats, bulgur wheat, rye, triticale, corn, barley, and buckwheat. And add tasty legumes (dried beans and peas) to your diet.

If you want to become really adept at choosing the most nutritious processed foods (and many are very good for you), learn to read the ingredient listing on package labels. Food additives are a complex and controversial subject, but the most important things to avoid are salt (sodium), sugar (such as sucrose, dextrose, and fructose), and fat (butter, lard, margarine, and any oil).

Eat Nutrient-Dense Foods. The Nutrient Density Chart on pages 334–335 can become an indispensable dietary tool (make a photocopy and carry it with you when you shop or dine out). Every time you favor a B food over a C, or an A food over a B, you're reducing fat, sugar, and salt, and increasing the number of nutrients you're eating per calorie.

Foods naturally high in fat are relatively easy to spot (for example, marbled meat or creamy salad dressing). It is more difficult to detect the amount of fat added in the course of food processing. If you eat mostly less-processed food, then you need only cut down on the salt, sugar, and fat you add in cooking and at the table.

Any cooking method that uses a lot of fat or oil adds fat to your food. Virtually every condiment is high in added sugar or salt or both (mustard, Worcestershire sauce, horseradish, and soy sauce are all high-salt condiments). Practice low-fat cooking methods (broil, bake, boil, poach, microwave), and stick as much as possible to condiments you can trust, such as natural herbs and spices, including pepper, and lemon juice or vinegar, instead of salt.

Restaurant meals may be the hardest place to avoid the hidden villains. But you can learn to eat out more wisely. You can ask for dressings and sauces to be brought on the side. You can choose the broiled fish over the pan-fried (sautéed) steak. You can eat the inevitable bread without butter. You can take a sip of water for every sip of wine. And so on.

Eat Moderate Amounts. Reducing the amount you eat is one of the most difficult new skills to learn. The basic rule that will help you keep the quantity down is to eat until you are satisfied, not until you are full. (It helps to pause a few minutes before you decide to have seconds or to order dessert.)

Some people in the study group found it effective to intentionally—and conspicuously—leave some food on their plates. This can be a very powerful message to your self. One participant who regularly attended a yoga ashram told her training group that disciples at the ashram were taught they should "leave a little on their plate (at meal's end) for the guru"! as a small, self-affirming act of self-discipline. Her cotrainees saw this as a wonderful strategy for introducing portion control. In week 2, they each began leaving a little on their plate (even though their mothers had always taught them to "clean their plate"). In week 3, they served themselves a little less *and* left a little more on the plate. In week 4, they left "a little something for the guru" in the pot on the stove. This group was uniformly delighted with the strong positive self-feedback this gave them: They experienced each small action as an act of self-mastery. In yogic thinking, as in the Body Age Program, the goal is to listen to, respect, and follow "the guru within."

Eat at Least Three Regular Meals, Including Breakfast. This guideline may seem simple, but for many of our program participants it proved a real roadblock. If you haven't been eating one of the three square meals you need each day, then you may find it very hard to change this habit, and initially very stressful. If this dietary change seems too threatening, we suggest you start elsewhere, or approach it as a slow and incremental process. Instead of suddenly "starting to eat breakfast," try phasing in a morning meal. In the first week, you might do nothing more than make yourself sit down and drink a glass of juice before dashing out the door. The next step (this was used by one of our study subjects) might be to make a whole-wheat bread peanut butter sandwich the night before (he didn't feel he had "time" for breakfast) and put it on top of the juice container in the fridge.

Practice Smart Snacking Patterns. Snacking is a major dietary obstacle for many people, yet quite often having a snack has little to do with needing that quick-energy "sugar boost" and a lot to do with the desire to change location and get some physical activity during a stressful day. Recognizing this, Sylvia, a secretary in the program, organized a "snack brigade" at work. Each of the five secretaries in her office agreed to be responsible for bringing in nutritious, tasty, interesting snack food one day per week. When you wanted a snack (that is, a break), you got up and went to the "snack marshall's" desk, and took a brief and nutritious breather. Some of the nutritious snacks were fresh fruit, yogurt, nuts, and raisins.

Smart snacks may require some planning. If the office coffee wagon contains only sweet and fatty delights such as donuts and danishes, come to work with your desired nutrient-dense snacks: a piece of fresh fruit, carrot sticks, or a slice of your favorite whole-grain bread. Just remember that your snacks are part of your total daily intake. Oversnacking plus three moderate meals can add up to the daily equivalent of three Roman feasts.

The ABCs of smart snacking are summarized on the chart below. Use it as your between-meal eating guide. (Refer also to the Nutrient Density Chart earlier in the chapter.)

Although you may not think of them as snacks, every beverage you drink between meals is part of your daily food intake. It's relatively easy for most people to replace soft drinks with fruit juice. And a glass of water is a filling snack. But the nonnutritious snack beverages most difficult for people to give up are those containing caffeine and alcohol.

Caffeine. By themselves, caffeinated drinks contain virtually no nutrients. We recommend that you drink no more than three caffeinated drinks a day, and none in the evening. Most people find it works to shift

THE ABCS OF SNACKING

A. Any Time	B. Occasionally	C. Seldom or Never
Fresh fruit	Dried fruit	Cookies
Raw vegetables	Vegetable with dip	Peanut-butter-and-
Whole-grain bread	Muffin (no butter)	jelly sandwiches
Low-fat yogurt/cheese	Cheese, flavored	Chips, french fries
	yogurt	Cake, pastries
	Nuts, seeds	All candy
Unsweetened juice,	Low-cal or caffeine	Soda pop (with sugar)
water, herbal tea	drinks	

COMMON SOURCES OF CAFFEINE

Food	Caffeine (average in mg.)
Coffee (6-oz. cup)	100
Weak tea (6-oz. cup)	35
Cola (10-oz. can)	35
Chocolate milk (7.5 oz.)	4
Hot cocoa (6 oz.)	15
Dark chocolate bar (2 oz.)	45
Milk chocolate bar (2 oz.)	15

to decaffeinated tea or coffee, or to drink caffeinated beverages only when they truly want their stress-raising properties. Drinking caffeine is not a good way to relax. When you want a cup of coffee, it's often the soothing, warm liquid and the companionship that you crave, not the caffeine.

Alcohol. Used in moderation, alcohol can be part of a healthy diet. But in excess it leads to serious health problems, including malabsorption of nutrients and the development of a fatty liver than can eventually result in cirrhosis. Heavy alcohol consumption also dramatically saps your energy by slowing down cell oxidation and energy production, and by slowing the discharge of fatigue acids. In nutritional terms, alcohol is second only to fat in calories per gram (7), and it delivers completely empty calories.

Use alcohol sparingly. A daily average of two glasses of wine or beer, or one ounce of hard liquor, is moderate consumption. Any more than that is too much. Remember: It takes your body approximately one hour to process 1½ ounces of hard liquor, a bottle of beer, or a glass of wine.

Here are a few basic guidelines for wise drinking. Always eat something before you drink (foods high in fat or protein are best at slowing down the body's alcohol absorption), then wait about fifteen minutes before your first sip. Drink slowly, to allow your liver to process the alcohol. Drink when you're relaxed, not in order to relax; under stress, your body absorbs alcohol more quickly.

Drink Six Cups of Fluid a Day, at Least Two of Them Water. In short, if you're feeling thirsty, pour yourself a glass of water. One side benefit of drinking more liquids is that you'll find it easier to eat moderate amounts.

Take a Broad-Based Vitamin-Mineral Supplement. The Your Vitality Quotient supplement we gave our study subjects is widely available through health food and drugstores, so that our readers may follow the Institute's program completely. The Your Vitality Quotient supplement contains the ten vitamins we identified as crucial. These are: Vitamin A (beta carotene form); vitamin C (ascorbate form); vitamin B_1 (thiamine); vitamin B_2 (riboflavin); vitamin B_3 (niacin); vitamin B_6 (pyridoxine); vitamin B_{12} (cyanocobalamin); vitamin E (d-alpha tocopherol); folic acid, and biotin. It also contains the seventeen essential minerals listed on page 351.

The ideal time to take a supplement is immediately after eating breakfast or dinner, when your digestive enzymes are fully activated and will make the most of the vitamins and minerals you've just ingested.

If our Vitality Quotient formula is not readily available to you, the Institute can provide you specific information on how the more common supplements can be combined to achieve anti-aging effects. Please write to us:

Nutrition Biochemistry
Canadian Institute of Stress
Suite 3100, Shipp Centre
3300 Bloor St. West
Toronto, Canada M8X 2X3

YOUR FOUR-WEEK START-UP PROGRAM

Week 1: Get Ready. Keep a daily diet diary, using the Nutrient Density Chart to rate the ABCs of your current diet. This information will help you refine your priority list of opportunities to eat better and to plan for concrete action in week 2.
Week 2: Take Your First Step. Change one priority eating behavior.
Week 3: Build on Your Success. Add to or deepen your week 2 change.
Week 4: Consolidating Your Gains. In one area, you are now eating a little better. Find ways to further improve your chosen change.

With nutrition, as with all five interventions, the key to success is choosing, affirming, and phasing in a series of small, concrete, and specific behavioral changes. The four-week program we describe below will help you introduce some new, self-affirming nutritional habits. Begin with one of the eight guidelines that seems relatively easy to follow (it might be improving your snacking, moderating the amount you eat, or starting to eat breakfast). Save the more intractable aspects of your daily diet until you've created a firm foundation of three square meals a day.

Within each guideline, there are specific problem areas you may have identified, any one of which can be an excellent place to start. Here are a few possibilities: too much refined sugar; too much salt; too much caffeine; too much alcohol; not enough fiber; too much fat (or a related area such as high-fat cooking).

Week 1: Get Ready

Fill out your Action Diary Planning Page. Your first step this week is to enter into a firm contract with yourself to introduce the following new behaviors:

1. *Begin with autogenic relaxation with affirmations and visualizations.* Find the twenty minutes of quiet time you need to do your first autogenic relaxation. While in this deeply relaxed state, repeat your one or two personalized nutrition affirmations. Then spend a few minutes visualizing successful nutrition behaviors. Repeat your autogenic practice at least four more times this week. Use your nutrition affirmations daily, ideally two or three times.

2. *Keep a diet diary.* While doing nothing to change your current eating habits, keep a thorough diet diary this week. The purpose of the diet diary is to make you even more aware of how, what, when, and where you eat.

In a notebook you carry with you throughout the day, record *every* item of food you consume, including water, tea, coffee, and alcohol. Be as detailed as possible, noting, for example, whether you added 2% milk or cream to your morning coffee, or if you put butter on your potato at supper. Note how the food was cooked. For example, were your vegetables steamed or fried? Remember: Don't change your habits yet; simply observe them. After a week of keeping your diary, you'll know your current nutritional practices intimately, and you'll be highly motivated to change.

At the end of each day, go over your diary entries and code each one according to the Nutrient Density Chart on pages 334–335. Rate each item as either A (nutrient dense), B (on the fence), or C (empty calories). Note that a moderately nutrient-dense ham and cheese sandwich (a B) becomes less nutritious (a C) when you have it with both butter and mayonnaise. As a general rule, if you add fat (butter, cream, cheese), sugar, or salt (or a condiment high in one or more of these three), an A becomes a B, and a B becomes a C. Similarly, if you add fat, salt, or sugar in cooking, the nutrient-density rating goes down.

Now take a look at your daily nutritional balance. Count up the number of servings under each food group. Unless you were eating big portions, don't worry too much about actual serving size. (For a reminder about serving sizes, see p. 336) Take a look at the rough proportion of fresh or unprocessed (and lightly processed) food versus processed food in your diet.

Finally, flag the items you know are high in fat, sugar, or salt, and count the number of cups of caffeine and the number of glasses of wine or liquor. Count the number of glasses of water.

See the accompanying sample for what a typical diary page might look like.

Follow this routine for seven days. On the seventh day, reread your whole diary, with an eye to evaluating the variety of your diet and looking for larger patterns and opportunities. Does a pork chop show up more than once? How many different fruits and vegetables do you consume? Do you eat them both raw (more vitamins) and cooked? Are there several servings of dark green and deep yellow vegetables in the mix? Reread your summary comments for each day. What patterns emerge?

Now look back at your scores in the "Rate Yourself" section. Were you being easy on yourself? Would you like to change any of them? Where are your clear priorities for behavior change?

3. *Prioritize and plan.* Refine your list of opportunities to eat better from the "Rate Yourself" section. These are the concrete behaviors you want to introduce in your action program, ranked in order of doability and desirability (your top priority should be something you want to change that doesn't seem too difficult). Your top choice is the single new eating behavior you will introduce next week.

4. *Check in with your partner.* Best of all, make a date to get together to go over each other's diet diaries. Your buddy may spot some patterns you've missed, or be able to bring some hidden fats, sugars, or salts out into the open.

5. *Record your daily progress in your Action Diary.* This is very important. Recording your progress gives you self-feedback and therefore a sense of accomplishment, and will allow you to spot patterns of success or shortfall. Eating should be enjoyable, not drudgery, so don't be hard on yourself when you're less than perfect. Take pleasure in the fact that you are now much more deeply aware of your eating habits and your opportunities to change them for the better.

SAMPLE DIET DIARY PAGE

Entry	Comments (Feelings, Behaviors, Patterns)
Monday	
Breakfast (7 A.M.) 1 glass orange juice (A) 1 slice whole-wheat toast with butter and jam (B) (fat, sugar) 1 cup coffee with cream (C) (fat)	Ate quickly. Drank coffee in two gulps. Felt urge to buy donut on way to work.
9 A.M. 1 cup coffee with cream (C) (fat, sugar) 1 donut (C) (fat, sugar)	Have to have coffee as soon as I arrive at work. Coffee trolley has danishes and donuts (which I can't resist).
10:30 A.M. 1 cup coffee with cream (C) (fat)	
Lunch (1 P.M.) 1 bowl cream-of-carrot soup (B) (fat, salt) 1 ham-and-cheese sandwich on rye bread with lettuce and tomato, mustard, butter, mayonnaise (C) (fat, salt) 1 apple (A) 1 chocolate chip cookie (C) (fat, sugar) 1 cup coffee with cream (C) (fat)	Felt slightly nauseated after this meal, which I ate too quickly. Didn't really enjoy the cookie.
3 P.M. 1 can of cola (C) (sugar) 1 granola bar (B?) (sugar)	
Dinner (7:30 P.M.) 1 pork chop (C) (fat) 1 baked potato with butter (B) (fat) 1 serving broccoli with butter (B) (fat) 1 bowl salad with thousand island dressing (B) (fat) 1 bowl chocolate ice cream (C) (fat, sugar) 2 glasses of wine (C) 1 cup coffee with cream (C) (fat)	Fell asleep in front of the TV after dinner.
10 P.M. 2 slices of cheddar cheese (B) (fat) 1 slice whole-wheat bread (A)	I wasn't really hungry, but I always have a snack before bed (it helps me sleep).

Summary
3 As; 7 Bs; 12 Cs. Too much fat and sugar; diet heavily tilted toward empty calories.

Bread and cereal group: 4 servings (including granola bar)
Meat group: 2 servings
Dairy group: 4 servings (including the bowl of ice cream and all that cream in coffee)
Fruit and vegetable group: 6 servings (including lettuce and tomato in sandwich)

Unprocessed food is about 50 percent of day's intake.

Cups of caffeine: 6 (including can of cola)

Glasses of water: 0

Alcohol: 2 glasses of wine

My Comments
Breakfast is too small and lacking representatives from all four food groups. Daily food balance is off, with bread and cereal group too low and dairy group too high. Diet is high in added fats (butter, cream) and in sugar (desserts, snacks). Too much caffeine. Salt looks okay as long as I don't add lots of salt at the table and don't use highly salted butter. No water consumed during entire day.

Overall, nutrient density is quite poor. Very few items are A, while there are many Bs and more Cs. My short-term goal is to move some of the Cs to Bs and some of the Bs to As.

Week 2: Take Your First Step

Fill out your Action Diary Planning Page. Agree to do the following during the coming week:

1. *Continue to practice autogenic relaxation with affirmations and visualizations.* Set aside quiet time at least four times this week for autogenic practice. In addition, use your affirmations daily to reinforce the changes you are making, ideally three or more times each day.

2. *Introduce one meaningful eating change.* Make this the easiest new eating behavior that affirms your nutritional goals. If you aren't now eating breakfast, are skipping lunch, or are skimping on one of the three meals, we strongly recommend that you concentrate first on eating three (more balanced) meals a day. If this seems too much to tackle, don't worry. After you've worked on some less ambitious changes, you'll likely find this one easier to face.

For nonbreakfast-eaters, beginning to eat breakfast is a powerfully self-affirming change. Since it is a significant alteration in your self-defeating eating habits, it may seem unpleasant at first. The first few bowls of cereal may seem quite unpalatable, or your spouse or family may resist the change if it threatens their schedule or eating habits. And it probably means you'll change your morning ritual, perhaps even getting up a few minutes earlier. (If this happens, be aware that negative and skeptical thoughts can be changed to positive and self-nurturing thoughts using your affirmations.) Like any meaningful change, eating breakfast is concrete and measurable: Either you.do it or you don't. And once you get into the habit, you will feel the positive effects of replenishing your body early in the morning. As an added benefit, you will have a new sense of control over your life.

One senior executive in the Body Age Program complained that by starting to eat breakfast, he was losing touch with his staff (he no longer felt the urge to head for the donut wagon as it rolled through his department in mid-morning). His solution to this roadblock was to have fresh fruit included on the wagon. The result was, in his words, "the best of both worlds."

If you are already regularly eating three meals, you may want to concentrate right away on the nutritional balance of what you are eating, by making sure you're getting the right ratio of servings from the four basic food groups. But remember: The smallest change is still significant. Substituting a nutritious snack for a sweet and fatty one each day this week is a very meaningful, concrete step toward high-performance nutrition.

3. *Check in with your partner*. Giving and getting support will help you through the rough spots. Don't be embarrassed to boast about your successes. You might even schedule a nutritious dinner date so that the two of you can compare notes (or practice your nutrient-dense cooking skills).

4. *Record your progress in your Action Diary*. Congratulate yourself for every success, and use this self-monitoring process to keep tabs on your overall nutritional progress. What areas are still problems for you?

Here is a sample Action Diary Planning Page for week 2 of High-Performance Nutrition. Your own planning page should suit your lifestyle and schedule. Find ways to introduce each specific behavior without major dislocations. If you find that your contract turns out to be too ambitious, modify it to reduce the load and lower the stress level that inevitably goes with change. Above all, remember to give each behavior you undertake on this self-care contract the SMART test. Ask yourself whether it is Specific, Measurable, Acceptable, Realistic, and Truthful.

ACTION DIARY FOR WEEK OF *April 9* TO *April 15*

Planning Page

Affirmations (My self-themes for this week in key words and phrases)

I *eat breakfast every day.*

I *feel food energy fueling my body.*

(Other) *My body is a health-seeking mechanism*

Opportunity Visualizations (I clearly see myself . . .)

I clearly see myself sitting down at the kitchen table and eating a relaxed breakfast. The breakfast consists of fresh juice, cereal, toast, skim milk, fresh fruit, and tea. Some of my favorite music is playing in the background, and while I'm eating I'm enjoying reading the entertainment section of the newspaper

I choose to deepen this Vital Life Skill as follows (My specific behavioral objectives this week)

I choose to *do a fifteen-minute autogenic relaxation followed by affirmation and visualization at least 4x's during the coming week*

Under the following circumstances: *Monday, Wednesday & Friday at home after work before dinner in the den with the door closed. Sunday morning before lunch.*

I choose to *repeat my nutrition affirmations at least 3x's each day this week*

Under the following circumstances: *In front of the mirror in the morning; as soon as I return to my desk after lunch; as soon as I get into bed at night. In addition, I will say my affirmations every time I am about to make a food choice (for example, when I'm tempted to eat a donut or choosing between canned and fresh vegetables at the market)*

I choose to *eat a full breakfast each workday morning this week*

Under the following circumstances: *sitting down at the kitchen table between 7:15 and 7:30 A.M.*

My other opportunity situations for skill practice are:

1. *Taking more time for lunch and eating lunch sitting down away from my desk*

2. *Substituting more nutritious snacks for the donuts and coffee I seem to be addicted to.*

3. *Drinking herbal tea instead of caffeine tea in the evening*

I have arranged to check in with my partner . . .

When?
On Monday, Wednesday and Friday evenings

About
How my breakfast eating is going

Week 3: Build on Your Success

Fill out your Action Diary Planning Page. Agree to do the following during the coming week:

1. *Practice autogenic relaxation with affirmations and visualizations.* Feel free to change your nutrition affirmations and visualizations as the weeks pass and your new nutritional habits take root. Continue to set aside four quiet times each week for autogenic practice. And use your affirmations daily, ideally two or three times per day.

2. *Continue practicing your new nutritional behavior.* Continue to take your vitamin-mineral supplement, and continue to explore the new nutritional behavior you introduced last week. If it was eating three meals a day, now may be the time to look more closely at the variety or the nutritional balance between the four food groups at each meal and to move toward the target ratio. If last week it was reducing the amount of sugar you add to tea and coffee, now try cutting down on foods (including condiments) that are high in refined sugar. If you reduced your alcohol consumption last week, experiment with reducing it further in each of the next two weeks. If you worked on increasing the amount of fiber, add additional high-fiber foods to your diet. Whatever you decide to do, continue to make small, specific changes.

3. *Check in with your partner.*

4. *Record your progress in your Action Diary.* As each week goes by, you should have more of a sense that you are choosing what you eat in ways that affirm the person you want to be. You are looking after yourself better by eating better. Congratulate yourself for every success and every new nutritional awareness.

Week 4: Consolidate Your Gains

Fill out your Action Diary Planning Page. Agree to do the following during the coming week:

1. *Continue to practice autogenic relaxation with affirmations and visualizations.* Use your affirmations daily to reinforce your more self-affirming nutritional style.

2. *Consolidate your new eating skill.* Whatever problem area you chose to work on, continue to address it in this final week. By now, it is beginning to become a habit instead of a novelty.

One participant reported that food planning and shopping had always been such a low priority that she typically left it until Saturday, when it became even more distasteful because it took up weekend time. In her program, she self-contracted to add more fresh fruits and vegetables to each day's diet, and made a visit to a greengrocer part of her late Saturday afternoon itinerary. But when she learned that the fresh produce arrived on Friday, she switched her shopping to Friday after work so that she could buy it at its best. The seemingly small decision to buy fresh fruits and vegetables had led her to discover that when she wanted to eat right she could find time to shop on a weekday.

3. *Check in with your partner.*

4. *Record your progress in your Action Diary.* At the end of this week, look back over your diary for the past four weeks. How much progress have you made? What small, concrete things are you doing differently? Congratulate yourself for your success.

Continuing Your Prescription

You have now laid the groundwork for high-performance nutrition. Do you want to continue looking after yourself better by eating better? If you do, you will quickly notice the increases in energy and the improvement in weight that so many of our study subjects experienced with this Vital Life Skill.

It takes about three weeks for a new behavior to become a self-affirming habit. A good way to continue is to pick one meaningful diet change and work on it for the next three weeks. Then choose another and another, until you are living a healthier life. Save the most difficult or troublesome areas of your diet for much later, after you've learned just how big a difference you can make with seemingly small, but concrete, changes.

As soon as you feel ready, but no sooner than week 8, begin phasing in the next intervention on your Prescription Pad. As you do so, continue to explore the possibilities of eating better.

Ernie, a Basket Case interior decorator (age 36, body age 48, appearance age 46), showed remarkable progress over the eight months of the program. He had been on just about every fad diet imaginable, even though he was not overweight; in fact, he was about ten pounds below his ideal. Despite his constant questing after nutritional nirvana, the only constant in his life was a steady decrease in his overall energy reserves.

As you can imagine, when nutrition turned out to be his top priority, Ernie had mixed emotions: He thought he'd exhausted this avenue for self-improvement but wanted to believe we might have "the answer" he'd been looking for. When he rated himself against our eight basic eating guidelines, he discovered to his amazement that he was the most poorly nourished person in his class. Although he had followed his fads "religiously, to the letter," he had never deeply believed in any of them and had never kept at any of them for more than a couple of months.

Above all, our program appealed to Ernie's common sense. In particular he liked "the psychological digestion" of our eating guidelines thorough autogenics, the diary-based commitment to action, and having a partner to help him along the way.

He set to work. First he tackled breakfast. Instead of his usual brown rice with liquified herbs and grasses, he began to eat complete protein in the morning: skim milk over whole-grain cereal—and even the occasional egg. And he started carrying fruit or nuts and raisins to work as snacks. Lunchtime for him had traditionally been either a protein-poor repast he culled from the office cafeteria (there were so many things he wasn't supposed to eat) or, rarely, a meal at a "group-approved vegetarian restaurant." He now began exploring other lunchtime possibilities, including some of the genuinely nutritious foods prepared in the cafeteria kitchen. (Ernie was also one of those in the study group who received the vitamin-mineral supplement, not the placebo.) In short, before long, Ernie was getting the calories he needed and eating them in a more nutrient-dense way.

After four months, Ernie reported that his energy level was consistently higher than before he started the program and that he wasn't "constantly getting over a cold, or coming down with the flu" (in fact, his immunoglobulin A level was markedly improved to within normal range). But he was beginning to feel alienated from some of his old friends, whose lives "seem to center on the latest diet or Oriental elixir." They pooh-poohed the Body Age Program as "too much like what our mothers used to tell us."

However, Ernie persevered with the help of his partner, who encouraged him to look at the evidence of his improved health and energy and not to listen to the criticism. Not long after the four-month checkup, Ernie turned his attention to exercise: He began supplementing his weekly yoga classes with regular routines for strength and stamina. By eight months, Ernie's weight was up fifteen pounds, well within his ideal weight range, and his appearance age was down from 46 to 35. His body age had dropped 10 years to 38, and both of his immune system measures were in the normal range.

Ernie seemed almost embarrassed by his success. As he put it, "I feel great. I can work the hours I want to. And my food bill—and my food shopping time—has been cut in half. I guess my mother was right: The basics work if you believe in them."

CHAPTER 13
Six Success Stories

In the foregoing chapters, we've introduced you to many of the people who successfully completed the Body Age Program. Their stories have provided glimpses of the five Vital Life Skills at work. Perhaps, however, you're still having trouble getting started. If so, you may be inspired by reading the success stories of six of our study subjects.

The case histories that follow complete the stories of six people (and six stressotypes) you met in chapter 4. They demonstrate how the individual elements of your prescription can interact to increase its effectiveness, with success in one area flowing into others.

CASE 1: Jim, Personnel Manager
Age 46, Body Age 55, Appearance Age 56
DOMINANT STRESSOTYPE: Speed Freak
SECONDARY STRESSOTYPE: Loner
PRESCRIPTION: 1) Relaxation, 2) Values/Goals, 3) Communication

Do you remember Jim, the man with a hundred irons in the fire and the entrenched belief that in order to succeed he had to give 110 percent all the time? Just before he entered the program, he'd experienced an apparent heart attack that turned out to be severe chest tension resulting from overstress. He simply didn't know how to slow down.

Like many Speed Freaks, Jim became an instant convert to relaxation skills and began to practice them almost obsessively. Initially, he used the autogenic tape every day, as soon as he got home from work, and on the weekends, too. This pattern continued while he phased in the next part of his prescription, Values/Goals Clarification.

During the training sessions, Jim had identified the following as his most fundamental core value: "I want my life to add up to something so I can really feel it adding up." As he examined the way his current lifestyle prevented the attainment of this ideal self, he became acutely aware that by scattering himself so widely, his life was in a hundred pieces, all demanding time and energy, and none delivering much satisfaction.

So Jim made the decision to commit himself full-time for at least a year to his work as the personnel manager at a food-processing company. This meant turning down an enticing job offer that would have meant moving (yet again), no more "constant fishing for new job offers," and no more outside consulting evenings and weekends.

In the first month, this narrower focus on one job quickly led Jim to find his work more enjoyable and more rewarding. He was still giving it 110 percent, but focusing on one job left him less exhausted than he'd been before. His stress level had gone down because his level of uncertainty had been reduced, and with it many of his customary vitality drains had disappeared. This new comfort with his job (and with himself) paved the way for his use of other relaxation techniques. He started to incorporate brief mind-focusing exercises (his favorite was the spiral relaxation) into his office routine. And he used similar techniques to help him make the transition when "changing hats" from work to home.

Jim chose as his affirmation a line from a Beatles song: "Let it be." He found himself humming the tune dozens of times a day, although he still found many other people "a little too laid back." As a visualization, he chose the following: "Life is like eating with chopsticks: taking care with a light touch. When I consume life this way, it seems to bring much more satisfaction."

At the end of his fourth week, although he didn't yet feel his life was "adding up," Jim had developed a clearly visualized sense of the things that subtracted from and the things that added to his energy level. He loved fast cars and used a racing image in his daily diary entries, summarizing his stress pattern as if it were a "tachometer readout": for example, "Orange: Watch it" or "Red today: Back off!" Like so many Speed Freaks, Jim wouldn't address the pattern itself—energy brinkmanship—until he had a solution, in his case the lower stress levels and increased sense of control that come with relaxation skills.

In the second month, Jim's diary entries began to reflect his new sense of focus and his increasing ability to relax. He later reported that, when he took stock at the end of each week, he could "see for the first time how what I do at work most days *is* adding up. I can feel the direction that I was missing. Maybe it was always there, but I never realized how important it was to relax, to back off, and see the bigger picture.'' Relaxation was for him a necessary first step to being able to look squarely at his values and goals.

With only one job to take care of, he also had more spare time, which set the table for the fulfillment of his top two leisure goals: ''to relax more often'' and ''to be closer to family.'' He started to go twice a week for an hour-long shiatsu massage, adding yet another relaxation technique to his arsenal. In the second month, he signed up for a shiatsu training course and practiced the skills he was learning at home with his wife. In this way a simple beginner's course in massage had provided a focus separate from his work and some much-needed balance in his life.

It had also, without his deliberately planning it, led to the early phasing in ''in spades'' of the communication part of his prescription, which he hadn't planned to tackle until the fifth or sixth month. Communication through touching (in the form of massage) quickly opened the door to a richer relationship with his wife: He felt good because he was doing something for himself that also helped someone he cared for. And because he felt more and more at ease with his spouse, he found he was able to more easily share with her his often conflicting feelings; for example, his doubts about committing to anything less than the ''ideal job.'' Massage even changed his relationships at work: He started practicing a form of self-massage, called Do-In, that you can use sitting at your desk, and several of his fellow executives were soon following his lead.

Before long, Jim's colleagues began to notice his new commitment to his job. One commented, ''I always thought you were a nice guy, but I never really believed you'd go the extra mile for us. I'm beginning to change my mind.'' Apparently the company's president agreed. When Jim came in for his eight-month checkup, he had just learned he was in line for a promotion to vice-president of industrial relations.

Jim had other reasons to feel good about himself. His body age was down by 13 years to 42, and he looked it (his appearance age had dropped to 41). He carried himself with more confidence and moved more fluidly. In addition, his blood pressure had improved from 134/85 to 118/81.

But the last word belongs to Jim: ''I still can't really believe it. I was trying so hard, moving so fast, I never caught a firm grasp on anything. Now I take time to enjoy the small things my wife and daughter do . . . maybe just a word or a gesture mean a lot more. I remember them more than the big, blow-out parties I used to think were the only way to have a good time. I've learned to use those chopsticks like a native Chinese.''

CASE 2: Harriet, Hospital Nursing Director
Age 45, Body Age 59, Appearance Age 56
DOMINANT STRESSOTYPE: Basket Case
SECONDARY STRESSOTYPE: Worry Wart
PRESCRIPTION: 1) Nutrition, 2) Relaxation, 3) Exercise

When we met Harriet in chapter 4, she was at the end of her tether, "on a frightening downward spiral toward a complete mental and physical breakdown." She was barely able to hold herself together at work; evenings and weekends she collapsed completely. And her marriage was a mess (she had no energy for sex, and her husband had lots of time for affairs).

Nutrition was Harriet's top priority and her nutritional self-analysis revealed two major opportunity situations: to eat breakfast (she always skipped it), and to eat a balanced lunch, not just a hasty piece of fruit or a sandwich.

As anyone who's ever tried a new diet knows, changing even the smallest nutritional habit can be very difficult—and stressful. This proved true in Harriet's case. When she started making breakfast—not only for herself but for the whole family (she wanted their support)—her three teenagers complained noisily and found all sorts of excuses not to eat it ("No time, Mom, I'll be late for school"), and her husband initially refused to have anything to do with this "superficial family get-together" (he interpreted the sudden appearance of breakfast as just another one of his wife's ploys to get him more involved in their failing marriage). Nonetheless, Harriet persisted. By the end of the first month, breakfast was becoming a routine her family rarely missed.

Although eating "right" leads almost inevitably to your weight returning to normal, this effect doesn't always appear right away. In week 4, Harriet almost "fell off the breakfast wagon" when she discovered she'd gained three pounds. But her eyes told her she was starting to look better (she was a daily practitioner of the naked mirror test recommended in the nutrition chapter). In her diary, she concluded, "I know I feel more energetic because of breakfast, and I'm really proud that my family is joining me. I guess the difference in the mirror is that my weight isn't just draped all over me. I'm carrying it better."

With breakfast under her belt, along with the extra food energy it provided to help her through the day, Harriet turned her attention to lunch. Again she met resistance to her new behavior, this time from her hospital colleagues who joked that she was "slacking off" or "maybe having an affair" when she began taking a full hour at lunchtime. Given her husband's constant infidelities, the irony of this remark wasn't lost on Harriet. But she later joked that in a way she *was* having an affair. "I began to feel a freedom and zest I hadn't experienced since my wilder days in college."

In the third month, Harriet experimented with the exercise part of her prescription by joining the staff aerobics class at the hospital. But she found it just didn't suit her to exercise in this intense way; she wanted something gentler. "Besides," she later commented, "I walk miles every day in my job. And now that I know more about exercise, I'm planning my rounds so I get a mild workout as I go."

In the third month, almost by accident, Harriet began working on the third component of her prescription: relaxation. From the start, she'd been using the autogenic tape regularly with the following affirmation: "I respect my energy." Lately she'd taken to visiting local health-food stores to look for more nutritious foods to add to her diet. On one such trip, she saw a poster for a Tai Chi class near the hospital. She signed up and began going to two classes a week. In addition to muscle stretching, Tai Chi gave her wonderful deep relaxation. "The breathing techniques are the same as they teach at the Institute," she commented. As she continued with Tai Chi, her husband began to get interested (he'd done karate in college). Soon he joined her class, and they began practicing together at home.

At her four-month checkup, Harriet's weight was down by fourteen pounds, and, even more noticeable, she was carrying herself in a more upright, energetic way.

At her eight-month checkup, Harriet's body age was down by 13 years to 46, the same as her calendar age when she finished the program. She had lost twenty-eight pounds (not by dieting but by eating more nutritiously) and was now near her ideal weight. She told us she was proud to be seen with her husband "on a night out, at Tai Chi, or sunbathing at the cottage."

In her final interview, Harriet reflected on the progress she'd made. "All my professional training as a nurse had taught me that it's the few, small things you do for patients that make a big difference in their recovery. But I never applied that wisdom to myself. I often joke about that now: 'Physician, heal thyself.' But it works. Just ask our hospital dietician. She still can't understand why I take such a strong interest in making the patients' breakfasts appetizing enough that they actually eat them."

Two years after she graduated from the program, Dr. Earle ran into Harriet at the hospital where she still worked as director of nursing. She looked great, even though she'd just emerged from a difficult meeting about cutbacks in her nursing staff. She was handling this by using the cognitive reappraisal technique and said that she had a plan that she was going to share with her head nurses that would give them "a little stress inoculation.'' Her changes, it seemed, had breathed new life into her marriage. Her husband, she now concluded, had been ''going through male menopause, and feeling pretty low energy and unattractive himself''; his affairs with younger women had only increased his sense of growing old and less physically in charge. Once he began exercising, his old self-confidence began to return.

In addition, Harriet's husband (a Speed Freak) had stumbled across the Values/Goals Clarification exercises from her Body Age Program manual and had done them on his own. This had led, in her words, to ''a real settling down, and more time at home, which actually made me a bit uneasy at first.'' But Harriet was now enjoying her job and her rejuvenated relationship, and spending time with her kids, who would soon be off to college.

At her four-month checkup, Harriet reported that she was eating a balanced breakfast (with her whole family) and lunch almost every day. It hadn't been easy: ''At first, it was really tough just getting up the energy to change those two habits. But I was determined to have breakfast—and I did. And gradually I actually had the energy, in the second month, to go out for a good lunch.'' She was exercising reasonably well, and she was practicing relaxation regularly, with Tai Chi as her favorite method. And she was able to reflect rather cogently on the differences between her old self and her new self. She summarized her old lifestyle as ''garbage in, garbage out,'' and commented, ''It's no wonder I often felt people put about as much value on me as on garbage. I wasn't respecting myself any more than that either.''

CASE 3: George, Stockbroker
Age 36, Body Age 44, Appearance Age 45
DOMINANT STRESSOTYPE: Cliff Walker
SECONDARY STRESSOTYPE: Speed Freak
PRESCRIPTION: 1) Nutrition, 2) Relaxation, 3) Exercise

You might say that George entered the Body Age Program more out of fear than genuine self-concern. His heart attack, chronic back problems, and persistent fatigue had him (and his doctor) pretty worried. But he still figured it was ''all in his genes,'' and he really wanted us to give him a pill that would take the pain away. For a while, it looked as though he would quit the program rather than face himself.

By the end of the first training session, George could ''see the writing on the wall'' in terms of his health. He coped with this revelation by going to a bar and drinking himself to oblivion. But he did turn up at the next class two days later, out of fear not only for his health but for his job; he had just learned that because of his most recent physical exam his disability insurance premium was about to double, and he worried that this information would reach the ears of his senior partners. However, George still saw the Body Age Program as a way to "hedge his bets."

George likely wouldn't have lasted through the training sessions if it weren't for his program partner. Leslie, a Loner-Drifter, was 12 years older and a recovering alcoholic who hadn't had a drink since his mid-thirties. Leslie began to meet George before each training session and to drive with him to the class. Then, once the program began, he was in touch several times every week. ·

Leslie was very supportive of George as he tackled his first nutritional goal: cutting down on his drinking and use of sedatives. In George's first self-care contract, he agreed to drink no more than a total of two beers (no hard liquor) a day. He also contracted with himself (and his partner) to use sleeping pills only if he lay awake for more than an hour. As part of his strategy to cope with his insomnia, George developed the affirmation "I sleep in comfort" and used the following affirmation with each session of autogenic relaxation: "I get into bed and when I turn off the light I feel 'cared for,' the way I felt when I was recovering in the hospital after my heart attack. I see myself with no responsibilities, being looked after."

As George began to get his drinking under some control (he still tended to get high at parties and occasionally with business associates while on the road), he "made it a matter of pride to find a balanced meal on even the most gluttonous menu in town." Unfortunately, his wife was no help in this, but Leslie was: They usually met once a week for a nutritious buddy lunch.

In week 4, George turned his first major corner. Until then, he'd had trouble coming up with any affirmations that seemed to help with his drinking. But one day, after listening to the autogenic tape, in his words, "I surfaced with an affirmation that had come to me almost magically." It was "No toxic waste." He didn't know what to make of it, but it felt right. And it "worked like a charm" in helping him turn down drinks. About a week after the muse descended, George suddenly realized consciously what his intuitive mind had already understood: Not only did booze and pills leave daily wastes in his body and give him hangovers, but, more important, his "life was a waste" because of his "toxic" body. As one result, he began drinking eight detoxifying glasses of water a day.

In the second month, George decided to shop for and cook three meals at home each week; his wife didn't object, since she seldom found time to cook. A fringe benefit of this new behavior was that George felt less need to drink after a day at work: "I unwind when I'm cooking," he later told us. "It's the only part of the day when I see clearly the exact results I'm aiming for." Inadvertently, George had discovered that cooking was a very useful relaxation technique for him. (He'd been using the autogenic tape since day one, but otherwise had ignored the relaxation skills he'd learned during the training sessions.)

At the beginning of the third month, George and Leslie signed up for Chinese cooking classes (George later attributed much of his weight loss to this cuisine). In the fourth month, he started to replace "useless" business lunches with at least three brisk walks at lunch hour each week, thus beginning to phase in the third part of his prescription: exercise.

One day in the fourth month, in the middle of a noon walk, George suddenly realized that he was unwittingly using the breathing techniques we'd taught him to pace himself and "to recover from adrenalin surges" going up hills. When he mentioned this to Leslie, who was an airline pilot, his partner immediately made a connection to his job (he used formal relaxation techniques frequently during flights, especially to keep his cool when waiting to land at a congested airport). George was so taken with this idea that he started to visualize himself as an airline pilot navigating his way through phone calls and meetings. And he began consciously to use self-pacing relaxation techniques at work.

At the beginning of the fifth month, George tried out some breathing techniques during an office day and began to use cognitive reappraisal with difficult situations that had previously been "driving me crazy." It wasn't long before he became known as "Mr. Cool" at the office—a level head under pressure. He found that, as a result, his demanding clients were easier to deal with: He found he could help them "keep perspective" through the roller coaster of playing the market.

At his eight-month checkup, George was a different person from the overweight Cliff Walker who'd shambled into the first training session. His body age was down 10 years to 34 (2 years younger than his calendar age). He'd lost twenty-four pounds (getting close to his ideal weight) and had totally eliminated the two rolls of antacids he'd used daily. According to our judges, he looked younger than his years: about 30. He admitted he still liked "his grog," but now mostly enjoyed it in moderation at the occasional party, and still took the occasional sleeping pill, primarily on business trips when he just couldn't come down from a stressful day.

George was particularly proud that his resting heart rate was down from 85 to 68 beats per minute. His blood pressure had also dropped below the target for his age to 118/80. When his physician asked if he was taking any blood pressure medication, George had taken delight in answering a firm no.

We saw George about six months after graduation. He told us that he and his wife were now separated: They had both "wanted out for years" but couldn't seem to schedule "a meeting to really look at the issue." He also mentioned (with a trace of guilt) that he'd just come back "from the best vacation I've ever had." His final words as he walked out of the Institute for the last time were that we would be hearing shortly from three juniors in his brokerage firm about whom he was "a little worried."

CASE 4: John, Lawyer
Age 43, Body Age 49, Appearance Age 49
DOMINANT STRESSOTYPE: Drifter
SECONDARY STRESSOTYPE: Loner
PRESCRIPTION: 1) Communication, 2) Values/Goals, 3) Relaxation

Dapper John, all dressed up with no clear idea where to go: successful but completely unhappy with his job, divorced from his wife, with a busy social life, but lonely. This was the man who entered the Body Age Program a very smooth operator who was "very good with words" but who rarely said anything that "really mattered very much," to him or to other people: "Just slip-sliding through the day, going through the motions, getting results but not feeling them."

John couldn't make much of the Values/Goals Clarification training sessions. He appeared to be a confirmed drifter. The sessions that really made sense to him were about Self-Affirming Communication; all those words he used so well had become an armor against, rather than an invitation to, others. As he reflected on his work and social life, he could see hundreds of opportunities to communicate better and in more self-respecting ways.

For one thing, at work his sloppiness and irregular hours had become an issue with his partners. He decided to start arriving at appointments on time and to keep the receptionist informed of his schedule. After doing this for three weeks (and noticing that taking his job more seriously made it more enjoyable and his colleagues more pleasant), he sat down with his secretary and then with his partners to arrange for feedback whenever they observed him falling into his old bad habits. To help him keep on track, he agreed to submit his docketed time with clients on a predictable weekly basis, something he hadn't done for years.

At first, John's secretary was suspicious of the changes she saw. One day she joked, "Who's suing you?" On another occasion, she asked, "What are you covering up now?" But as her boss's new behavior persisted, she began to trust his transformation; eventually she was willing to take steps to help him (previously his "sloppiness" had frustrated her so much that she had simply "done her job" and withheld any real support). For the first time, they actually began to enjoy working together.

By week 4, however, John was in a mild state of panic and free-floating anxiety, which often sets in when a person realizes he actually can make a significant change. As he put it, "A part of me wanted to go back to playing it off the wall at the office. As I became more organized and predictable, I feared I was turning into a boring person—my worst fear in life." Yet John felt good, more solid. The event that seemed to get him back on track was a summary note he made in his diary at the end of week 4: "I feel 'up' because I didn't let anyone 'down' all week at the office—it's that simple."

In the second month, John began to experiment with better communication outside the office; above all, in better managing his "social whirl." During his autogenic sessions, he started visualizing himself saying a polite but firm no to some of the countless invitations that came his way (he usually accepted every one because of "a vague sense of panic" that he might miss "something or someone really important"). He also used the affirmation "I say no, when I mean no." Then, when he began turning down those dinner parties and receptions he really didn't want to attend, he deliberately used the pronoun "I" more frequently. And he began experimenting with more self-affirming language when talking to his friends.

In the third month, John got in touch with Frank, an old friend he hadn't seen for years but with whom he'd always been able to talk openly, including about his feelings. Frank was a civil servant, a class of individual John had always dismissed as "a bit lackluster and boring." But Frank turned out to be a breath of fresh air who "believes what he's doing is important, and he enjoys it, even though he's not paid very well." As so often happens with Drifters, this relationship with someone "who does have his feet on the ground" opened the door to Values/Goals Clarification.

And in the third month, John decided to declare a "year's moratorium on any more knee-jerk career decisions" while he concentrated on his core leisure values, the most important of which turned out to be an unrealized interest in nature. His other key values were to do something completely different from work and to spend time with stimulating people.

As a first step, John bought several books about wildflowers, the aspect of nature that most attracted him. With their help, he soon identified "an astounding number of types of wildflowers" around his summerhouse. When he learned that a chapter of the National Wildflower Association (founded by Lady Bird Johnson) was being formed in his area, he went to the first meeting. There he offered to do the legal incorporation work for the new chapter but, consciously practicing his self-affirming communication skills, declined to become a director. He wanted to spend his time in the countryside, not in boring meetings. The association field trips were very satisfying, not only of his need for nature but of his desire to be with people. He described his fellow flower enthusiasts as "the most mixed bag of people I've ever met" and was soon inviting some of his new friends to his summerhouse.

When John came into the Institute for his eight-month reassessment, he was dressed as fashionably as when we'd first met him. But this time the patent leather briefcase had been left at the office, replaced by a wildflower calendar being sold to raise money for the Wildflower Association. Although his body age was down by 8 years to 41 and his appearance age to an impressive 39, the most dramatic change was measured by the psychological tests for "comfort with self" and "comfort with others." His scores in both areas had moved from the twentieth percentile (very low) to well above the ninetieth percentile.

John, ever the wordsmith, summed up his success rather eloquently as "the story of the social butterfly who came to light on a wildflower."

CASE 5: Garry, Chain Store Manager
Age 37, Body Age 48, Appearance Age 45
DOMINANT STRESSOTYPE : Worry Wart
SECONDARY STRESSOTYPE: Drifter
PRESCRIPTION: 1) Relaxation, 2) Values/Goals, 3) Communication

When Garry entered the Body Age Program, he was about to worry himself out of his latest job managing a chain of convenience stores, and his most recent relationship, only a few months old, was already "worrying him to death." His worrying had been formalized into a daily ritual, a way of life.

Garry's attitude was obvious in the way he approached the program. In the initial interview, he listened too attentively, leaning forward in his chair at a 45-degree angle. He answered questions too quickly and expansively, always trying to appear highly motivated, anxious to impress with everything he had read, which was considerable. His chances of dropping out seemed high: Our prognosis was that he would set unrealistic goals and then use his failure to achieve them as an excuse for leaving.

Fortunately, Garry discovered relaxation in the first training session. In fact, you could almost say it was love at first sight. Even before the training period was complete, he was using the autogenic tape and practicing a number of breathing techniques. He told his second class that the tape got him so relaxed that, even though he knew "he should get up and begin worrying," his "body didn't want to." Nonetheless, this early success provided him with new material for worry. He complained that the tape was "too powerful," and then worried aloud that he couldn't decide when was the best time to use it—morning, lunch, evening, or some other time of day.

At this point, one of the women in the class interrupted him with a suggestion. She recalled that in the initial training session Garry had described "his stress" as a kind of "whirring inside." She suggested that for Garry the best time to relax was whenever he felt the whirring feeling. And she proposed an ingenious visualization: Garry should see the "whirr" as a "WRRRR" and imagine that the letters WR represented the message "Worry-Relax."

Garry got the message. He loved rituals, so he thought this idea was terrific and built it into his first self-care contract. Thus in one stroke he turned his worst enemy—his obsessive and mechanistic response to any troublesome event—into his greatest ally.

In the first month, Garry was so successful at relaxing instead of WRRRing that he was a little like a chain smoker who has just quit cold turkey; Garry missed the worry just as a smoker discovers endless unfilled hours when he no longer "relaxes" with a cigarette. Previously, he had filled every blank moment with angst and anguish. Now he began to worry that all this relaxation was preventing him from concentrating on his elusive "goals in life," especially finding the right career, what he referred to as "his bread-and-butter issues." Clearly he was now ready for some Values/Goals Clarification. At the end of week 4, Garry reported, "It's like somebody added four hours to my day. And I think it's about time I found out what I want to do with them."

In the second month, as Garry got in touch with his core career values, he was shocked to discover that his first career choice six jobs ago (as an economics teacher at a junior college) had provided more opportunities for valued self-expression than anything he'd done since. But the new, more relaxed Garry didn't follow true to his old form: He didn't quit his current job and go straight back to teaching. Instead, he backed off to "take a more detached look at the options," using the technique of cognitive reappraisal. This helped him see that, in his current job, he was getting some of the things he valued. He liked selling, he was fascinated by computers and electronics (in his previous job, he'd sold computers), and he enjoyed administration (lots of this in his present managerial position).

This led him, in the third month, to get in touch with two teacher friends who were still in the academic world. Not only did they give him a realistic picture of what teaching would be like for him now, he also renewed long-dormant friendships and found himself spending pleasant hours with people he really liked but hadn't seemed to have time for before. Inadvertently, Garry was putting the third component of his prescription, communication/relationships, into action. Meanwhile, he decided to design the kind of teaching job that would be perfect for him.

In the fourth month, he approached the Dean of Business at his old junior college and proposed two new courses on starting and managing small retail businesses or franchises in the high-tech area. Too quickly for Garry to worry, the dean offered him a job beginning in the fall semester (it was then late spring). Garry accepted and gave his current employer ample notice, staying on with the retail chain until just before classes were to start. In his spare time, he did background reading and wrote his course outlines.

Garry's eight-month checkup fell in August, just before his new job was to start. But the stress of this career change hadn't aged him—just the opposite. His body age had dropped 11 years to 37 (he'd turned 38 during the program), and his appearance age was even lower at 33. The Institute receptionist, who remembered him from eight months before, commented, ''It looks like someone lifted the weight of the world off his shoulders.''

At his final interview, we asked Garry if the transition period had been worrisome for him. He replied that he ''hadn't found much time for worrying in the past month'' because he was so busy doing his day job, preparing for his fall classes, and ''hanging out'' with his old college friends. He did admit to wondering occasionally how his new-old career would go, but he was so busy either problem solving or enjoying himself that whenever he heard the WRRRing sound he would just get up and do something else.

CASE 6: Ruth, Social Worker
Age 36, Body Age 50, Appearance Age 48
DOMINANT STRESSOTYPE: Loner
SECONDARY STRESSOTYPE: Drifter
PRESCRIPTION: 1) Values/Goals, 2) Communication, 3) Relaxation

Ruth, the self-styled Lone Ranger, was outwardly a very tough cookie, but it didn't take long for her resistance to crumble. This happened at the training session at which she was introduced to Values/Goals Clarification. As soon as she listed on a piece of paper the work experiences she really valued, she was hit with the enormity of the gap between her Real Self (what she was currently doing) and her Ideal Self (who and how she would like to be). It was very sobering for her to discover how little her chosen career of helping other people was giving back to her. No wonder she had dropped in and out of the work force so often.

Ruth's list of core career interests and values was as follows:

To be of service to others.
To organize things from the grassroots up.
To be a leader/motivator, but not a manager.

To have flexible hours and working conditions (not to be "in
a 9 to 5 cage"), although she was quite willing to work
long hours.

To be able to see "progress, improvements in the system,
not just helping people to adjust to substandard conditions."

Ruth then had the courage to take the leap of faith, even though she
felt as though there was nothing she could do as a social worker to get
closer to her ideal. She made a contract with herself to use this list of
values as a place from which to start. As she put it, "I have some solid
skills and, heaven knows, a breadth of experiences. But, in terms of a
pattern, building in a clear direction, I'm starting from ground zero. But
I'm prepared to work from there."

As Ruth considered her values list, she kept thinking back to the most
stable period in her career, when she'd lasted 5 years in the same job.
This had coincided with her active involvement in the union, eventually
as shop steward for her local in a large welfare organization. That union
activity had given her some of the experiences she was now missing.

In the first month, Ruth decided to find out what kinds of union positions
were available in her city. Then she sent off her resumé to the organizations that sounded interesting. While she was working quietly toward
a possible career change, she got involved with her union local. She
immediately discovered "how great it is to spend time with people who
are putting in more than just their eight hours, spending their personal
time to try to change the status quo." Soon she was involved in a couple
of union projects, and she started going out with the group after meetings
for a couple of beers. In this fashion, acting on an important value had
led her directly to explore the second part of her prescription: commu-
nication/relationships. Without really noticing the transition, she found
she was no longer "sitting around home sipping a drink alone." One
day when she dropped in to her local liquor store, the familiar face behind
the counter asked if she'd been away on vacation.

As a Loner, Ruth found her relationship with her program partner very
difficult at first, but ultimately very rewarding. Her buddy was Jennifer,
a Drifter-Basket Case (age 47, body age 52) who came to represent for
Ruth the life path she had rejected in adolescence. In her words, Jennifer
was "the immaculate, perennial debutante"; she had married young to
an already rich man and never worked. Ruth later commented, "It was
as though we were twins separated at birth and living in totally reverse-
image worlds," worlds in which neither of them found much satisfaction.

At first, Ruth and Jennifer were wary of each other; only in the second
month did they move beyond sharing the bare essentials of their self-care

contracts. The turning point came when they discovered that the affirmations they had developed separately were strikingly similar. Ruth: "My life begins anew each day" (taken from a Moody Blues song she loved). Jennifer: "I am the rising sun." These affirmations reflected a basic theme common to both women: "Better a little bit late than never at all," as Ruth put it.

Subsequently, their relationship blossomed, although almost exclusively at a distance: They rarely met but talked frequently and intimately by telephone. Later they each remarked that, by having sympathy for the other (the loneliness in Ruth; the emptiness in Jennifer), they began to value their countless everyday opportunities for self-expression, and to take advantage of some of them.

In week 4, Ruth was puzzled and a little upset: "I should be tired, beat. I'm spending so much more time doing things with people—the Institute classes, the union meetings, plus my job—but I have more energy, not less. It's strange. It's not right." Like Speed Freaks, Loners often feel they are fish out of water in the anxious early stages of change. For most, as for Ruth (and Jim), it is usually the contrast between their old and new lives that keeps them going. Here's how Ruth described it: "If it hadn't been for Jennifer, who represented my worst fears about a wasted life, I might not have hung in with my new choices. But I felt needed at the union. And my diary told me, in undeniable black and white, that I was going in the right direction for me."

In the second month, Ruth started deliberately to try out active listening skills—her favorite training session—with her union friends. For her, active listening was "just shutting up and letting other people have their say," something she'd been unaccustomed to in her big sister-little sister relationships. As she later reflected, although this keeping quiet was very hard for her to do, it was better than being the "lonely center of attention, the strong mother who looks after everyone."

By the fourth month, Ruth felt ready to phase in the third component of her prescription: She began to use several of the relaxation skills she'd been practicing at home. The breathing exercises turned out to be particularly useful when she ran a weekend workshop for the union's negotiating committee on how to keep cool at the negotiating table. The seminar was a big success, leading the union's regional president to offer her a full-time job as health and safety officer.

Ruth was hesitant to leave her new group of friends (she was also enjoying her social work job more). So she went back and did the career values exercises again, especially the Career Values Achievement Form. That clinched her decision, confirming her perception that the union position gave her "an even fuller chance to be who I am." She took the job.

When Ruth came to the Institute for her eight-month checkup, we noticed a lot of changes. Her manner could still be gruff, but the old distance wasn't there, and genuine warmth was now close to the surface. And her face looked much softer and friendlier. She was also taking much better care of herself: Gone were the sloppy clothes and unbecoming haircut. Her appearance age was down to 36 and that improvement was echoed in her body age score, down to 39.

Just before her final visit to the Institute, Ruth had started the new job with the union. She told us she had hung two pictures on the wall of her new office. One was a portrait of the Lone Ranger (mask and all). Next to this, enlarged to twice the size of the image of her former self, was a photo of her with several dozen friends taken at the farewell party at her old job. In summarizing her success, Ruth again quoted from the Moody Blues: "Take your share of the gifts that are there. They all belong to you."

SUMMING UP SUCCESS

These real-life examples demonstrate that there are many ways to put your prescription into practice, but certain things stand out in the experience of our study subjects.

   In every case, small steps led to major changes.

   The prescription works interactively, success in one area feeding success in another. Often, as you phase in one intervention, you'll inadvertently discover a useful way to start phasing in another.

   No one is perfect and no one follows his or her prescription to the absolute letter. Yet the more of your prescription you follow, the more success you'll likely have.

   A partner makes a big difference in providing support when you need it and a useful sounding board along the way.

   People found many different ways to use visualization and affirmation, but almost everyone found these techniques powerful aids to self-actualization (especially in the context of autogenic relaxation).

Measuring Your Progress

   After four months on your Vitality Action Program, you are ready to retest for body age and retake the Vitality Quotient Test. This is sufficient time for your new behaviors to have become self-affirming habits that have led to measurable biochemical changes in your body. You can retake the tests sooner, but it's unlikely any significant difference will show up. When you compare your results with your original scores, you will have objective confirmation of what you already know: that you feel better and have more energy.

You may also wish to follow the example of the Body Age Study and retest after eight months. This target "final exam" may help keep you on track and motivated to continue practicing your prescription and refining your newly honed Vital Life Skills.

You can keep track of your rising Vitality Quotient and your diminishing body age in appendix B, "Your Vitality Record."

A Few Last Words about First Principles

We'd like to leave you with a few thoughts about our book and its proven program for achieving vitalizing change. Like most good advice, we believe it can be boiled down to some very simple essentials:

1. *Energy efficiency equals good health and vitality.* Stress-energy efficiency means a slow rate of aging (inefficiency in your body systems is what the aging process is all about). Making priorities and choosing where you most want to make a behavior change is an efficient use of your personal resources. In sum, if you always aim for maximum energy efficiency, you will tend to make the right choices.

2. *Balance is your ultimate goal.* Just as true physical fitness results from a balance between sound nutrition and effective exercise, and just as a healthy balance between your work and your leisure increases your zest for life, so true vitality is the result of a balanced lifestyle in which you are using and honing all five Vital Life Skills. The idea of living in balance is nothing new: It was the ancient Greeks who first came up with the motto "Nothing to excess" and who talked about the "golden mean."

But the Body Age Program not only confirms this age-old truth; it also provides you with the concrete framework and the specific tools to bring your life into a vital balance. Whatever your stressotype profile, it is an expression of imbalance within your personal ecosystem. The purpose of your personal prescription is to reverse wasteful vitality drains and help you achieve balance. Only then can you discover what it means to experience maximum bodily efficiency and vital good health.

3. *Your feelings are as important as your logical, rational mind.* Most self-help books appeal almost exclusively to your sense of logic: Overweight? Here's how you lose it. Stressed out? Here are the techniques of stress management. Middle-aged flab or lower-back pain? Here's the exercise program that you've been waiting for. They give you lots of information and then set you adrift in a sea of uncertainty. Because they appeal primarily to your rational mind, most of the time they fail, unless you bring to them your own strong sense of self-motivation.

Underlying our success in helping our 602 study participants reduce their body ages was their use of positive affirmations and visual images, mental techniques that engage your emotions as well as your intellect, that tap into the right side of your brain, where creativity and intuition reside. These enable you to make each behavior change a positive expression of your ever more solid sense of self-esteem. You may decide to replace your relaxation tape with your favorite form of deep relaxation, or you may find that you can visualize and affirm successfully without continuing to use this formal technique. But affirmation and visualization are the keys to maximum success.

To these three basic principles we can only add that ultimately it all comes down to you. We have provided you with the tools to live a more vital life. Like those exceptional people who die young at an old age and those exceptional patients who confound a terminal cancer diagnosis with "spontaneous remission," only you can decide whether you want to be a 10 out of 10 on the well-being scale every day for the rest of your life.

Hans Selye would have found in this book a powerful elaboration of the philosophy he developed and refined over his long and vital life. It seems appropriate to leave the last words of *Your Vitality Quotient* to him: "If we learn to attune our lives to the natural laws which govern us all, just as water at sea level must always boil at 100 degrees centigrade and freeze at 0 degrees centigrade, so our bodies will respond to the demands we make upon them in equally predictable ways. Our choice is to become aware of and live in harmony with these basic laws, or to live in conflict with them. My life's work as a scientist has been to understand the demands we place on our limited supply of personal 'adaptation energy' in pursuing our purposes. My aim . . . has been to translate my understanding into a set of guidelines for robust, harmonious living, in which distress and ill health play a minor role."

APPENDICES

APPENDIX A
Your Action Diary (for photocopying)

ACTION DIARY FOR WEEK OF _____ TO _____

Planning Page

Affirmations (My self-themes for this week in key words and phrases)

I _____

I _____

(Other) _____

_____

Opportunity Visualizations (I clearly see myself . . .)

_____

_____

_____

_____

_____

_____

I choose to deepen this Vital Life Skill as follows (My specific behavioral objectives this week)

I choose to _____

_____

Under the following circumstances: _____

_____

I choose to _____

_____

Under the following circumstances: _____

_____

I choose to _____

_____

Under the following circumstances: _____

_____

I choose to _____

_____

Under the following circumstances: _____

_____

I choose to _____

_____

Under the following circumstances: _____

_____

My other opportunity situations for skill practice are:

_____

_____

_____

_____

I have arranged to check in with my partner . . .

When?   About

_____   _____

_____   _____

_____   _____

ACTION DIARY FOR WEEK OF _____ TO _____

Progress Recording Page

Vital Life Skills Being Mastered: _____

	Congratulations on Vital Actions	Opportunities for Doing It Better
Monday	_____	_____
	_____	_____
	_____	_____
	_____	_____
Tuesday	_____	_____
	_____	_____
	_____	_____
	_____	_____
Wednesday	_____	_____
	_____	_____
	_____	_____
	_____	_____
Thursday	_____	_____
	_____	_____
	_____	_____
	_____	_____
Friday	_____	_____
	_____	_____
	_____	_____

Saturday _____   _____
_____   _____
_____   _____
_____   _____
_____   _____
_____   _____

Sunday _____   _____
_____   _____
_____   _____
_____   _____
_____   _____
_____   _____

My Summary of Progress at End of Week (Have any patterns emerged?
Does my self-care contract require modification?)

APPENDIX B
Your Vitality Record

This section is for you to record your vital progress from the time you begin your personalized Body Age Program. We've designed it to parallel the four-month and eight-month checkup points of the original Body Age Study.

NOTE: **If you want to participate in the Body Age Study II, turn to Appendix D.**

1. Program Entry

Calendar Age _____

Body Age _____

Vitality Quotient _____

Stressotype Subscores:

Speed Freak _____

Basket Case _____

Cliff Walker _____

Drifter _____

Worry Wart _____

Loner _____

PRESCRIPTION:

Intervention #1 _____

Intervention #2 _____

Intervention #3 _____

2. Four-Month Checkup

Calendar Age _____

Body Age _____

Vitality Quotient _____

Stressotype Subscores:

Speed Freak _____

Basket Case _____

Cliff Walker _____

Drifter _____

Worry Wart _____

Loner _____

PRESCRIPTION PROGRESS:

Intervention #1 _____

Intervention #2 _____

Intervention #3 _____

General Comments on Progress (Body age gain? V.Q. improvement? How are you feeling? What important changes are you aware of?)

_____

_____

_____

3. Eight-month Checkup

Calendar Age _____   Stressotype Subscores:

Body Age _____

Vitality Quotient _____   Speed Freak _____

Basket Case _____

Cliff Walker _____

Drifter _____

Worry Wart _____

Loner _____

PRESCRIPTION PROGRESS:

Intervention #1 _____

Intervention #2 _____

Intervention #3 _____

Summary Comments (Body age gain, V.Q. improvement, and major signs of success)

_____

_____

_____

APPENDIX C
How to Order Your Autogenic Relaxation Tape

Many people find their own recorded voice even more effective than a professional's, but if you wish to use the Institute's Body Age Autogenic Tape instead of recording your own, fill out the order form below.

The Body Age Tape is a two-sided, studio-quality cassette narrated by Dr. Earle. Side 1 is a fifteen-minute autogenic relaxation, with soothing background music, designed to deepen the autogenic rooting of your Vital Life Skills. On side 2, Dr. Earle guides you through an exercise for getting your second wind during fatiguing or unusually demanding times.

We will send you your tape by first-class mail within three days of receiving your order. All mail or FAX orders must be accompanied by a credit card number (VISA or MasterCard only). Please do not send cash or checks. The price per cassette is $14 (U.S.) or $17 (Canadian). If you and your program partner both want a tape, you can order two for $24 (U.S.), $28 (Canadian).

ORDER FORM

Please send me _____ Body Age Autogenic Tape(s) at a total cost of $ _____ and bill me as follows:

VISA number _____   Expiration Date _____

MasterCard number _____   Expiration Date _____

My name _____

Address _____

Send this order form to: Audio Visual
                            Canadian Institute of Stress
                            Suite 3100, Shipp Centre
                            3300 Bloor Street West
                            Toronto, Canada M8X 2X3

                            FAX # 1–416–239–9526

APPENDIX D
How to Join Body Age II: An International Study of Body Age Reversal

The Canadian Institute of Stress invites you to become part of Body Age II, the next step in our study of the most powerful methods for lowering body age and increasing vitality. If you want to help us learn more about stress and aging, complete the confidential Registration Form opposite and mail it to us. You incur absolutely no obligation by doing so, and confidentiality is guaranteed.

After four months of following your personal vitality prescription, take the Body Age and Vitality Quotient tests again. Then fill out the Body Age Progress Report and mail it to the Institute. Again, your confidentiality is guaranteed, and no further obligation is involved.

Your progress will become part of our ongoing study of stress and aging. We will conduct detailed analyses of the success enjoyed by our readers and the factors contributing to this success. You will be joining a study group that includes readers from Canada, the United States, and the United Kingdom, as well as other countries around the world.

If you would like to receive a copy of our summary report *Body Age II: Results and Recommendations*, enclose a money order for $6 (U.S.) or $7 (Canadian) —to cover printing, postage, and handling—when you mail us your Progess Report.

Please send your Registration Form—as soon as you begin your Body Age Program—to:

> Body Age Tracking Center
> Canadian Institute of Stress
> Suite 3100, Shipp Centre
> 3300 Bloor Street West
> Toronto, Canada M8X 2X3
>
> Attn: Dr. Richard Earle

BODY AGE II
REGISTRATION FORM (CONFIDENTIAL)

1. Name _____

2. Address _____

   _____

3. Sex: M ____ F ____   4. Your age ____

5. Single ____   Married ____
   Separated ____   Divorced ____

6. Do you have children living with you? Yes ____ No ____

7. Your occupation _____

8. Highest school grade or degree achieved _____

9. Your present body age ____ years

10. Your present V.Q. Score (0–600) ____

11. Your six stressotype scores at present:
    Speed Freak ____   Drifter ____
    Loner ____   Worry Wart ____
    Basket Case ____   Cliff Walker ____

12. Which one of the five interventions are you starting with?

    _____

13. Which will be your second intervention?

    _____

14. Within how many weeks do you plan to start the second intervention? In
    ____ weeks

15. Will you be working with a program partner? Yes ____ No ____

16. How is your partner related to you (spouse, friend, co-worker)?

    _____

17. Are you recording your own autogenic tape or using the Institute's?
    My own ____   Institute tape ____

18. Beyond a reduced body age and an improved V.Q., what *specific* changes or benefits do you want to achieve from following your personal Vitality Quotient program?

I plan to achieve _____

_____

_____

_____

_____

_____

_____

_____

_____

_____

_____

_____

_____

_____

_____

_____

BODY AGE II
PROGRESS REPORT (CONFIDENTIAL)

(Return after four months on your program)

1. Name _____

2. Address _____

_____

3. Sex: M ____ F ____   4. Your age ____

5. How many weeks have you been following your Body Age Program? ____
   weeks.

6. Your body age now ____ years; when you started program ____ years.

7. Your present V.Q. score (0–600) ____; when you started (0–600) ____

8. Your six stressotype scores at present:
   Speed Freak ____   Drifter ____
   Loner ____   Worry Wart ____
   Basket Case ____   Cliff Walker ____

9. What are the five most effective changes you've made to date in following
   your Body Age Program (listed in order of their effectiveness: "a" = the most
   effective for you)?

   a) _____

   b) _____

   c) _____

   d) _____

   e) _____

10. What signs of progress did you notice first? When?

   a) _____

   b) _____

   c) _____

   d) _____

   e) _____

11. What roadblocks or difficulties did you experience in putting your program into practice?

    a) _____

    b) _____

    c) _____

12. On average, how many times per week have you used your autogenic tape? _____ times per week.

13. On average, how many times per day have you repeated your affirmations? _____ times; used your visualizations? _____ times.

14. How often did you check in with your program partner about your and his/her progress? _____ times per week.

15. What were several of your most powerful affirmations and visualizations?

    _____

    _____

    _____

    _____

    _____

    _____

    _____

    _____

    _____

    _____

    _____

16. Do you wish a copy of the summary *Body Age II: Results and Recommendations* mailed to you upon its completion? Yes _____ No _____ (If Yes, enclose $6 U.S. or $7 Canadian.)

ABOUT THE AUTHORS

Although his name doesn't appear on the cover, in a very real sense Hans Selye is one of the authors of this book. Selye was the renowned Austrian-born Canadian doctor who revolutionized the way we think about disease. It was his pioneering work on human stress—dating from his first publication of the stress concept in the journal *Nature* in 1936—that led ultimately to the aging research on which *Your Vitality Quotient* is based. Although many researchers have elaborated on his theories and expanded our knowledge of the biochemistry of the human stress reaction, no one has challenged Selye's fundamental assumptions about the way the body behaves under stress.

Richard Earle, Ph.D., cofounded the Canadian Institute of Stress with Dr. Selye in 1978 and has been its director ever since. Before joining the Institute, he was a senior civil servant with Ontario's Ministry of Health; his last position was as Director of Research and Development Programs. At the University of Toronto's Faculty of Medicine, where he is Adjunct Professor in the Department of Health Administration, Dr. Earle teaches research methodology. He is an advisor in industrial psychology to the Japan Management Association.

In his role as director of the Institute, Dr. Earle has helped corporations and their employees cope with stress, has lectured at several dozen North American and Japanese universities on stress and aging in human performance, and has consulted to dozens of private and public television programs. He is a popular guest on radio and television. As well, he has written numerous academic papers on the subjects of stress and aging.

Dr. Earle has found that the Body Age Program has worked well for him in practice. (He is 43 years old, but his body age is 34.) His dominant stressotype (that is, the category that indicates the way he is most prone to deal poorly with stress) is the Loner, for whom the priority area of work is clarifying his values and goals. Dr. Earle makes a point of regularly sitting down with pencil and paper to review his key life values and actions, including how well he's using his time. A core value for him, and most Loners, is enriching personal relationships, and he is careful not to confuse his professional contacts with the more basic relationships he needs. As he says, "I plan for social get-togethers with friends, encourage my wife, Margaret, to encourage me to spend time with friends, and use time on airplanes to write letters to people I care about but don't get to see often." He also enjoys newspaper cartoons and often clips out a favorite one to share with friends.

Having taught stress management for so many years, Dr. Earle now follows much of the advice in this book without thinking. But he is still learning. He often tells the following story in his stress management seminars because it represented a turning point for him. "It happened about eight years ago. I was in downtown Toronto around eight o'clock at night after teaching all day, and I was carrying a heavy briefcase as I got onto a two-story escalator going up. I was about to start walking up the moving steps when a little voice in the back of my mind said, 'Richard, you don't have to carry that briefcase.' This message seemed to make sense, so I put the briefcase down and let the escalator carry me and it up the two floors.

"I was on cloud nine for the rest of the evening: This seemingly insignificant event made me ecstatically happy. At long last, I was automatically practicing what I had been preaching about stress-energy efficiency. I was doing what I knew made perfect sense. That was the first time I really saw clearly that it's the small, specific, incredibly mundane changes that add up to lasting change. My preaching had taken root in me."

David Imrie, M.D., began his medical practice as a family physician, but he soon began to realize that many of his patients' complaints were not due to a specific organic disease but resulted from controllable psychosocial and behavioral factors. For example, back problems often confound conventional medical diagnosis but can be successfully treated if, as often happens, they result from too much stress and too little exercise. It was this perception that led him to found the Back Care Centre in 1978 and to develop his highly successful Back Power Program, now widely used in North American industry. His message on back problems is that, like stress, they can be controlled and managed if a person is willing and knowledgeable. He has produced a number of films on his back-reconditioning technique, which are shown throughout North America and the United Kingdom. His "Working Back" film series won the prestigious U.S. National Safety Council Film Award. He has lectured on the subject of back care to many organizations, including the U.S. National Safety Council and the American Occupational Nursing Association. His Back Power Program was recently adopted by the Workers Compensation Board of Ontario (covering 4.5 million workers) and will soon be adopted by several other Canadian provinces. The program has also been adopted by the U.S. National Safety Association and has been endorsed by a number of state and local safety councils. Dr. Imrie spends much of the year on the road giving lectures and seminars and consulting to a number of major Canadian companies. His Back Power Program has helped hundreds of thousands of people.

He is the author of *Good-Bye Backache* and the forthcoming *Back Power Program*, the first book on the management of back problems that is a collaboration between a physician and a chiropractor.

Dr. Imrie believes that *Your Vitality Quotient* will be of great interest to physicians. Doctors are trained to identify and manage specific diseases but are less well equipped to deal with the nonspecific factors that contribute to disease, the predominant being chronic high stress. As he says, "This book provides a framework that doctors can use to help their patients make the fundamental lifestyle changes that will deal with the root cause of their problems—not just treat the symptoms."

Dr. Imrie has found that this book's prescription for his stressotype suits him: Although his chronological age is 43, his body age is 37. David belongs to the stressotype called Speed Freak, someone who likes to have ten projects going at once and who never stops from morning until night. A typical day for him starts at 6:30 A.M. with a half-hour run and usually includes a game of squash, tennis, or hockey. As he says, "One of the things that was missing in my very active life was deliberate relaxation. Despite all my exercise, I was finding that I was usually quite tired at the end of the day and would wake up after a full night's sleep feeling unrefreshed. I also suffered from frequent acid indigestion and nasal allergies."

The priority intervention for David's stressotype is relaxation. As he says, "When I started to use some of the relaxation techniques that are part of our prescription for Speed Freaks, I discovered two things: I slept better and had more energy for all the things I wanted to do, and I was more focused and efficient while doing them. I've lost weight (without consciously dieting), the indigestion and the allergies are gone, and even my squash game has improved. I now regularly beat players who are 'better' than me. I'm spending less time keeping fit, yet I feel fitter. By learning to focus and pace my energy expenditure better, I am accomplishing more and feeling better doing it."

The Canadian Institute of Stress is a nonprofit organization that is a world leader in the fields of personal and industrial stress management. Its staff members run personal stress-management programs, teach courses in stress reduction for physicians and other health professionals, advise companies on how to set up employee counseling programs, and act as consultants to major corporations going through periods of stressful transition. More than 2,200 men and women have completed the Institute's Body Age Program, on which this book is based.

The Institute's Body Age research is continuing. It is currently tracking and analyzing the progress made by a group of more than 300 patients with chronic fatigue syndrome (yuppie flu) who were put through a specially tailored Body Age Program. The autogenic skills used so effectively by the original Body Age Study subjects (autogenic relaxation, visualization, and affirmation) are being further explored in work with professional and amateur champion athletes. And the Institute is now beginning to train business executives in "vitality skills" that focus on the demands of rapidly changing companies doing business in the Pacific Rim countries—especially Japan—where North American executives typically experience dramatically accelerated aging. As of this writing, the Institute has collected data on 5,600 individual businesspeople.

ACKNOWLEDGMENTS

The authors would like to thank the following people for their contribution to the successful completion of *Your Vitality Quotient*:

Leslie Rose of the Canadian Institute of Stress, an inspiring teacher whose commitment to being the best possible is constant, for his help with many aspects of this work, including reading and commenting on the manuscript at several stages.

Ann Rittenberg, literary agent, for her enthusiastic and professional handling of the book at every stage from auction to editing.

Bob Miller, formerly of Warner Books, who believed in our idea from the start.

Liv Blumer, of Warner Books, for her sensitive and pragmatic editing and her effective subsidiary rights savvy.

Harvey-Jane Kowal, managing editor at Warner Books, for piloting us cheerfully through countless production complexities.

Pat Fogarty, our copy editor, for polishing the prose and clarifying the confusions.

Peter Catt, assertiveness trainer and Gestalt therapist, for his help with the communications chapter and bibliography.

John Griffin, fitness specialist, for reading and commenting on the exercise chapter.

Dr. Edmund Li, of the University of Toronto Department of Nutritional Sciences in the Faculty of Medicine, for his extensive help in the revision of the chapter on nutrition.

Sharon and Barry Cooke and Paul Simpson, for their help in refining our suggestions for further reading.

Emma Hesse, for her simple and graceful illustrations.

Sharon Gignac, for transcribing taped interviews.

We would also like to thank the many people at Warner Books, New York; Random House, Canada; and Macmillan, U.K., who have believed in our book and published it with conviction.

Richard Earle would particularly like to acknowledge the following:

My wife, Margaret, whose love led me home.

My mother and father, who provided deep roots for the sunny as well as the stormy days.

The friends whose constancy has helped me learn that "When the student is ready, the teacher will appear."

Hans Selye, Norm Bell, and Naoharu Fujii, who taught me more than they knew.

The many colleagues whose insights, enthusiasm, and long hours made the Body Age Program itself a case study of vitality in action.

David Imrie would particularly like to acknowledge the following:

My wife, Sue, who shares my stress load.

Dr. Wilf Auger, a simple, wise man.

My sister, Jan, a physiotherapist who taught me the importance of muscles, the forgotten part of our bodies.

Gord Stewart, who taught me the importance of stretching.

Lyman Johnson, Doctor of Chiropractic, for his original thoughts on stress.

Jeremy Brown, publisher, who taught me the power of words.

Rick Archbold would particularly like to acknowledge the following:

Rick Feldman, for his enduring friendship and support.

Carol Morris, for her love and guidance through good times and bad.

FURTHER READING

Many of you will want to explore further some of the subjects presented in *Your Vitality Quotient*, particularly the five interventions, or Vital Life Skills. The following selected list for further reading will help you do this efficiently. The list is divided into two sections: books for deepening your understanding of the five Vital Life Skills, as well as the overall process of behavior change; and books that apply to the areas of stress, aging, and the Body Age Study.

We have listed two basic types of books: popularly written books that we recommend highly and that you should find fairly easily in your bookstore or library; and more academic or scholarly tomes. The latter, which are generally less easy to read and more difficult to find, but which contain very valuable material, are indicated with a dagger. In many cases, we've included a brief comment on the book, highlighting its most interesting or useful aspects.

Within each section, the books are listed alphabetically by author. For the popular books, we provide the most recent (or easily available) and least expensive edition of which we are aware.

407

EXPLORING THE VITAL LIFE SKILLS

General Books

These books relate to two or more interventions or to the overall process of behavior change.

†Burton, Arthur. *What Makes Behavior Change Possible?* New York: Bruner-Mazel, 1976.

Carson, Richard D. *Taming Your Gremlin: A Guide to Enjoying Yourself.* New York: Harper and Row, 1986. Carson claims that 95 percent of psychotherapy consists of teaching people to enjoy themselves. Thanks to the author's tremendous sense of humor, this book helps you do just that.

De Bono, Edward. *Six Thinking Hats.* Toronto: Key Porter, 1985; Boston: Little, Brown, 1986. This exploration of the untapped potential of the mind to solve problems using lateral thinking—a proven technique that yields novel and creative solutions and often leads to powerful results—is of particular relevance to Values/Goals Clarification.

Farquhar, John W. *The American Way of Life Need Not Be Hazardous to Your Health.* Reading, Mass.: Addison-Wesley, 1987. Dr. Farquhar identifies seven major risk factors (among them smoking, poor nutrition, and lack of exercise) and suggests realistic, step-by-step action plans for behavior change.

Feldenkrais, Moshe. *Awareness Through Movement: Health Exercises for Personal Growth.* New York: Harper and Row, 1972. This simple, powerful approach to releasing the holding patterns in your body, which can provide surprising insights into your psyche, is of particular relevance to our exercise and relaxation chapters.

†Fisch, Richard, et al. *The Tactics of Change: Doing Therapy Briefly.* San Francisco: Jossey-Bass, 1982.

Gendlin, Eugene. *Focusing.* New York: Bantam, 1981.

Gordon, Thomas. *P.E.T. [Parent Effectiveness Training] in Action.* New York: Peter Wyden, 1976. Useful for the values/goals and the communications interventions, this is a book and training manual about values, relationships, and clear communicating for parents and children. But its lessons about learning to listen for and communicate feelings are applicable to all relationships.

Kassorla, Irene C. *Go for It!* New York: Dell, 1984.

Maltz, Maxwell. *Psycho-Cybernetics.* New York: Pocket Books, 1983. This is one of the earliest—and best—examinations of self-hypnosis as a means to enhanced performance.

Morehouse, Laurence E., and Leonard Gross. *Maximum Performance*. New York: Simon and Schuster, 1977.

†Ostrander, Sheila, and Lynn Schroeder. *Superlearning*. New York: Delacorte, 1979.

Schuller, Robert H. *Tough Times Never Last But Tough People Do!* New York: Bantam, 1984. This book, which is about looking for the opportunities in your problems, reaffirms your ability to confront and conquer challenges.

Waitley, Denis. *Seed of Greatness*. New York: Pocket Books, 1983.

Watson, David L., and Roland G. Tharp. *Self-Directed Behavior: Self-Modification for Personal Adjustment*. Monterey, Calif.: Brooks-Cole, 1985. For professionals and laymen alike, this wonderful book provides practical strategies for changing self-defeating thought and behavior patterns.

Wheelis, Allen. *How People Change*. New York: Harper and Row, 1974.

Autogenic Training (Affirmations, Visualization, Autogenic Relaxation)

In addition to the books listed here, those by Carl Simonton and Bernie Siegel listed below under "Stress, Aging, and the Body Age Study" contain much useful information about using visualization to help the healing process.

Bry, Adelaide, and Marjorie Bair. *Directing the Movies of Your Mind: Visualization for Health and Insight*. New York: Harper and Row, 1978. This practical guide puts you in the director's chair as the director of your own life's story.

Gallwey, W. Timothy. *The Inner Game of Golf*. New York: Random House, 1981. In perhaps the most useful of Gallwey's "Inner Game" books, the roles of deep relaxation, visualization/mental rehearsal, and physical-mental-emotional harmony for peak athletic performance are presented in a practically useful way.

Gawain, Shakti. *Creative Visualization*. New York: Bantam, 1982. This is our favorite book on visualization. Many useful exercises and examples of visualization at work are presented in a format that involves the reader while clearly teaching simple techniques that can further profound goals of self-change.

Shone, Ronald. *Creative Visualization: How To Use Imagery and Imagination for Self-Improvement*. Rochester, Vt.: Thorsons, 1984. This easy-to-read book captures research highlights as well as a wide variety of practical applications and how-to techniques.

Wolberg, L. *Hypnosis: Is It for You?* New York: Basic Books, 1978.

Values/Goals Clarification

Bolles, Richard. *The Three Boxes of Life, and How To Get Out of Them.* Berkeley, Calif.: Ten Speed Press, 1981. This book is by the author of *What Color Is Your Parachute?*, a very good guide to coping with career change. Both volumes emphasize the importance of clarified values in the development of concrete strategies for dealing with several of life's major stressors, such as job loss, career change, and uncertainty.

Hill, Napoleon. *Think and Grow Rich.* (Rev. ed.) New York: Hawthorn, 1967.

Kavanaugh, Terence. *Heart Attack? Counter-Attack! A Practical Plan for a Healthy Heart.* New York: Van Nostrand Reinhold, 1976. This inspiring story of a doctor who rehabilitated heart attack recovery patients through exercise and diet and entered them in the Boston Marathon contains useful tips for the nutrition and exercise interventions.

Koberg, Don, and Jim Bagnall. *The Universal Traveler: A Soft-Systems Guide to Creativity. Problem-Solving, and the Process of Reaching Goals.* (Rev.ed.) New York: Kaufman, 1981.

Lakein, Alan. *How To Get Control of Your Time and Your Life.* New York: Signet, 1974. This classic and very practical how-to book does just what its title says.

Levinson, Daniel, et al. *The Seasons of a Man's Life.* New York: Ballantine, 1979.

Maslow, Abraham. *Toward a Psychology of Being.* New York: Van Nostrand Reinhold, 1968. Only when your most basic needs for food, shelter, and other comforts are taken care of can you begin to ascend the pyramid of self-actualization toward "peak experiences" of fulfillment growing out of an integrated, balanced self.

Scholz, Nelle T., et al. *How To Decide: A Guide for Women.* (Rev.ed.) New York: College Entrance Exam Board, 1976.

Sheehy, Gail. *Passages: Predictable Crises of Adult Life.* New York: Bantam, 1977.

†Simon, Sidney B., et al. *Values Clarification: A Handbook of Practical Strategies for Teachers and Students.* New York: Dodd, Mead, 1978.

Von Oech, Roger. *A Whack on the Side of the Head: How To Unlock Your Mind for Innovation*. New York: Warner Books, 1983. By one of the original creative consultants to Silicon Valley, this is a book about how to play and generate creative ideas through lateral thinking.

Winston, Stephanie. *Getting Organized: The Easy Way To Put Your Life in Order*. New York: Warner Books, 1985.

Effective Relaxation

Beech, H. R. *A Behavioral Approach to the Management of Stress: A Practical Guide to Techniques*. New York: Wiley, 1982.

Benson, Herbert, and Miriam Z. Klipper. *The Relaxation Response*. New York: Avon, 1976. Based on a now-famous study of the positive physiological effects of deep relaxation, this is useful advice on how to train your body to achieve them.

Davis, M. *The Relaxation and Stress Reduction Workbook*. Richmond, Calif.: New Harbinger, 1980.

Girdano, D., and G. Everly. *Controlling Stress and Tension*. Englewood Cliffs, N.J.: Prentice-Hall, 1979.

Goleman, D. *The Meditative Mind*. Los Angeles: Tarcher, 1988. This panoramic integration of philosophy and technique provides Eastern and Western perspectives on meditation.

†Green, Elmer, and Alyce Green. *Beyond Biofeedback*. New York: Delacorte, 1977.

Hendricks, C. G., and Russell Wills. *The Centering Book: Awareness Activities for Children, Parents and Teachers*. Englewood Cliffs, N.J.: Prentice-Hall, 1975.

Hofstadter, Douglas, and Daniel C. Dennett, eds. *The Mind's I: Fantasies and Reflections of Self and Soul*. New York: Bantam, 1982.

LeShan, Lawrence. *How To Meditate: A Guide to Self-Discovery*. New York: Bantam, 1986.

†Shapiro, Deane H., and Roger N. Walsh, eds. *Meditation: Classical and Contemporary Perspectives*. New York: Aldine de Gruyter, 1984.

†Wilber, Ken, et al. *Transformations of Consciousness: Conventional and Contemplative Developmental Approaches*. Boston: Shambhala, 1986.

Zi, Nancy. *The Art of Breathing: Thirty Simple Exercises for Improving Your Performance and Well-Being*. New York: Bantam Books, 1986. This outline of how-to advice and specific benefits and results is one of the best presentations of breathing techniques yet published.

Self-Affirming Communication

Alberti, Robert E., and Michael L. Lemmons. *Stand Up, Speak Out, Talk Back.* New York: Pocket Books, 1975.

Bach, George R., and Peter Wyden. *The Intimate Enemy: How To Fight Fair in Love and Marriage.* New York: Avon, 1981.

Berne, Eric. *What Do You Say After You Say Hello?* New York: Bantam, 1975.

Cawood, Diana. *Assertiveness for Managers: Learning Effective Skills for Managing People.* Vancouver: International Self-Counsel Press, 1983. Good on both sides of the communication coin—receiving skills and message skills—this book looks at assertive behavior not as a set of techniques, but as the key to building successful relationships.

Cohen, Herb. *You Can Negotiate Anything.* New York: Bantam, 1982.

Fensterheim, Herbert, and Jean Baer. *Don't Say Yes When You Want To Say No.* New York: Dell, 1975. These highly effective guidelines will help you defuse self-defeating communication patterns.

Fisher, Roger, and William Ury. *Getting to Yes: Negotiating Agreement Without Giving In.* Boston: Houghton Mifflin, 1981.

Jakubowski, Patricia, and Arthur J. Lange. *The Assertive Option: Your Rights and Responsibilities.* Champaign, Ill.: Research Press Company, 1978. One of the best and most focused examinations of the subject, this book is written by the authors of one of the standard texts for assertiveness trainers.

†Jourard, S. *The Transparent Self.* Princeton, N. J.: Van Nostrand Reinhold, 1971.

†Laing, R. D. *The Politics of the Family and Other Essays.* New York: Pantheon Books, 1969.

Miller, Sherod, et al. *Straight Talk: A New Way To Get Closer to Others by Saying What You Really Mean.* New York: New American Library, 1982. Especially good on different self-defeating types of talk (small talk, control talk, and heavy control talk), this book explains how to replace them with straight talk, in which control is not a goal.

Perls, Frederick S. *Gestalt Therapy Verbatim.* New York: Bantam, 1971. Any of Perls's books on the Gestalt approach contain useful insights into the communications process. This is one of the more accessible and easy to read.

Pirsig, Robert. *Zen and the Art of Motorcycle Maintenance*. New York: Bantam, 1976. This novel provides as many compelling insights as any how-to book into the way relationships and personal values evolve and can be changed.

Rogers, Carl. *Client-Centered Therapy: Its Current Practice, Implications and Theory*. Boston: Houghton Mifflin, 1965. Our discussion of active listening owes much to Rogers and his ideas about effective listening. His client-centered psychotherapy is based on the assumption that people are basically good and that empathy, which requires respectful listening, is the best approach.

†Simenaur, Jacqueline, and David Carroll. *Singles: The New Americans:* New York: Simon and Schuster, 1982.

Viscott, David. *How To Live with Another Person*. New York: Pocket Books, 1983. This realistic and caring discussion presents many guidelines for a fulfilling intimate relationship (including marriage) that almost all "successful" couples wish they had known, and shared with each other, *sooner*.

Wyckoff, Hogie. *Solving Problems Together*. New York: Grove, 1980.

Essential Exercise

Anderson, Bob. *Stretching*. Bolinas, Calif.: Shelter Publications, 1980. Excellent illustrations of stretching exercises appropriate for specific sports.

†Astrand, Per-Olof, and Kaare Rodahl. *Textbook of Work Physiology: Physiological Basis of Exercisers*. New York: McGraw-Hill, 1977.

†Bloch, George J. *Body and Self: Elements of Human Biology, Behavior and Health*. Lost Altos, Calif.: Kauffmann, 1985.

†Cacioppo, John T., and Richard E. Petty, eds. *Perspectives in Cardiovascular Psychophysiology*. New York: Guilford Press, 1982.

Cooper, Kenneth. *The New Aerobics*. New York: Bantam, 1970. This widely acknowledged classic launched "aerobics" as a household word.

†Fotherby, K., and S.B. Pal, eds. *Exercise Endocrinology*. New York: Walter de Gruyter, 1985.

†Lamb, David R. *Physiology of Exercise: Responses and Adaptations*. New York: Macmillan, 1984.

†Leonard, George B. *The Ultimate Athlete: Re-Visioning Sports, Physical Education and the Body*. New York: Viking, 1975.

†Milvy, Paul, ed. *The Marathon: Physiological, Medical, Epidemiological and Psychological Studies*. New York: New York Academy of Sciences, 1977.

Morehouse, Laurence E., and Leonard Gross. *Total Fitness in Thirty Minutes a Week*. New York: Pocket Books, 1987.

Sheehan, George A. *Dr. Sheehan on Running*. Mountain View, Calif.: World, 1975. "At the age of forty-five, I pulled the emergency cord and ran out into the world. It was a decision that meant no less than a new life, a new course, a new destination. I was born again in my forty-fifth year." The modern medical guru of running also explores the philosophical and spiritual aspects of exercise. We also recommend his other books on running.

Stewart, Gordon W. *Every Body's Fitness Book*. Garden City, N. Y.: Doubleday, 1980. This explanation of the importance of balanced exercise puts stretching in its rightful place, as of primary importance for people over thirty.

High-Performance Nutrition

†Beasley, J. D. *The Impact of Nutrition on the Health of Americans: A Report to the Ford Foundation by the Medicine and Nutrition Project*. Annandale-on-Hudson, N. Y.: Bard College, 1981. This report is available by writing to the Ford Foundation, 320 East 43rd St., New York, New York, 10017.

Berger, Stuart M. *Dr. Berger's Immune Power Diet*. New York: Signet, 1986.

†Brewster, Letitia, and Michael Jacobson. *The Changing American Diet: A Chronicle of American Eating Habits from 1910–1980*. Washington, D.C.: Center for Science in the Public Interest, 1983.

Brody, Jane. *Jane Brody's Nutrition Book*. New York: Bantam Books, 1982. This is a thorough and readable compendium of current thinking on sound nutrition, although some of Brody's information is somewhat out of date. (Also highly recommended is *Jane Brody's Good Food Book*.)

DeBakey, Michael, et al. *The Living Heart Diet*. New York: Fireside (Simon and Schuster), 1986.

Hendler, Sheldon S. *The Complete Guide to Anti-Aging Nutrients*. New York: Simon and Schuster, 1986. This thorough and well-organized book reviews what we know and don't yet know on solid scientific grounds concerning these often-controversial vitamins and minerals.

Mayer, Jean. *A Diet for Living*. New York: Pocket Books, 1977.

Ornish, Dean. *Stress, Diet and Your Heart*. New York: Signet, 1984.

Pauling, Linus. *How To Live Longer and Feel Better*. New York: Avon, 1987.

†Pfeiffer, Carl C. *Mental and Elemental Nutrients: A Physician's Guide to Health Care*. New Canaan, Conn.: Keats, 1975.

†Philips, M., and A. Baetz, eds. *Diet and Resistance to Disease, Advances in Experimental Medicine and Biology*. New York: Plenum, 1981.

†Selvey, Nancy, and Philip L. White, eds. *Nutrition in the 1980s: Constraints on Our Knowledge*. New York: Allen R. Liss, 1981.

Stuart, Richard B., and Barbara Davis. *Slim Chance in a Fat World*. Champaign, Ill.: Research Press, 1978.

STRESS, AGING, AND THE BODY AGE STUDY

†Ader, Robert, ed. *Psychoneuroimmunology*. New York: Academic Press, 1981.

†Antonovsky, Aaron. *Health, Stress and Coping: New Perspectives on Mental and Physical Well-Being*. San Francisco: Jossey-Bass, 1979.

†Appley, Mortimer, ed. *Psychological Stress*. New York: Appleton-Century-Crofts, 1981.

†Becker, W. *Energy and the Living Cell: An Introduction to Bioenergetics*. Philadelphia: Lippincott, 1977.

†Behnke, John A., et al., eds. *The Biology of Aging*. New York: Plenum Press, 1978.

Benson, Herbert. *The Mind Body Effect: How Behavioral Medicine Can Show You the Way to Better Health*. New York: Simon and Schuster, 1979. This landmark book is based on research—both clinical and observations of everyday experiences—suggesting the existence of the body, mind, and emotions as a single integrated system.

Borysenko, Joan. *Minding the Body, Mending the Mind*. Reading, Mass.: Addison-Wesley, 1987. The author is one of the leading researchers in the growing field of psychoneuroimmunology.

Bressler, D. *Free Yourself from Pain*. New York: Simon and Schuster, 1979.

†Breznitz, Shlomo. *The Denial of Stress*. New York: International Universities Press, 1983.

Brown, Barbara B. *Supermind: The Ultimate Energy*. New York: Harper and Row, 1980. A pioneer in the field of biofeedback shares insights concerning the mind's abilities to direct and enhance physical functioning.

†Cheraskin, Emmanuel, et al. *The Vitamin C Connection*. New York: Harper and Row, 1983.

Chopra, Deepak. *Creating-Health: Beyond Prevention, Toward Perfection*. Boston: Houghton Mifflin, 1987. This personally and philosophically provocative book by a practicing physician leads readers to question the limits they may be unnecessarily imposing on how fully healthy they can be.

Cousins, Norman. *Anatomy of an Illness as Perceived by the Patient*. New York: Bantam, 1981. This is probably the most famous account of a patient's recovery from a "terminal" illness with the aid of mental and spiritual resources medicine often overlooks.

Dossey, Larry. *Space, Time and Medicine*. Boston: Shambhala, 1982. A fascinating integration of a physician's clinical experience with Eastern philosophy and the "new physics" that opens new frontiers in our thinking about self-healing.

Dunlop, Marilyn. *Body Defenses: The Marvels and Mysteries of the Immune System*. Toronto: Irwin, 1987. A professional science writer provides a very readable update on the organization and intricate functioning of the immune system in disease and disease treatment.

†Erickson, Milton H., et al. *Hypnotic Realities: The Induction of Clinical Hypnosis and Forms of Direct Suggestion*. New York: Irvington, 1976.

†Finch, C.E., and L. Hayflick. *Handbook of the Biology of Aging*. New York: Van Nostrand Reinhold, 1977.

Friedman, Meyer, and Ray H. Rosenman. *Type A Behavior and Your Heart*. New York: Fawcett, 1981. This classic study of behavior that increases the risk of heart disease—something the authors call "hurry sickness"—demonstrates that disease is often the result of nonspecific behavioral factors.

Glassman, Judith. *The Cancer Survivors, and How They Did It*. New York: Doubleday, 1983.

†Goldberger, Leo, and Shlomo Breznitz, eds. *The Handbook of Stress: Theoretical and Clinical Aspects*. New York: The Free Press, 1982.

Jampolsky, Gerald G. *Teach Only Love: The Seven Principles of Attitudinal Healing*. New York: Bantam, 1983.

†Knowles, John H., ed. *Doing Better and Feeling Worse: Health in the United States*. New York: Norton, 1977.

LeShan, Lawrence. *You Can Fight for Your Life: Emotional Factors in the Treatment of Cancer*. New York: Evans, 1977.

†Levi, Lennart. *Preventing Work Stress*. Reading, Mass.: Addison-Wesley, 1981.

Lewis, Howard R., and Martha E. Lewis. *Psychosomatics: How Your Emotions Can Damage Your Health*. New York: Pinnacle Books, 1975.

†Locke, Steven, and Mady Hornig-Rohan. *Mind and Immunity: Behavioral*

Immunology (1976–1982). An Annotated Bibliography. New York: Institute for the Advancement of Health, 1983.

†Matarazzo, Joseph D., et al., eds. *Behavioral Health: A Handbook of Health Enhancement and Disease Prevention.* New York: Wiley, 1984.

†Morgan, Robert. *Interventions in Applied Gerontology.* Dubuque, Iowa: Kendall-Hunt, 1981.

Pearsall, Paul. *Superimmunity: Master Your Emotions and Improve Your Health.* New York: Fawcett, 1987. This is one of the best overviews of the links between the mind and the immune system.

Pelletier, Kenneth R. *Mind as Healer, Mind as Slayer.* New York: Dell, 1977. This landmark book concerns stress as a causal factor in a number of common diseases.

———. *Holistic Medicine: From Stress to Optimum Health.* New York: Dell, 1980.

†Rockstein, Morris, ed. *Theoretical Aspects of Aging.* New York: Academic Press, 1974.

†Segre, D., and L. Smith. *Immunologic Aspects of Aging.* New York: Dekker, 1980.

Selye, Hans. *Stress Without Distress.* New York: Signet, 1975. Of Selye's many books, this is the best summary of his life and work, including both a thorough explanation of stress—the nonspecific bodily response to demands and challenges—and a discussion of his philosophy of altruistic egoism, a two-way integration and application of biochemical functioning with our values, goals, and beliefs.

———. *The Stress of My Life: A Scientist's Memoirs.* Toronto: McClelland and Stewart, 1976; Reading, Mass.: Butterworths, 1976. Dr. Selye's autobiography, including details of his discovery of the stress mechanism, which he first perceived as the "syndrome of simply being sick." By chronicling in a very personal way the step-by-step progress of his work, Selye offers readers an understanding of a complex scientific and medical subject rarely available to laymen.

†———. *The Stress of Life.* New York: McGraw-Hill, 1976.

†———. *Stress in Health and Disease.* Reading, Mass.: Butterworths, 1976.

Siegel, Bernie S. *Love, Medicine and Miracles.* New York: Perennial Library (Harper and Row), 1988. In this inspiring book, Dr. Siegel describes his work with exceptional cancer patients, including the use of imagery and artwork in the healing process.

Simonton, O. Carl, et al. *Getting Well Again*. New York: Bantam Books, 1980. This is the Simontons' first book about their revolutionary use of imaging and other mind-over-body techniques with cancer patients.

†Strehler, B. *Time, Cells and Aging*. New York: Academic Press: 1977.

†Taché, Jean. et al., eds. *Cancer, Stress and Death*. New York: Plenum, 1979.

†Thomas, Lewis. *The Lives of a Cell: Notes of a Biology Watcher*. New York: Viking, 1974.

†Underwood, E. J. *Trace Elements in Human and Animal Nutrition*. New York: Academic Press, 1977. This clear presentation of the role of trace elements highlights how much more we know about the nutritional requirements of pets and livestock than we do about human requirements.

†United States Office of the Assistant Secretary for Health and the Surgeon General. *Healthy People: The Surgeon General's Report on Health Promotion and Disease Prevention*. Washington, D.C.: U.S. Department of Health, Education, and Welfare, Office of the Surgeon General, 1979. Available from the U.S. Government Printing Office, Superintendent of Documents, 26 Federal Plaza, Room 110, New York, New York, 10278.

†Walford, R.L. *The Immunologic Theory of Aging*. Copenhagen: Minksgaard, 1969.

†Walsh, Roger N., and D. Shapiro, eds. *Beyond Health and Normality*. New York: Van Nostrand Reinhold, 1983.

†Winick, Myron., ed. *Nutrition and Aging*. New York: Wiley, 1976.

INDEX